AGING AND DECISION MAKING

AGING AND DECISION MAKING

EMPIRICAL AND APPLIED PERSPECTIVES

Edited by

THOMAS M. HESS

JONELL STROUGH

CORINNA E. LÖCKENHOFF

ELSEVIER

AMSTERDAM • BOSTON • HEIDELBERG • LONDON
NEW YORK • OXFORD • PARIS • SAN DIEGO
SAN FRANCISCO • SINGAPORE • SYDNEY • TOKYO
Academic Press is an imprint of Elsevier

Academic Press is an imprint of Elsevier
32 Jamestown Road, London NW1 7BY, UK
525 B Street, Suite 1800, San Diego, CA 92101-4495, USA
225 Wyman Street, Waltham, MA 02451, USA
The Boulevard, Langford Lane, Kidlington, Oxford OX5 1GB, UK

ISBN: 978-0-12-417148-0

British Library Cataloguing-in-Publication Data
A catalogue record for this book is available from the British Library

Library of Congress Cataloging-in-Publication Data
A catalog record for this book is available from the Library of Congress

For Information on all Academic Press publications
visit our website at http://store.elsevier.com/

Typeset by TNQ Books and Journals
www.tnq.co.in

Contents

Contributors xi
Foreword xv
Preface xxv

1. The Present, Past, and Future of Research on Aging and Decision Making

JONELL STROUGH, CORINNA E. LÖCKENHOFF, THOMAS M. HESS

Basic Issues in the Study of Aging and Decisions 2
Book Overview 8
Conclusion 12
References 13

1
NEUROBIOLOGICAL MECHANISMS

2. Modeling Cost–Benefit Decision Making in Aged Rodents

B. SOFIA BEAS, BARRY SETLOW, GREGORY R. SAMANEZ-LARKIN, JENNIFER L. BIZON

Introduction 17
Individual Differences and Cognitive Aging 18
Cross-Species Comparisons of Neural Circuitry Relevant for Decision Making 19
Cross-Species Considerations of Reinforcers 20
Intertemporal Decision Making 21
Probabilistic (Risky) Decision Making 28
The Role of Age-Related Memory Impairment in Decision Making 31
Conclusion 33
References 34

3. Decision Neuroscience and Aging

GREGORY R. SAMANEZ-LARKIN

Overview of Frontostriatal Neural Circuitry 41
Gains and Losses 44
Intertemporal Decision Making 45
Risky Decision Making 47

Learning 50
Conclusions 53
References 55

4. Towards a Mechanistic Understanding of Age-Related Changes in Learning and Decision Making: A Neuro-Computational Approach

BEN EPPINGER, RASMUS BRUCKNER

Age-Related Decline in the Dopamine System 62
Age Differences in Learning from Experience 65
Conclusions 71
References 74

5. Age-Associated Executive Dysfunction, the Prefrontal Cortex, and Complex Decision Making

NATALIE L. DENBURG, WILLIAM M. HEDGCOCK

Guiding Observations, Theoretical Frameworks, and Key Empirical Tests 81
Research on Aging 85
Conclusions and Implications 96
References 98

2

BEHAVIORAL MECHANISMS

6. Adaptive Decision Making and Aging

RUI MATA, ANIKA K. JOSEF, PATRICK LEMAIRE

An Ecological Perspective on Life-Span Changes in Strategy Use 105
Cognitive Aging: The Role of Cognitive Control and Reward Processing 108
Aging and Strategy Use 109
Aging and Strategy Use in Decision Making 114
Implications of Age Differences in Strategy Selection and Execution 120
Summary and Conclusion 121
References 122

7. Aging, Memory, and Decision Making

FABIO DEL MISSIER, TIMO MÄNTYLÄ, LARS-GÖRAN NILSSON

Introduction 127
Age-Related Changes in Memory Functioning and Their Influence on Judgment and Decision Making 128
Aging, Memory, and Decision Making: Where Do We Go From Here? 141
References 142

8. Complementary Contributions of Fluid and Crystallized Intelligence to Decision Making Across the Life Span

LISA ZAVAL, YE LI, ERIC J. JOHNSON, ELKE U. WEBER

Better or Worse Off? 149
Cognitive Capabilities and Decision Making Across the Adult Life Span 150
Complementary Cognitive Capabilities 153
Practical Decision Making and the Role of Domain-Specific Experience 157
Implications for Public Policy and Effective Decision Environments 161
Summary 164
References 164

9. Aging, Emotion, and Decision Making

JOSEPH A. MIKELS, MICHAEL M. SHUSTER, SYDNEY T. THAI

Age-Related Changes in Cognition, Emotion, and Motivation 170
Theoretical Perspectives on the Role of Affect in Judgment and Decision Making 172
Decision Making Across the Adult Life Span 178
Conclusions and Future Research Directions 182
References 184

10. A Prospect Theory-Based Evaluation of Dual-Process Influences on Aging and Decision Making: Support for a Contextual Perspective

THOMAS M. HESS

Dual-Process Perspectives on Decision Making 190
Dual-Process Influences and Prospect Theory 192
Conclusions 206
References 209

11. Age Differences in Time Perception and Their Implications for Decision Making Across the Life Span

CORINNA E. LÖCKENHOFF, JOSHUA L. RUTT

Age Differences in Global Time Horizons and Mental Representations of Time 214
Mechanisms 217
Implications for Decision Making 220
Future Directions and Practical Implications 225
References 227

12. Understanding Life-Span Developmental Changes in Decision-Making Competence

JONELL STROUGH, ANDREW M. PARKER, WÄNDI BRUINE DE BRUIN

Overview 235
Defining Decision-Making Competence 236
Deliberation, Affect, and Decision-Making Competence 238

Aging and Decision-Making Competence 239
Motivational Model of Aging and Decision-Making Competence 242
Current Challenges and Directions for Future Research 246
Summary and Conclusions 251
References 252

3

APPLIED PERSPECTIVES

13. Decision Making and Health Literacy among Older Adults
DANIEL MORROW, JESSIE CHIN

Introduction 261
Older Adults and Health Decisions 262
Aging, Health Literacy, and Health-Related Decisions 268
Conclusions 276
References 278

14. Decisions and Actions for Life Patterns and Health Practices as We Age: A Bottom-up Approach
HOWARD LEVENTHAL, JENNA HEROLD, ELAINE A. LEVENTHAL, EDITH BURNS, MICHAEL A. DIEFENBACH

Overview 283
Themes for Modeling Health Preferences and Decisions 284
Modeling the Processes Underlying Health Decisions and Actions 285
Executive Function in a Common-Sense Framework: Selective Evidence 295
Summary and Thoughts for the Future 303
References 306

15. Choice and Aging: Less is More
PI-JU LIU, STACEY WOOD, YANIV HANOCH

Introduction 309
Choice Preference and Size in Decision Making 310
Dual-Process Models and Implications for Decision Making in Older Adults 312
An Empirical Study Testing the Mediating Effect of Cognitive Ability on Choice Preference 314
Numeracy and Choice Set Size in Decision Making 317
Additional Factors in Relation to Choice Set Size and Preference 319
Summary 321
References 324

16. Financial Decision Making across the Adult Life Span: Dynamic Cognitive Capacities and Real-World Competence

DOUGLAS A. HERSHEY, JAMES T. AUSTIN, HELEN C. GUTIERREZ

Fluid Abilities, Crystallized Abilities, and Financial Knowledge 330
The Nature of Financial Decision-Making Tasks 332
Reasons Why Individuals Make Poor Financial Decisions 336
Interventions Designed to Improve Financial Decision Making 342
Summary and Conclusion 344
References 345

17. Aging and Consumer Decision Making

STEPHANIE M. CARPENTER, CAROLYN YOON

Age Differences in Basic Decision Skills and Strategies 351
Age Differences in Consumer Choice and Decision Making 354
Moderating Influences on Aging and Decision Making 357
Conclusions 365
References 366

18. A Framework for Decision Making in Couples across Adulthood

TARA L. QUEEN, CYNTHIA A. BERG, WILLIAM LOWRANCE

A Framework for Understanding Dyadic Decision-Making Processes 372
Existing Literature on Dyadic Decision Making 379
Future Directions 385
Conclusion 387
References 388

Index **393**

Contributors

James T. Austin College of Education and Human Ecology, Ohio State University, Columbus, OH, USA

B. Sofia Beas Department of Neuroscience, University of Florida College of Medicine, Gainesville, FL, USA

Cynthia A. Berg Department of Psychology, University of Utah, Salt Lake City, UT, USA

Jennifer L. Bizon Department of Neuroscience, University of Florida College of Medicine, Gainesville, FL, USA; Department of Psychiatry, University of Florida College of Medicine, Gainesville, FL, USA

Rasmus Bruckner Department of Psychology, Humboldt-Universität zu Berlin, Germany

Wändi Bruine de Bruin University of Leeds, West Yorkshire, England; Carnegie Mellon University, Pittsburgh, PA, USA

Edith Burns Department of Medicine, Medical College of Wisconsin, Milwaukee, WI, USA

Stephanie M. Carpenter Department of Psychology, University of Michigan, Ann Arbor, MI, USA

Jessie Chin Department of Educational Psychology, University of Illinois at Urbana-Champaign, Champaign, IL, USA

Fabio Del Missier Department of Life Sciences, Psychology Unit, University of Trieste, Trieste, Italy; Department of Psychology, Stockholm University, Stockholm, Sweden

Natalie L. Denburg Department of Neurology, Carver College of Medicine, Iowa City, IA, USA; Interdisciplinary Graduate Program in Neuroscience, Iowa City, IA, USA

Michael A. Diefenbach Department of Medicine and Urology, North Shore-Long Island Jewish Health System, NY, USA

Ben Eppinger Department of Psychology, Technische Universität Dresden, Germany

Helen C. Gutierrez Department of Psychology, Oklahoma State University, Stillwater, OK, USA

Yaniv Hanoch School of Psychology, Plymouth University, Plymouth, Devon, UK

William M. Hedgcock Department of Marketing, Tippie College of Business, Iowa City, IA, USA; Interdisciplinary Graduate Program in Neuroscience, Iowa City, IA, USA

Jenna Herold Department of Psychology, Rutgers University, NJ, USA

Douglas A. Hershey Department of Psychology, Oklahoma State University, Stillwater, OK, USA

Thomas M. Hess Department of Psychology, North Carolina State University, Raleigh, NC, USA

Eric J. Johnson Center for Decision Sciences, Columbia University, New York, NY, USA

Anika K. Josef Max Planck Institute for Human Development, Berlin, Germany

Patrick Lemaire Université de Provence, Marseille, France; Centre National de la Recherche Scientifique, Paris, France

Howard Leventhal Institute for Health & Department of Psychology, Rutgers University, New Brunswick, NJ, USA

Elaine A. Leventhal Department of Medicine, Robert Wood Johnson School of Medicine, Rutgers University, New Brunswick, NJ, USA

Ye Li School of Business Administration, University of California, Riverside, CA, USA

Pi-Ju Liu Psychology Department, University of San Francisco, San Francisco, CA, USA

Corinna E. Löckenhoff Department of Human Development, College of Human Ecology, Cornell University, Ithaca, NY, USA

William Lowrance Huntsman Cancer Institute, University of Utah, Salt Lake City, UT, USA

Timo Mäntylä Department of Psychology, Stockholm University, Stockholm, Sweden

Rui Mata Department of Psychology, University of Basel, Basel, Switzerland; Max Planck Institute for Human Development, Berlin, Germany

Joseph A. Mikels Department of Psychology, DePaul University, Chicago, IL, USA

Daniel Morrow Department of Educational Psychology, University of Illinois at Urbana-Champaign, Champaign, IL, USA

Lars-Göran Nilsson Department of Psychology, Stockholm University, Stockholm, Sweden; ARC, Karolinska Institutet Stockholm, Stockholm, Sweden; UFBI, Umeå University, Umeå, Sweden

Andrew M. Parker RAND Corporation, Pittsburgh, PA, USA

Tara L. Queen Department of Psychology, University of Utah, Salt Lake City, UT, USA

Joshua L. Rutt Department of Human Development, College of Human Ecology, Cornell University, Ithaca, NY, USA

Gregory R. Samanez-Larkin Department of Psychology, Yale University, New Haven, CT, USA

Barry Setlow Department of Neuroscience, University of Florida College of Medicine, Gainesville, FL, USA; Department of Psychiatry, University of Florida College of Medicine, Gainesville, FL, USA

Michael M. Shuster Department of Psychology, DePaul University, Chicago, IL, USA

JoNell Strough Department of Psychology, West Virginia University, Morgantown, WV, USA

Sydney T. Thai Department of Psychology, DePaul University, Chicago, IL, USA

Elke U. Weber Center for Decision Sciences, Columbia University, New York, NY, USA

Stacey Wood Department of Psychology, Scripps College, Claremont, CA, USA

Carolyn Yoon Marketing Department, Stephen M. Ross School of Business, University of Michigan, Ann Arbor, MI, USA

Lisa Zaval Department of Psychology, Columbia University, New York, NY, USA; Center for Decision Sciences, Columbia University, New York, NY, USA

Foreword*

DECISION MAKING AND AGING: EMERGING FINDINGS AND RESEARCH NEEDS

We are approaching a major demographic shift in the United States and globally, such that the number of individuals over the age of 65 will exceed the number under the age of 5, with no outlook for reversal of this trend in the foreseeable future (National Institute on Aging/World Health Organization, 2011). Contrary to popular stereotypes of aging, the majority of these older adults (at least in the United States) will be living at home, in the community, and will be free of dementia and major disability well into their 70s and early 80s (U.S. Census, 2014). Moreover, as many research and community surveys have revealed, as long as individuals remain in reasonably good health, life satisfaction and emotional well-being improve with age (Carstensen et al., 2011; Mroczek & Kolarz, 1998; Stone, Schwartz, Broderick, & Deaton, 2010). These observations suggest that the older adult population represents a large and potentially untapped resource in our society. But it also poses significant challenges.

Societies have begun to take a serious look at the implications of this demographic shift for policies related to health care, pensions, and retirement, among other domains. Individuals, in turn, are increasingly reminded—through the media, but also in workplaces and health-care contexts—that remaining independent into their later years will require careful planning and decision making in an array of financial and health domains. For example, the decisions that working-age adults make about retirement savings and insurance coverage in their 40s and 50s will determine their ability to sustain current lifestyles, buffer against health shocks, and provide for long-term care needs. Individuals also face decisions about health care and illness management—for themselves and for their family members—as well as decisions regarding preferences for end-of-life care in anticipation of future infirmity or incapacity. The ability to make sound decisions for the short and long term is also essential to optimal functioning in the workplace, as more individuals seek ways to extend their productive working lives into older age. These are the consequential decisions that first come to mind when considering the major decision-making challenges associated with aging.

Perhaps less salient, but no less consequential, are the multiple, small decisions taken over the course of adulthood that collectively impact quality of life at older ages. How well individuals age—and how long they live depends in part on a series of daily decisions, often taken without much deliberation, regarding engagement in and adherence to health behaviors and regimens, or about small expenditures of financial resources, social capital, and cognitive effort, all of which exist in finite supply. These are decisions that draw on individuals' capacity for self-regulation and self-control, their ability to keep long-term goals in mind, and their willingness to place appropriate value on their future well-being. The cumulative impact of these small choices can constrain future choices and make the difference between arriving at older age in good health, with cognitive capacity intact, and with the resources permitting the exercise of these assets in pursuit of well-being, versus encountering older age with compromised health and cognitive function, or without the financial wherewithal to address age-related challenges. How well equipped are middle-aged and older adults to make adaptive decisions across these many domains?

The chapters in this volume represent an effort to identify both the strengths and weaknesses of decision making in, and in anticipation of, older age. The authors represent perspectives on decision making that derive primarily from psychology and neuroscience, where the key questions concern the cognitive, emotional, and motivational capacities older adults bring to the decision context, and age-related changes in these processes and the neural systems that support them. This kind of basic science orientation lays essential groundwork for the design of decision-supportive interventions for adaptive aging. Throughout the volume, there is also a deep appreciation of the broad range of domains (e.g., health care, finances) and contexts (e.g., with intimate partners and family members, with health-care providers, in the consumer marketplace) in which decisions take place, and of the need for an appreciation of the interaction between individual capacities and context variables in the design of interventions.

OPEN QUESTIONS

Psychologists who study aging have postulated that negotiating the challenges of later life requires careful balancing of strengths gained through years of life experience and accumulated expertise, against vulnerabilities associated with the normal declines that accompany older age (Baltes, 1997; Carstensen, Isaacowitz, & Charles, 1999; Charles, 2010). Over the past decade or so, there has been a clear recognition, common across the decision sciences, of the interdependence among—and trade-offs between—cognitive capacities (which support the processing of information about alternatives, probabilities, risks, and rewards) and emotional functions (which reflect subjective values and preferences and are involved in forecasting the impact of choices on subjective well-being in the long term) (Coricelli, Dolan, & Sirigu, 2007; Rolls & Grabenhorst, 2008; Weber & Johnson, 2009). Aging throws a unique light on this interaction, as the balance of strengths and vulnerabilities shifts. There is evidence that as cognitive flexibility of youth wanes, individuals may increasingly draw on expertise, learned heuristics, and emotional maturity to tackle decisions. Whether these shifts in capacity enhance or undermine decision making is a topic of considerable research attention (Hess & Kotter-Grühn, 2011; Morrow et al., 2009). The more we learn about the specific cognitive and affective processes that account for age-related changes in decision making, the more precisely we can target interventions to compensate for vulnerabilities and leverage strengths.

Older age is also associated with both shifts in social goals and changes in social relationships and contexts. Yet our understanding of the impact of these changes on decision making remains limited. It is possible that changes in both goals and contexts affect the extent to which interpersonal processes, such as coercion, trust, competition, generativity, and empathy, influence decisions in health and financial domains (see, for example, Beadle et al., 2012; Castle et al., 2012). Age groups may also differ in the degree to which self-regarding versus other-regarding motives take priority, and in their susceptibility to the influence of peers, family members, the media, professional advisors, or service providers. Sociodemographic factors may moderate these influences, with differences in wealth, education, and occupational status exerting powerful effects both on the ability to make sound choices and on the array of choices available.

Several of the chapters in this volume highlight the importance of strategies and strategy selection for adaptive decision making. This area of inquiry holds considerable potential for research on decision making in aging. For example, research has suggested that older age is associated with improvements in emotion regulation, and that emotional regulatory strategies may underlie some age differences in decision making, yet psychologists are only beginning to explore the precise strategies that older adults bring to bear to regulate emotions (Isaacowitz & Blanchard-Fields, 2012; Urry & Gross, 2010). There is evidence to suggest that older adults are capable of employing strategies along the full emotion-regulation continuum (Gross, 1998). They engage in early-stage situation selection (Robenpor, Skogsberg, & Isaacowitz, 2013)—including avoiding situations that will lead to adverse outcomes and choosing those that promise to yield emotional rewards. They are also able, when immersed in a choice context, to selectively attend to certain information (Lohani & Isaacowitz, 2014; Löckenhoff & Carstensen, 2007). And they exhibit the ability to engage in later-stage reappraisal involving the potentially more cognitively taxing "reframing" of current experiences to facilitate better coping

(Lohani & Isaacowitz, 2014; Mather, Shafir, & Johnson, 2000). Effective decision supportive interventions may require careful analysis of decision context features and individual emotional regulatory strengths, while also accounting for biases of particular age groups—that is, a person-by-context-by-strategy framework rather than a "one size fits all" approach (Tucker, Feuerstein, Mende-Siedlecki, Ochsner, & Stern, 2012).

A RESEARCH AGENDA FOR THE FUTURE

Interdisciplinary research on the cognitive, affective, and social influences on decision making in aging has been growing over the past decade, encouraged, in part, by research initiatives at the *National Institute on Aging* (2006, 2010c, 2011) and the *National Institutes of Health* (2010, 2012). These include efforts to stimulate research in neuroeconomics and behavioral economics of aging, as well as basic research on decision making and on mechanisms of behavior change. The integration of approaches from psychology, economics, and neuroscience in neuroeconomics is shedding new light on foundations of decision making and choice behavior and how these processes unfold developmentally. Important questions remain concerning the origins and degree of age-related changes in reward sensitivity and in the function of neural systems for reward processing, intertemporal choice, self-control, and attitudes toward risk. Behavioral economic approaches hold promise for elucidating the influence of social, cultural, institutional, and situational contexts on decision making to shape the design of interventions, and for offering insights regarding individual differences in susceptibility to context effects. The *National Institute on Aging* (2011, 2014) continues to be interested in research at the intersection of these fields, as application of these approaches to aging has the potential to inform the development and refinement of integrative life-span economic theories of utility, learning, habit formation, behavior change, and strategic choice.

As we come to understand more about how individual predispositions interact with environments to shape trajectories of aging, there is also increasing recognition of the need for improved measurement of the core behavioral, psychological, and intermediate biological phenotypes (Lenzenweger, 2013) that account for individual variation in decision making and choice behavior over the life span (National Institute on Aging, 2007, 2010b, 2014). Psychometrically sound measures of "economic phenotypes" hold potential at many levels. If integrated into population-based studies, they could be useful for pooling data for genetic analyses, as well as for linking data on basic psychological capacities to real-world outcomes. Efforts to connect with population-based surveys providing administrative data on savings and insurance may be particularly fruitful in this regard. In intervention contexts, such measures may hold promise for identifying individuals for whom particular decision-supportive strategies are more or less likely to be successful (Sheffer et al., 2014).

In the years ahead, the *National Institute on Aging* (2014) will continue to encourage research on both the basic mechanisms and processes that impact choice as well as on the design of interventions to support adaptive decisions regarding savings, insurance, health care, timing of retirement, time use, and health behaviors, all of which have consequences for successful aging. The Institute continues to encourage research examining the neurobiological mechanisms and processes involved in decision making and aging, and in translation of basic science insights into interventions. While the past decade has seen progress in developing behavioral economic interventions for health, more attention to age differences is needed in those efforts. Research on social influences on decision making also remains a priority, including the role of family members, advisors, and social networks. As noted previously, consequential life decisions are rarely made in a social void, and we are only beginning to understand the impact of such social forces on choice.

Stronger links between basic decision science and applied research on health-related decision making are also needed. Recent work in applied health domains, such as advance care planning, illustrates that preferences evolve as individuals accommodate to new health circumstances, new sets of symptoms and probabilities, and that decisions need to be made and remade in light of those changes (Fried, O'Leary, Van Ness, & Fraenkel, 2007). One of the major challenges in the field of medical decision making concerns the objective definition of a "good" decision. As values change with age, or with changes in health state (Fried & Bradley, 2003), the criteria for classifying decisions as good may require reevaluation. Understanding the factors that influence decision making under these dynamic circumstances may aid in tailoring health-related decision aids to the particular needs and values of older adults.

The *National Institute on Aging*'s interest in basic and applied research on financial decision making remains strong because of the tight link between finances and health. In 2010, the U.S. government estimated the average cost of long-term care to be approximately $3300/month for care in assisted living, or $229/day for care in a nursing home (Department of Health and Human Services, http://longtermcare.gov/). These long-term care costs are not covered by Medicare, the insurance upon which the majority of older Americans rely. Such out-of-pocket health expenditures must be covered by retirement savings or supplemental insurance, and many older adults are ill prepared. Data from the NIA-supported *Health and Retirement Study* (National Institute on Aging, 2010a) reveal that more than one-third of U.S. adults have saved nothing for retirement, and the majority report not having saved enough. Indeed, in 1996, the median amount saved over 10 years was about $10,000. Recent analyses suggest that a substantial portion of the older population ends life with assets below $10,000, with no housing assets and little capacity to deal with unanticipated health expenditures or other financial shocks (Poterba, Venti, & Wise, 2012). Analyses of HRS data also reveal the extent to which health, social circumstances, and finances are closely intertwined. For example, an unexpected health event can take a large bite out of savings and have a long-term impact on earnings, with total income loss ranging from about $8700 for a minor health event to nearly $37,000 for a major health event. Widows and divorced women are especially vulnerable to losses in wealth that reduce the ability to cope with health shocks (NIA, 2010a).

Finally, there is emerging evidence that poverty and early adversity change trajectories of aging in profound ways, that these changes are evident early in life and compounded over the life course, and that these changes extend to ways that impact momentary decisions and the cognitive resources available to grapple with them (Haushofer & Fehr, 2014; Mani, Mullainathan, Shafir, & Zhao, 2013). Future research in large samples will be needed to explore the influences of early and later life socioeconomic conditions on decision making over the life course. This would be an important first step in bringing research on aging and decision making into a health disparities framework. Typically, we are not reaching the very poor in our studies, and that remains a significant gap. In addition, more work is needed on the influences of acute and chronic psychosocial stressors on the ability to make adaptive decisions in real time. Indeed, many important health decisions are made under time pressure, and under circumstances of considerable uncertainty and ambiguity. Older adults may be especially compromised under these circumstances, as well as more likely to find themselves in such situations.

CONCLUSION

Decisions large and small play a fundamental role in shaping life-course trajectories of health and well-being. It is encouraging to see a growing number of research teams engaged in exploring cutting-edge approaches in the burgeoning field of research on decision making and aging. The chapters in this volume collectively underscore the point that choice is a ubiquitous component of everyday functioning. How we invest our limited social, temporal, psychological, financial, and physical resources has implications for many important aging relevant outcomes. Adequate preparation for later-life health and financial security involves making multiple small and consequential decisions early in life with an eye to an uncertain and distant future need. How individuals negotiate this complex terrain can serve either to shore up or to undermine the foundations for a healthy older age. There is also a need for lifelong maintenance of strategic decision-making skills in the workplace, as adults extend working lives and remain in active leadership roles that determine the short- and long-term fate of the organizations they serve. These are decisions that matter, and that affect future options and starting conditions, not only for ourselves but for others in our social spheres.

Lisbeth Nielsen
Division of Behavioral and Social Research
National Institute on Aging, MD, USA

References

Baltes, P. B. (1997). On the incomplete architecture of human ontogeny: Selection, optimization, and compensation as foundation of developmental theory. *American Psychologist, 52*(4), 366–380.

Beadle, J. N., Paradiso, S., Kovach, C., Polgreen, L., Denburg, N. L., & Tranel, D. (2012). Effects of age-related differences in empathy on social economic decision-making. *International Psychogeriatrics, 24*(5), 822–833.

Carstensen, L. L., Isaacowitz, D. M., & Charles, S. T. (1999). Taking time seriously: A theory of socioemotional selectivity. *American Psychologist, 54*(3), 165–181.

Carstensen, L. L., Turan, B., Scheibe, S., Ram, N., Ersner-Hershfield, H., Samanez-Larkin, G. R., et al. (2011). Emotional experience improves with age: evidence based on over 10 years of experience sampling. *Psychology and Aging, 26*(1), 21–33.

Castle, E., Eisenberger, N. I., Seeman, T. E., Moons, W. G., Boggero, I. A., Grinblatt, M. S., et al. (2012). Neural and behavioral bases of age differences in perceptions of trust. *Proceedings of the National Academy of Sciences, 109*(51), 20848–20852.

Charles, S. T. (2010). Strength and vulnerability integration: A model of emotional well-being across adulthood. *Psychological Bulletin, 136*(6), 1068–1091.

Coricelli, G., Dolan, R. J., & Sirigu, A. (2007). Brain, emotion and decision making: The paradigmatic example of regret. *Trends in Cognitive Science, 11*(6), 258–265.

Department of Health and Human Services, LongTermCare.gov. http://longtermcare.gov/.

Fried, T. R., & Bradley, E. H. (2003). What matters to seriously ill older persons making end-of-life treatment decisions? A qualitative study. *Journal of Palliative Medicine, 6*(2), 237–244.

Fried, T. R., O'Leary, J., Van Ness, P., & Fraenkel, L. (2007). Inconsistency over time in the preferences of older persons with advanced illness for life-sustaining treatment. *Journal of the American Geriatrics Society, 55*(7), 1007–1014.

Gross, J. J. (1998). Antecedent- and response-focused emotion regulation: Divergent consequences for experience, expression, and physiology. *Journal of Personality and Social Psychology, 74*, 224–237.

Haushofer, J., & Fehr, E. (2014). On the psychology of poverty. *Science, 344*(6186), 862–867.

Hess, T. M., & Kotter-Grühn, D. (2011). Social knowledge and goal-based influences on social information processing in adulthood. *Psychology and Aging, 26*(4), 792–802.

Isaacowitz, D. M., & Blanchard-Fields, F. (2012). Linking process and outcome in the study of emotion and aging. *Perspectives in Psychological Science, 7*(1), 3–17.

Lenzenweger, M. F. (2013). Endophenotype, intermediate phenotype, biomarker: Definitions, concept comparisons, clarifications. *Depression and Anxiety, 30*(3), 185–189.

Löckenhoff, C. E., & Carstensen, L. L. (2007). Aging, emotion, and health-related decision strategies: Motivational manipulations can reduce age differences. *Psychology and Aging, 22*(1), 134–146.

Lohani, M., & Isaacowitz, D. M. (2014). Age differences in managing response to sadness elicitors using attentional deployment, positive reappraisal and suppression. *Cognition and Emotion, 28*(4), 678–697.

Mani, A., Mullainathan, S., Shafir, E., & Zhao, J. (2013). Poverty impedes cognitive function. *Science, 341*(6149), 976–980.

Mather, M., Shafir, E., & Johnson, M. K. (2000). Misremembrance of options past: Source monitoring and choice. *Psychological Science, 11*(2), 132–138.

Morrow, D. G., Miller, L. M., Ridolfo, H. E., Magnor, C., Fischer, U. M., Kokayeff, N. K., et al. (2009). Expertise and age differences in pilot decision making. *Neuropsychology, Development, and Cognition. Section B, Aging Neuropsychology, and Cognition, 16*(1), 33–55.

Mroczek, D. K., & Kolarz, C. M. (1998). The effect of age on positive and negative affect: A developmental perspective on happiness. *Journal of Personality and Social Psychology, 75*(5), 1333–1349.

National Institute on Aging. (2006). *Neuroeconomics of aging RFA.* http://grants.nih.gov/grants/guide/rfa-files/RFA-AG-06-011.html.

National Institute on Aging. (2007). *NIA workshop on refining economic phenotypes.* http://www.nia.nih.gov/ResearchInformation/ExtramuralPrograms/BehavioralAndSocialResearch/Psychology.htm.

National Institute on Aging. (2010a). *Growing older in America: The Health and Retirement Study.* http://hrsonline.isr.umich.edu/index.php?p=dbook.

National Institute on Aging. (2010b). *Workshop on economic phenotypes.* http://www.nia.nih.gov/about/events/2011/workshop-economic-phenotypes.

National Institute on Aging. (2010c). *Health aging through behavioral economic analyses of situations.* http://grants.nih.gov/grants/guide/rfa-files/RFA-AG-10-008.html.

National Institute on Aging. (2011). *Social neuroscience and neuroeconomics of aging PAR.* http://grants.nih.gov/grants/guide/pa-files/PAR-11-337.html.

National Institute on Aging. (2014). *National advisory council on aging 2013 BSR review committee report.* http://www.nia.nih.gov/research/announcements/2014/03/naca-evaluation-bsr-report-2013.

National Institute on Aging/World Health Organization. (2011). *Global health and aging.* NIH Publication. no. 11-7737, October 2011.

National Institutes of Health. (2010). *Science of behavior Change: Finding mechanisms of change in the laboratory and the field RFA.* http://grants.nih.gov/grants/guide/rfa-files/RFA-RM-10-002.html.

National Institutes of Health. (2012). *Basic research on decision making RFA.* http://grants.nih.gov/grants/guide/rfa-files/RFA-MH-12-130.html.

Poterba, J. M., Venti, S. F., & Wise, D. A. (2012). *Were they prepared for retirement? Financial status at advanced ages in the HRS and AHEAD cohorts.* NBER Working Paper 17824. http://www.nber.org/papers/w17824.

Rolls, E. T., & Grabenhorst, F. (2008). The orbitofrontal cortex and beyond: From affect to decision-making. *Progress in Neurobiology, 86*(3), 216–244.

Rovenpor, D. R., Skogsberg, N. J., & Isaacowitz, D. M. (2013). The choices we make: An examination of situation selection in younger and older adults. *Psychology and Aging, 28*(2), 365–376.

Sheffer, C. E., Christensen, D. R., Landes, R., Carter, L. P., Jackson, L., & Bickel, W. K. (2014). Delay discounting rates: A strong prognostic indicator of smoking relapse. *Addictive Behaviors, 39*(11), 1682–1689.

Stone, A. A., Schwartz, J. E., Broderick, J. E., & Deaton, A. (2010). A snapshot of the age distribution of psychological well-being in the United States. *Proceedings of the National Academy of Sciences, 107*(22), 9985–9990.

Tucker, A. M., Feuerstein, R., Mende-Siedlecki, P., Ochsner, K. N., & Stern, Y. (2012). Double dissociation: Circadian off-peak times increase emotional reactivity; aging impairs emotion regulation via reappraisal. *Emotion, 12*(5), 869–874.

Urry, H. L., & Gross, J. J. (2010). Emotion regulation in older age. *Current Directions in Psychological Science, 19*(6), 352–357.
U.S. Census Bureau, P23-212. (2014). *65+ in the United States: 2010*. Washington, DC: U.S. Government Printing Office.
Weber, E. U., & Johnson, E. J. (2009). Mindful judgment and decision making. *Annual Review of Psychology, 60*, 53–85.

Preface

Research on cognitive aging has accumulated decades of evidence documenting age-related shifts in basic components of cognitive functioning, but until the turn of the century, age differences in more complex processes drawing on multiple cognitive abilities or integrating affect and reason remained relatively unexplored. Decision making in particular had attracted very little research attention in spite of its momentous implications for older adults' health and well-being. In two influential reports, the National Research Council (NRC, 2000, 2006) outlined an agenda for aging research in the new millennium, and a recurring theme was the need to better understand the impact of aging on decision making, acknowledging both the multitude of contexts in which important decisions are made and the myriad of age-correlated influences on such decisions. Responding to this call to action, the three editors—both individually and collectively—have been involved in a series of symposia focused on decision making and aging that were presented at the annual scientific meetings of the American Psychological Association, the Gerontological Society of America, and the Society for Judgment and Decision Making over the past 15 years. The goal of some of the earlier presentations was to increase the visibility of work in this area and highlight the significance of decision-making processes for understanding and promoting functioning in later life with the related aim of generating interest in the topic among other researchers. Later symposia—organized by the editors and others—promoted further maturation of the field by highlighting programmatic research efforts across different research groups and fostering cross-disciplinary collaborations.

This book is a natural extension of these efforts. Noting the high degree of interest in these symposia and the growing number of related panels at recent meetings, we believed that it was the right time to compile an edited volume, which provides a status report on the field. A related impetus for the book was the burgeoning interest in research on decision making and aging reflected in the growth in empirical studies on the topic across a wide array of disciplines representing both applied and basic researchers. Although certainly not complete, a quick *PsychInfo* search of articles published in peer-reviewed journals using the key words "decision making" and either "aging" or "older adults" identified only 23 articles published during the 5-year period from 2000 to 2004 versus 142 from 2010 through the completion of this book in Fall 2014. Thus, the increase in research activity is quite dramatic.

Our goal in developing this volume was to provide a state-of-the-art review of current perspectives and empirical work relating to psychological perspectives on the study of aging and decision making. The coverage is quite broad, including chapters on animal studies, brain functions, behavioral processes, experience, cognitive abilities, affective processes, social influences, and practical applications of this research for consumer, medical, and financial decision making. Our aim was to offer a representative sampling of the major topics of interest, prominent conceptual frameworks, diverse methodologies, and multiple levels of analysis. Accordingly, we recruited authors representing laboratories whose research is at the forefront of work in the field.

We acknowledge, however, that we do not cover some important topics highlighted in the NRC reports. For some areas, this is due to an underrepresentation in the research literature. Others were excluded because they were considered outside the scope of this book. For example, there is little discussion of changes in decision making associated with pathological aging (e.g., mild cognitive impairment, Alzheimer's disease) because the present volume focuses on normative patterns seen in healthy aging.

In sum, we consider this volume as a sort of progress report on the agenda laid out by the NRC. It reviews current research and theory relevant to the topics identified in those reports, and identifies areas in need of further study. We also believe that the chapters in this volume will update the NRC reports through theoretical insights and the identification of new sets of issues that will continue to move the field forward. We hope our work will prove valuable to researchers and graduate students in the field, as well as to practitioners who deal with older adults and their families as they grapple with important life decisions.

We would like to acknowledge the valuable assistance of Emily Ekle and Barbara Makinster at Elsevier during the development of the proposal and eventual production of the book. We would also like to acknowledge the assistance of many of the chapters' authors in the volume who assisted in reviewing other authors' chapters—most chapters were reviewed by at least two of the editors and one other contributor. Their commentaries were invaluable in helping to shape and focus each contribution. Finally, we would like to acknowledge specific sources of support received by each of us that aided greatly in preparation of this volume. Hess was supported, in part, by funding from the National Institute on Aging (NIA; R01 AG05552 and R01 AG020153) and also greatly benefitted from a sabbatical leave granted by North Carolina

State University. Strough benefitted from a sabbatical leave granted by West Virginia University, and a visiting professorship at the Centre for Decision Research, Leeds University Business School. Löckenhoff was supported in part by NIA grant 1R21AG043741.

Thomas M. Hess
JoNell Strough
Corinna E. Löckenhoff

CHAPTER

1

The Present, Past, and Future of Research on Aging and Decision Making

JoNell Strough[1], *Corinna E. Löckenhoff*[2], *Thomas M. Hess*[3]

[1]Department of Psychology, West Virginia University, Morgantown, WV, USA; [2]Department of Human Development, College of Human Ecology, Cornell University, Ithaca, NY, USA; [3]Department of Psychology, North Carolina State University, Raleigh, NC, USA

Two volumes published by the National Research Council in the United States at the beginning of the twenty-first century (National Research Council, 2000, 2006) emphasized that the "aging of America" created an immediate need to understand and promote effective functioning of older adults in their everyday lives—a need that is still urgent today (see Nielsen, this volume). The 2000 volume emphasized cognitive aging and the need for research addressing neural health, cognition in context, and the structure of the aging mind. The 2006 volume emphasized the importance of motivation, socioemotional functioning, and social contextual influences, including cultural attitudes about aging as well as ethnicity, race, and culture. Central to both reports was a call for a better understanding of age-related influences on decision making. Together, these two volumes set an agenda for studying aging and decision making that is reflected in much of the contemporary research on this topic, including the chapters in this book.

Since the turn of the millennium, the field of aging and decision making has dramatically expanded. Theoretical frameworks now incorporate affective, motivational, interpersonal, and neuroscience perspectives (to name just a few) in addition to cognition, and researchers have begun to consider a wide array of outcomes ranging from markers of neurological activation

http://dx.doi.org/10.1016/B978-0-12-417148-0.00001-7

tracked over the course of seconds, to savings rates and long-term health trajectories tracked over the course of decades. For the purpose of this book, we broadly group this rich body of work into three sections devoted to neurobiological mechanisms, behavioral mechanisms (including cognition, affect, and motivation), and applied perspectives, although many of the chapters touch on multiple areas. We first consider some of the major issues within each of these broad areas in more detail and then provide a brief description of the individual chapters. The chapters themselves trace how research in each area has progressed since the publication of the volumes by the National Research Council (2000, 2006) and outline important new directions, as well as open questions and methodological challenges.

BASIC ISSUES IN THE STUDY OF AGING AND DECISIONS

Neurobiological Mechanisms

Mather's (2006) paper for the National Research Council called for greater integration of work on decision making with work on cognitive neuroscience. Neurobiological perspectives on aging and decision making have seen rapid development between 2000 and 2010 propelled in part by unprecedented progress in brain-imaging techniques. Our understanding of age-related structural changes in gross anatomy (often examined postmortem) is now enriched by functional images of the living brain available at increasingly higher spatial and temporal resolution.

Concomitant changes in theoretical frameworks have left their mark as well. The nascent field of decision neuroscience integrates neuroscience perspectives with disciplines traditionally associated with decision science including economics and psychology. Inspired by initiatives such as the Scientific Research Network on Decision Neuroscience and Aging (www.srndna.org), researchers have begun to apply this interdisciplinary perspective to the aging brain. As a result, research interest has expanded beyond attention and memory processes located in medial temporal and lateral cortical regions that have traditionally been the focus of cognitive aging research. In particular, Mather's (2006) report targeted the dorsolateral prefrontal cortex and orbitofrontal cortex as areas that could yield important insights because changes in these two regions of the brain are differentially linked to aging (see Raz & Rodrigue, 2006). Today, regions of growing interest for aging and decision making include prefrontal networks associated with executive functioning (Harlé & Sanfey, 2012), frontostriatial pathways linked to reward processing (Samanez-Larkin, Levens, Perry, Dougherty, & Knutson, 2012), and affective processes in the limbic system (Schott et al., 2007).

Many of the specific topics investigated from a neurobiological perspective reflect areas of interest outlined in the National Research Council reports (2000, 2006). For instance, neurobiological approaches have been used to address the role of motivation in older adults' decision making by investigating the neural representation of rewards (e.g., Samanez-Larkin et al., 2007). Neuroimaging studies have also advanced our understanding of age differences in intertemporal choice (Eppinger, Nystrom, & Cohen, 2012), probabilistic decisions (Samanez-Larkin et al., 2012), and the ability to integrate novel information in complex decision scenarios (Eppinger, Hämmerer, & Li, 2011).

Although these recent developments have yielded large amounts of new data, the interpretation of this information is not without challenges. One basic hurdle is a lack of integration across methods and levels of analysis. How do age-related structural changes in gross anatomy, variations in neurotransmitter levels and receptors, and shifts in neural activity relate to each other, and how are they associated with behavioral changes in decision strategies and—ultimately—decision outcomes? Even more challenging is the search for underlying causal pathways. If we see empirical evidence for age differences in brain activation during a given decision task, does it reflect passive loss due to biological aging, active efforts at compensation, age-related increases in access to experience-based knowledge, or a motivated shift toward decision strategies that benefit emotion regulation? To further complicate matters, several of these mechanisms may operate at the same time and interact with one another. Researchers represented in this volume have begun to tackle these questions using a variety of strategies ranging from controlled experiments in animal models to the development of novel theoretical frameworks that allow for the integration of age patterns across tasks, brain regions, and levels of analysis.

Behavioral Mechanisms: Cognition, Affect, and Motivation

Much of the early research on age-related shifts in decision-making strategies and outcomes was informed by a cognitive aging perspective and focused on behavioral responses observed in laboratory settings (Yates & Patalano, 1999). In their paper for the National Research Council, Peters, Finucane, MacGregor, and Slovic (2000) noted a need for research investigating whether aging is associated with greater reliance on heuristic processing due to increases in experience and declines in cognitive abilities necessary for deliberative processing. Heuristic processing reflects using cognitive shortcuts such as availability (judging probabilities by how easily something comes to mind) instead of more effortful deliberation of facts. Although heuristics can be useful because they save time, reduce effort, and often yield "good enough" decisions (Epstein, 1994;

Gigerenzer, 2008), they can also produce decisions that are systematically biased (Tversky & Kahneman, 1974). In addition to prompting research on aging and heuristic processing, Peters et al. (2000) also noted a need for research on affect and decision making, a point that was elaborated on by Mather in her 2006 paper for the National Research Council. Mather (2006) further suggested that older adults' decisions might be enhanced by effective control of emotions and focusing on emotionally salient goals.

An influential article published by Peters, Hess, Västfjäll, and Auman in 2007 expanded on these ideas by combining ideas from "dual-process" models of decision making (which posit two interacting decision modes, one based on reason and deliberation and another based on intuitions and heuristics arising from affect and experience; see Evans, 2008 for a review) with decades of basic research on age-related changes in cognition and affect to outline potential trajectories of decision making over the life span. This paper represented the fusion and cross-fertilization of ideas from two types of literature, adult development and behavioral decision making. Building on this, researchers increasingly focused on the implications of older adults' cognitive and affective strengths and vulnerabilities for decision processes and outcomes. As the chapters in this volume show, this is a vigorous area of research. Recent work establishes that cognitive and affective mechanisms are both important for understanding decision making in later adulthood, and there is increasing appreciation that, in some contexts, experience and improvements in affect regulation can offset age-related cognitive declines, whereas in other contexts, relying on affect can have detrimental consequences for decisions.

The publication of the Peters, Hess, Västfjäll, and Auman's (2007) article occurred alongside growing recognition by behavioral decision-making researchers that findings based solely on undergraduate college students may suffer from limited generalizability and thus have limited utility for addressing key societal issues presented by an aging population. Accordingly, investigators began to broaden the populations studied to include people of diverse ages. At about the same time, adult development and aging researchers began to adopt many of the standard tasks that decision scientists developed for laboratory research. Merging methods, theories, and findings from the adult development and aging and behavioral decision-making literature has proved fruitful. The number of studies addressing aging and decision making has increased substantially over the past decade, and a basic understanding of age differences in key decision-making competencies has begun to emerge.

In their 2000 paper for the National Research Council, Peters and colleagues pointed to a need to develop a reliable measure of decision-making competence to be used with older adults. Many of the standard laboratory tasks designed by decision scientists were originally created to reveal key decision biases and deviations from models of "rational" or "normative" decision making (models originating from economic theories and principles addressing how to maximize favorable outcomes). These standard tasks often pit decisions based on logic and reason against decisions based on emotions and intuition. This makes them ideal not only for testing ideas about cognitive and affective underpinnings of decisions, but also ideas about aging and decision-making competence. Researchers have begun to address how some of the key aspects of decision-making competence described by Peters et al. (2000)—such as the ability to resist irrelevant variations in how information is presented (i.e., "framing effects") and the ability to effectively integrate information—differ by age, and how performance on standard tasks can be used to reliably measure decision-making competence (see Bruine de Bruin, Parker, & Fischhoff, 2007; Finucane & Gullion, 2010). Chapters in this volume discuss necessary next steps in this area of research.

The chapters in this volume also address other research topics identified by the National Research Council (2000, 2006) to varying degrees. For instance, one theme that cuts across several chapters is the importance of taking age differences in motivation and goals into account, and the associated need to examine contextual influences on older adults' decisions. Age differences in risky decisions and older adults' ability to learn from repeated decisions are starting to be better understood (e.g., Mather et al., 2012; Rolison, Hanoch, & Wood, 2012; Weller et al., 2014), but much is still unknown. For instance, in her 2006 paper for the Council, Mather suggested that in some cases what might appear to be greater risk aversion in older adults might instead reflect avoiding making a decision. Current paradigms used to examine risky decision making do not facilitate testing this idea. Other topics highlighted by the National Research Council (2000, 2006) have received relatively little attention, such as affective forecasting or the ability to predict future feelings and the role of specific emotions such as regret (cf. Bjälkebring, Västfjäll, & Johansson, 2013; Nielsen, Knutson, & Carstensen, 2008).

In sum, research on cognitive, affective, and motivational mechanisms has facilitated significant advances in our basic understanding of aging and decision making over the past decade. Yet much of this work is still in its early stages, and significant gaps exist with some topics having received almost no attention. New research that builds on existing knowledge to fill key gaps in our basic understanding of aging and decision making is necessary to facilitate translational efforts aimed at improving older adults' daily lives.

Applied Research

Applied decision-making research, the third broad area considered in this volume, has begun to address the challenge of applying basic research by acknowledging that the strengths and vulnerabilities of the aging decision maker may be more or less apparent depending upon context-related demands and supports. Although a thorough understanding of the basic neural and behavioral mechanisms behind age effects in decision making is important, it is perhaps equally important to understand behavior in the specific contexts in which older adults function. Examination of performance within these contexts provides a means for testing the generalizability of factors identified in research that might be considered more in the realm of basic science. In addition, context-specific investigations are likely to identify important moderating factors that may not necessarily be considered or even relevant in more traditional experimental studies and theoretical models. The National Research Council (2000) identified specific domains of everyday life where a better understanding of decision-making processes and outcomes was needed in order to promote effective functioning. These included health, finances, and end-of-life care, and the social context in which these decisions are made.

The everyday contexts in which decisions about health and finances occur involve a level of complexity that may be difficult to study in the lab, further highlighting the importance of applied research in determining the extent to which basic science results can be applied to real-world contexts. A prime example of these issues can be seen in studies of decision making regarding medical matters. Decisions about health may be emotionally charged (e.g., choices involving trade-offs between quality of life and survival), complex (e.g., involving comparisons between multiple insurance plans varying along many dimensions), and involve the use of numerical information (e.g., outcomes associated with treatments, costs associated with procedures). In many respects, these factors can easily map onto the types of concepts that researchers study in the lab. For example, one could manipulate the complexity of information, number of choices, and emotional content of options to examine hypothesized age differences involving the interplay between affect and deliberation. In everyday life, however, such decisions are likely to be complicated and influenced by a number of other factors that may not be considered in traditional models. For example, medical decisions—particularly in later life—are rarely made absent consultation with spouses, children, and other family members, as well as with physicians involved in treatment (Dy & Purnell, 2012). These individuals may provide emotional support, information, and assistance in comprehending information, potentially compensating for normative age-related declines in ability. They may also, however, attempt to influence outcomes in a manner that may not always be in the best interests of the individual.

Knowledge and beliefs are also likely to play an important role in determining choices regarding health. For example, the ability to understand and communicate information related to health—often referred to as health literacy—is positively associated with health outcomes (Bostock &

Steptoe, 2012), and the extent to which health literacy is negatively affected by aging is likely to impact decision making in a manner not accounted for in theoretical models (e.g., Mõttus et al., 2014). Specific experiences with and lay-beliefs about diseases will also influence the effectiveness of health-related decisions (Kim, 2014). Individuals may possess ideas about the effectiveness of treatments based on the experiences of familiar others (e.g., a friend who has cancer and did not respond to radiation) or schemas about specific diseases and symptoms that may not be accurate and are discrepant from those of knowledgeable health-care professionals. These factors may steer decisions in unforeseen and idiosyncratic ways that are, nonetheless, important to understand because they may result in poor choices.

Finally, an understanding of "aging" influences on decision making is further complicated by the fact that many of these moderating influences may actually reflect cohort-based effects as opposed to aging-related phenomena. It is possible that older adults of the future (i.e., today's young adults) will be more knowledgeable about health, have more sources of information available—along with the ability to access this information—and possess different ideas and attitudes regarding interactions with health-care professionals. This highlights the importance of not only understanding context in terms of types of decisions, but also in broader terms that are consistent with life-span contextual views of development and the multiple factors influencing behavior (e.g., Baltes, Staudinger, & Lindenberger, 1999).

Applied research on aging and decision making has increased our understanding of key research topics identified by the National Research Council (2000, 2006). In particular, we now are beginning to have a better understanding of the potential detrimental consequences of age-related cognitive declines for older adults' decisions about health and finances. However, we know relatively little about other applied topics identified by Peters et al. (2000) in their paper for the Council, such as how people make decisions about end-of-life care (Raijmakers et al., 2012) and what influences older adults' decisions to discontinue driving (Choi, Mezuk, & Rebok, 2012). In addition, basic research on age differences in risky decision making has yet to be translated to applied settings to understand whether older adults are more susceptible to financial scams, a topic of importance noted by Mather (2006) in her paper for the Council. Somewhat inconsistent with popular perceptions, recent work suggests that aging is not associated with greater susceptibility to financial fraud (Ross, Grossmann, & Schryer, 2014), and basic research on risky decision making could be useful in understanding protective factors. At a broader level, there is very little understanding of the long-term consequences of decisions made earlier in life, reflecting that cross-sectional rather than longitudinal designs have typically been used. Finally, little research has considered how features of the social context such as culture, race, and ethnicity may influence decision-making processes and outcomes. Such issues are important given well-documented health and financial disparities. Thus, while important steps have been made toward understanding decision making in everyday contexts, much research remains to be done.

Summary

In sum, across the last decade there has been considerable progress in advancing knowledge of aging and decision making in areas targeted by the National Research Council (2000, 2006). Continued progress will depend on filling remaining gaps and using ideas and findings from each of the three broad research areas considered in this volume—neurobiological perspectives, behavioral mechanisms, and applied research—to inform research in the other areas. Doing so will facilitate the development of interventions for improving functioning and quality of life in an aging population.

BOOK OVERVIEW

Neurobiological Mechanisms

The chapters in this section provide an overview of current knowledge about the neurobiological mechanisms behind age-related shifts in decision making and highlight emerging research methods and directions in this rapidly developing field. Beas, Setlow, Samanez-Larkin, and Bizon argue that animal models provide unique advantages for studying the influence of brain aging on decision processes since they offer high levels of experimenter control over contextual variables and prior experience—factors that are often difficult to account for in human studies. Beas and colleagues illustrate the promise of this approach by reviewing the literature on rodent models of age-related shifts in cost–benefit decision making. Although specific paradigms and reinforcers vary across species, findings indicate remarkable similarities in age effects for intertemporal and probabilistic decision making in rats and humans, suggesting that homologous age-associated changes in neural circuitry may be driving such effects.

Turning to reward-related decision making in humans, Samanez-Larkin focuses on the role of frontostriatal brain systems responsible for the anticipation and processing of reward-related signals. Research on age-related changes in these regions has documented structural atrophy and lower neurotransmitter levels, but the functional implications of such effects remain poorly understood. Samanez-Larkin's review of the available literature shows little evidence for age differences in basic neural reactivity to monetary gains and losses, but suggests that deficits in communication across frontostriatial networks may impair complex decision tasks that require the integration of novel feedback over time.

Also focusing on reward-based decision making, Eppinger and Bruckner propose a neuro-computational approach to understanding neural mechanisms at the root of age effects in behavioral preferences. They suggest that age-related deficits in reinforcement learning contribute to age differences in decisions from experience where the expected value of alternative choice options needs is learned over time. Drawing on a growing literature documenting age-related changes in the dopamine system, they suggest that older adults may experience specific deficits in updating reward values in response to positive and negative feedback—especially when outcomes are probabilistic.

Denburg and Hedgcock conclude this section of the book by examining empirical support for the frontal aging hypothesis, which proposes that brain structures in the frontal lobe are disproportionately affected by age-related changes. They focus on the well-established Iowa Gambling Task, which requires decision makers to forgo immediate gains to avoid delayed, probabilistic losses. Patients with prefrontal lesions are known to perform poorly on this task, and the authors present behavioral, psychophysiological, and functional imaging data indicating that about one-third of seemingly healthy older adults show substantial deficits in this task even though they perform normally on standard tests of cognitive aging.

Behavioral Mechanisms

The research reviewed in this section represents the "state of the art" in terms of current knowledge of behavioral mechanisms relevant to understanding aging and decision making. These chapters also point out that this research is still very much in its infancy. Several chapters focus primarily on cognitive mechanisms. Mata, Josef, and Lemaire argue that core cognitive abilities of cognitive control and reward processing facilitate adaptation to distinct ecological niches through their influence on strategy selection and execution. Mata and colleagues' chapter also provides a bridge between the neural mechanisms discussed in the first section of the book by highlighting the neural correlates of behavioral strategies. The ecological perspective that guides Mata, Josef, and Lemaire's ideas about age differences in strategy selection and execution is consistent with other chapters in this section that conceptualize decision making as a contextually embedded process.

Del Missier, Mäntylä, and Nilsson home in on one cognitive mechanism—memory. The authors review research investigating distinct types of memory (working, episodic, semantic, implicit) as mediating performance on judgment and decision-making tasks corresponding to key facets of decision-making competence such as the ability to accurately apply decision rules. Del Missier and colleagues argue that declines in working memory play a pivotal role in explaining why older adults perform worse on cognitively demanding decision-making tasks, while noting that these declines must be understood in the context of other cognitive and noncognitive changes.

Zaval, Li, Johnson, and Weber not only consider the implications of age-related cognitive declines for decision making but also suggest a remedy. Their framework posits that older adults compensate for declining fluid cognitive abilities by using domain-specific knowledge and experience. They apply their framework to review research from diverse domains such as job performance and consumer decisions, and suggest implications for public policy and the design of effective decision interventions for older adults.

In contrast to the focus on cognitive mechanisms that pervades several chapters, Mikels, Shuster, and Thai focus on the role of emotion in aging and decision making. The authors argue that emotions and affect are central to the study of aging and decision making because these mechanisms explain age differences in decisions, even after accounting for age differences due to cognitive mechanisms. Further, Mikels and colleagues highlight that incidental positive affect in later adulthood is a double-edged sword that can be beneficial or detrimental for older adults' decision making.

Hess builds on dual process models and uses four theories of the changing interplay of affect and cognition with age—relative preservation of affective processing, heightened focus on affect, selective focus on affect, and selective deployment of cognitive resources—to derive predictions about aging and risky decisions from the perspective of prospect theory. Lacking support for predictions derived from any single theory, Hess argues that older adults' decision making is multidirectional and multidimensional, and thus best approached from a contextual theoretical perspective.

Löckenhoff and Rutt draw attention to an aspect of the decision context that has been relatively under-investigated: the temporal context within which all decisions take place. The authors review cognitive and affective mechanisms that may underlie age differences in mental representations of time, including objective and subjective remaining life-expectancy. Building on this, Löckenhoff and Rutt argue that consideration of age differences in temporal horizons is essential for understanding decision strategies and outcomes across the life span.

The final chapter in this section, by Strough, Parker, and Bruine de Bruin, addresses how older adults may maintain and potentially improve their decision-making competence despite cognitive declines by drawing on experience and affect-regulation skills. The authors consider how to measure decision-making competence using a portfolio of laboratory tasks. Strough and colleagues then argue that motivation and contextual demands influence how much older adults use deliberative, experiential, and affective skills important for performing well on these tasks. The authors also discuss barriers to translating laboratory research to improve older adults' real-world financial and health decisions, and make recommendations about how to overcome these barriers.

Applied Contexts

The chapters in the final section reflect a more applied approach to the study of decision making and aging in that they review research involving particular everyday contexts and the factors that may be operative within those contexts. Morrow and Chin examine how health literacy impacts older adults' abilities to make effective decisions about health care; that is, how does aging affect the ability to access, comprehend, and use health information? Of particular interest is the degree to which normative changes in ability interact with experience and age-relevant goals, and how our understanding of such factors can be used to design more effective tools for promoting adaptive decision making in later life.

The chapter by H. Leventhal, Herold, E.A. Leventhal, Burns, and Diefenbach addresses medical decision making as well, but from a slightly different perspective. Specifically, the focus here is on how representations (i.e., mental models) of illnesses and symptoms affect the types of decisions we make, and how these representations are influenced by diverse factors such as knowledge, prior experiences, bodily sensations, and context. These authors frame their discussion within the context of a specific model of medical decision making—the Common Sense Model—and focus on how age-related changes in factors such as executive functioning may affect specific components of the model and resulting outcomes.

Liu, Wood, and Hanoch also focus on health-related decisions, but with a specific emphasis on how aging influences the choices we make about insurance plans. They frame their discussion within the context of decisions regarding Medicare Part D prescription drug plans, the variety of which has posed real challenges to older adults' ability and willingness to make decisions. An important point of concern here is the degree to which a variety of choices may overwhelm decision making, and the degree to which ability—including numeracy skills—and personal relevance moderate older adults' abilities to effectively deal with this variety.

The chapter by Hershey, Austin, and Gutierrez continues with the general theme of consumer decision making, but focuses more broadly on making decisions relating to finances. The authors emphasize the importance of normative changes in cognitive ability in determining effective decision making, but they also highlight the fact that the specific types of financial tasks that people encounter covary with age and life stages. Critically, the contexts associated with financial decision making become more complex with age in adulthood, and outcomes are associated with greater uncertainty. This proposes unique challenges for older adults, and the authors make recommendations regarding ways in which we might facilitate effective decision making in later life.

Carpenter and Yoon also address consumer decision making, but take a broader focus that attempts to characterize the particular aspects of relevant tasks that may determine age differences in performance. In addition to interactions between cognitive skills and task complexity, they argue that factors such as meaningfulness and personal relevance of the decision context, as well as an individual's expertise, may moderate the effectiveness of older adults' decisions. Thus, once again, the context of the specific task—in this case, the product domain—needs to be considered to fully understand age effects.

Finally, harkening back to a theme highlighted earlier with respect to medical decisions, Queen, Berg, and Lowrance examine the social context surrounding everyday decision making by exploring how couples make decisions. Recognizing the reality that many decisions of consequence—as well as more mundane ones—are made in consultation with a significant other, these authors explore the factors that influence dyadic decision making and associated outcomes. Although research in this area is relatively sparse, Queen and colleagues present a specific framework for understanding potential influences and identifying ways in which dyads might optimize decision making at different points in the life span.

CONCLUSION

In conclusion, although the chapters in this book do not necessarily reflect an exhaustive review of research on aging and decision making, they provide a good representation of the major areas of research and the diversity of current "state-of-the-art" approaches to the topic. Thus, they can be viewed as a progress report on the themes outlined by the National Research Council reports. Each chapter also builds on these themes by highlighting more specific issues that have arisen as a result of recent growth in this body of research. In combination, the chapters in this volume provide the necessary background for researchers and practitioners with an interest in aging and decision making and update the agenda for future studies exploring this field.

References

Baltes, P. B., Staudinger, U. M., & Lindenberger, U. (1999). Lifespan psychology: Theory and application to intellectual functioning. *Annual Review of Psychology, 50*, 471–507.

Bjälkebring, P., Västfjäll, D., & Johansson, B. (2013). Regulation of experienced and anticipated regret for daily decisions in younger and older adults in a Swedish one-week diary study. *Geropsych: The Journal of Gerontopsychology and Geriatric Psychiatry, 26*(4), 233–241.

Bostock, S., & Steptoe, A. (2012). Association between low functional health literacy and mortality in older adults: Longitudinal cohort study. *British Medical Journal, 344*.

Bruine de Bruin, W., Parker, A. M., & Fischhoff, B. (2007). Individual differences in adult decision-making competence. *Journal of Personality & Social Psychology, 92*(5), 938–956.

Choi, M., Mezuk, B., & Rebok, G. W. (2012). Voluntary and involuntary driving cessation in later life. *Journal of Gerontological Social Work, 55*(4), 367–376.

Dy, S. M., & Purnell, T. S. (2012). Key concepts relevant to quality of complex and shared decision-making in health care: a literature review. *Social Science & Medicine, 74*(4), 582–587.

Eppinger, B., Hämmerer, D., & Li, S.-C. (2011). Neuromodulation of reward-based learning and decision making in human aging. *Annals of the New York Academy of Sciences, 1235*(1), 1–17.

Eppinger, B., Nystrom, L. E., & Cohen, J. D. (2012). Reduced sensitivity to immediate reward during decision-making in older than younger adults. *PloS One, 7*(5), e36953.

Epstein, S. (1994). Integration of the cognitive and the psychodynamic unconscious. *American Psychologist, 49*(8), 709–724.

Evans, J. St B. T. (2008). Dual-processing accounts of reasoning, judgment, and social cognition. *Annual Review of Psychology, 59*, 255–278.

Finucane, M. L., & Gullion, C. M. (2010). Developing a tool for measuring the decision-making competence of older adults. *Psychology and Aging, 25*(2), 271–288.

Gigerenzer, G. (2008). Why heuristics work. *Perspectives on Psychological Science, 3*(1), 20–29.

Harlé, K. M., & Sanfey, A. G. (2012). Social economic decision-making across the lifespan: An fMRI investigation. *Neuropsychologia, 50*(7), 1416–1424.

Kim, H. (2014). The impacts of vicarious illness experience on response to gain- versus loss-framed breast cancer screening (BCS) messages. *Health Communication, 29*(9), 854–865.

Mather, M. (2006). A review of decision-making processes: Weighing the risks and benefits of aging. In L. L. Carstensen, & C. R. Hartel (Eds.), *When I'm 64* (pp. 145–173). Washington D.C.: The National Academies Press.

Mather, M., Mazar, N., Gorlick, M. A., Lighthall, N. R., Burgeno, J., Schoeke, A., et al. (2012). Risk preferences and aging: The "certainty effect" in older adults' decision making. *Psychology and Aging, 27*(4), 801–816.

Mõttus, R., Johnson, W., Murray, C., Wolf, M. S., Starr, J. M., & Deary, I. J. (2014). Towards understanding the links between health literacy and physical health. *Health Psychology, 33*(2), 164–173.

National Research Council (2000). *The aging mind: Opportunities in cognitive research. Committee on Future Direction for Cognitive Research on Aging*. In P. C. Stern & L. L. Carstensen (Eds.), *Comission on Behavioral and Social Sciences and Education*. Washington D.C.: The National Academies Press.

National Research Council (2006). *When I'm 64. Committee on Aging Frontiers in Social Psychology, Personality, and Adult Developmental Psychology*. In L. L. Carstensen & C. R. Hartel (Eds.), *Board on Behavioral, Cognitive, and Sensory Sciences, Division of Behavioral and Social Sciences and Education*. Washington D.C.: The National Academies Press.

Nielsen, L., Knutson, B., & Carstensen, L. L. (2008). Affect dynamics, affective forecasting, and aging. *Emotion, 8*(3), 318–330.

Peters, E., Finucane, M. L., MacGregor, D. G., & Slovic, P. (2000). The bearable lightness of aging: Judgment and decision making processes in older adults. In P. C. Stern, & L. L. Carstensen (Eds.), *The aging mind: Opportunities in cognitive research* (pp. 144–165). Washington D.C.: The National Academies Press.

Peters, E., Hess, T. M., Västfjäll, D., & Auman, C. (2007). Adult age differences in dual information processes: Implications for the role of affective and deliberative processes in older adults' decision making. *Perspectives on Psychological Science*, *2*, 1–23.

Raijmakers, N. H., van Zuylen, L., Costantini, M., Caraceni, A., Clark, J. B., De Simone, G., et al. (2012). Issues and needs in end-of-life decision making: An international modified Delphi study. *Palliative Medicine*, *26*(7), 947–953.

Raz, N., & Rodrigue, K. M. (2006). Differential aging of the brain: Patterns, cognitive correlates and modifiers. *Neuroscience and Biobehavioral Reviews*, *30*(6), 730–748.

Rolison, J. J., Hanoch, Y., & Wood, S. (2012). Risky decision making in younger and older adults: The role of learning. *Psychology and Aging*, *27*(1), 129–140.

Ross, M., Grossmann, I., & Schryer, E. (2014). Contrary to psychological and popular opinion, there is no compelling evidence that older adults are disproportionately victimized by consumer fraud. *Perspectives on Psychological Science*, *9*(4), 427–442.

Samanez-Larkin, G. R., Gibbs, S. E. B., Khanna, K., Nielsen, L., Carstensen, L. L., & Knutson, B. (2007). Anticipation of monetary gain but not loss in healthy older adults. *Nature Neuroscience*, *10*(6), 787–791.

Samanez-Larkin, G. R., Levens, S. M., Perry, L. M., Dougherty, R. F., & Knutson, B. (2012). Frontostriatal white matter integrity mediates adult age differences in probabilistic reward learning. *The Journal of Neuroscience*, *32*(15), 5333–5337.

Schott, B. H., Niehaus, L., Wittmann, B. C., Schütze, H., Seidenbecher, C. I., Heinze, H.-J., et al. (2007). Ageing and early-stage Parkinson's disease affect separable neural mechanisms of mesolimbic reward processing. *Brain*, *130*(Pt. 9), 2412–2424.

Tversky, A., & Kahneman, D. (1974). Judgment under uncertainty: Heuristics and biases. *Science*, *185*(4157), 1124–1131.

Weller, J. A., Buchanan, T. W., Shackleford, C., Morganstern, A., Hartman, J. J., Yuska, J., et al. (2014). Diurnal cortisol rhythm is associated with increased risky decision-making in older adults. *Psychology and Aging*, *29*(2), 271–283.

Yates, J. F., & Patalano, A. L. (1999). Decision making and aging. In D. C. Park, R. W. Morrell, & K. Shifren (Eds.), *Processing of medical information in aging patients: Cognitive and human factors perspectives* (pp. 31–54). Mahwah, NJ, US: Lawrence Erlbaum Associates Publishers.

SECTION 1

NEUROBIOLOGICAL MECHANISMS

CHAPTER

2

Modeling Cost–Benefit Decision Making in Aged Rodents

B. Sofia Beas[1], *Barry Setlow*[1,2], *Gregory R. Samanez-Larkin*[3], *Jennifer L. Bizon*[1,2]

[1]Department of Neuroscience, University of Florida College of Medicine, Gainesville, FL, USA; [2]Department of Psychiatry, University of Florida College of Medicine, Gainesville, FL, USA; [3]Department of Psychology, Yale University, New Haven, CT, USA

INTRODUCTION

An emerging literature indicates that multiple aspects of decision making change with advancing age. Given that progress in medical science and healthier lifestyles have contributed to unprecedented numbers of individuals living to advanced ages, it is becoming increasingly important to elucidate how brain aging influences decision making, and to develop strategies for maintaining optimal decision making across the life span. Animal models offer several advantages for understanding how brain aging influences decision-making processes. In particular, the high degree of experimenter control that is achievable in rodent studies circumvents challenges in dissociating age-related neurobiological influences on decision making from the influences of experiential factors that often stratify by age cohort in humans. In addition, the relatively short life span of rodents (2–3 years) can allow realistic longitudinal evaluation of decision making across the full life span. This chapter will highlight different approaches for investigating decision making in rodents and how these approaches can be optimized for aging studies. We will describe

Aging and Decision Making
http://dx.doi.org/10.1016/B978-0-12-417148-0.00002-9

recent findings regarding cost–benefit decision making in aged rats and will review some of the neural and cognitive factors that may contribute to altered decision making across species.

INDIVIDUAL DIFFERENCES AND COGNITIVE AGING

Many cognitive capacities decline as a function of age in rodents (Bizon, Foster, Alexander, & Glisky, 2012; Burke, Ryan, & Barnes, 2012; Foster, Defazio, & Bizon, 2012). Such findings closely parallel those in human aging, in that old rats exhibit deficits on behavioral paradigms that assess learning, memory, and executive function (Alexander et al., 2012; Roberson et al., 2012). Notably, in humans there is often considerable variability with respect to the presence and severity of age-related cognitive alterations, with some individuals demonstrating marked cognitive deficits and other individuals maintaining cognitive abilities akin to much younger subjects (Morrison & Baxter, 2012). Such individual differences can also be reliably observed in both inbred and outbred rat strains, with some aged rats performing mnemonic tasks on par with young adult rats whereas others perform well outside the range of the young, demonstrating impairment (Barense, Fox, & Baxter, 2002; Beas, Setlow, & Bizon, 2013; Bizon et al., 2009; Gallagher, Burwell, & Burchinal, 1993). In rodents, these individual differences are reliable; for example, aged rats classified as "memory-unimpaired" or "memory-impaired" relative to a young adult cohort in a spatial learning task continue to demonstrate performance consistent with their original classification several months later (Gallagher et al., 1993).

Individual differences in rodent mnemonic abilities have been leveraged in order to distinguish those genetic, epigenetic, neurobiological, and environmental factors that specifically contribute to memory decline from factors that change more generally as a function of chronological age. For example, individual performance of aged rats on the hippocampal-dependent Morris water maze has been used to identify NMDA, GABAergic, and cholinergic receptor dysfunction, as well as changes in gene expression as important contributors to memory decline at advanced ages (Banuelos et al., 2013; Bizon et al., 2001; Haberman et al., 2011; Kumar & Foster, 2013; Zhang, Watson, Gallagher, & Nicolle, 2007). Building on the behavioral paradigms described below for assessing cost–benefit decision making in rodents, similar approaches could be used to elucidate the neural mechanisms that govern age-related alterations in cost–benefit decision making. Indeed, one advantage of rodent models is that neural factors identified using correlational approaches can then be specifically manipulated (e.g., using pharmacological or genetic tools) to test their role in choice behavior in both young and aged subjects.

CROSS-SPECIES COMPARISONS OF NEURAL CIRCUITRY RELEVANT FOR DECISION MAKING

Across species, neuroimaging studies as well as findings from lesion and brain inactivation studies have strongly implicated prefrontal corticostriatal circuitry as critical for cost–benefit decision making (Bechara & Van Der Linden, 2005; Floresco, St Onge, Ghods-Sharifi, & Winstanley, 2008; Kable & Glimcher, 2009). Distinct components of this circuitry have been linked to processing of information related to different aspects of decision making, including reward valuation, risk, and time delays (Peters & Buchel, 2011; Platt & Huettel, 2008). In humans, the dorsolateral prefrontal cortex (PFC) is important for mediating specific executive functions such as working memory and behavioral flexibility, which may help maintain current reward–cost contingencies and optimize choice behavior (Miller & Cohen, 2001). In contrast, the orbitofrontal cortex (OFC) and striatum are critical for reward valuation, and particularly in the case of OFC, in assigning outcome value when it must be inferred rather than directly experienced (Jones et al., 2012; Levy & Glimcher, 2012). The rodent PFC is not as anatomically complex as the primate; however, many of the critical neuroanatomical and functional characteristics present in primates are preserved in rodents, enabling meaningful cross-species comparisons relevant to the study of decision making. Indeed, there is substantial evidence indicating that rodents have neuroanatomical and functional cortical homologues of primate PFC subregions, and that rodents are capable of a wide variety of complex goal-directed behaviors that are supported by these systems (for review, see Bizon et al., 2012; Brown & Bowman, 2002; Kesner & Churchwell, 2011; Uylings, Groenewegen, & Kolb, 2003). As shown in Figure 1, the rodent medial PFC (which includes the anterior cingulate, infralimbic, and prelimbic cortices) is considered the homologue of the primate dorsolateral PFC, whereas the rodent OFC is considered the homologue of the primate OFC. As in primates, rodent mPFC and OFC share strong reciprocal connections with the mediodorsal thalamus (Rose & Woolsey, 1948), as well as similar patterns of innervation by ascending modulatory systems (e.g., Gaykema, van Weeghel, Hersh, & Luiten, 1991). Moreover, selective damage to these PFC subregions in rodents produces distinct patterns of behavioral deficits that correspond to functional distinctions between these cortical regions in primates. For example, medial PFC lesions in rodents impair performance in tests of set-shifting and working memory in a manner that is comparable to similar studies in nonhuman primates following dorsolateral PFC damage (Birrell & Brown, 2000; Bizon et al., 2012; Dias, Robbins, & Roberts, 1996). Similarly, OFC damage in both rodents and primates produces behavioral deficits in reversal learning and reward revaluation tasks (Baxter, Parker, Lindner, Izquierdo, & Murray, 2000; Gallagher, McMahan, & Schoenbaum, 1999;

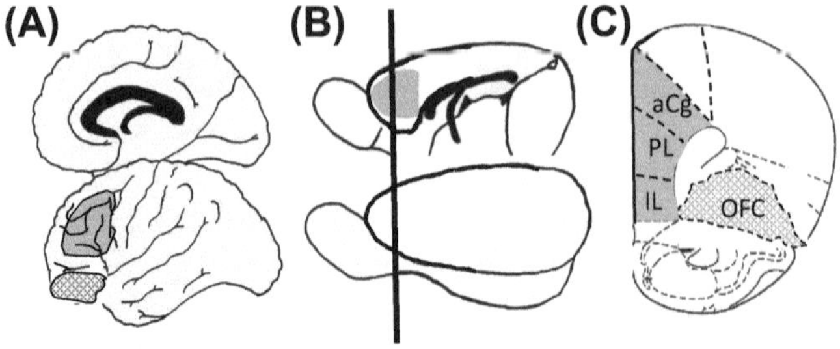

FIGURE 1 (A) Schematic of the human brain in which prefrontal cortical areas important for decision making have been indicated. These include the dorsolateral prefrontal cortex (Brodmann's area 46, solid gray) and the orbitofrontal cortex (Brodmann's areas 10, 11, and 47, stippled gray). The dorsolateral prefrontal cortex has been implicated in executive function, including working memory and cognitive flexibility, whereas the orbitofrontal cortex has been implicated in reward valuation. (B), (C) Schematic of the rat brain in which the functional homologues to the primate prefrontal cortex are indicated. The black line in (B) shows the approximate plane of section for the coronal view shown in (C). In rats, the coronal plane is the best orientation for appreciating the subdivisions of the medial prefrontal cortex (including prelimbic, infralimbic, and anterior cingulate cortices, solid gray) and the orbitofrontal cortex (stippled gray). (aCg, anterior cingulate cortex; PL, prelimbic cortex; IL, infralimbic cortex; OFC, orbitofrontal cortex.) (*The coronal section shown in* (C) *is adapted from Paxinos and Watson (1998), and this figure is modified from Bizon et al. (2012), Frontiers in Aging Neuroscience.*)

Rudebeck & Murray, 2011; Schoenbaum, Nugent, Saddoris, & Setlow, 2002). Beyond the dorsolateral PFC and OFC, other functional and anatomical rodent homologues of primate PFC subregions have been identified and reviewed (Kesner & Churchwell, 2011).

Homologies between rodent and primate striatum are more straightforward. The striatum and its afferents from the dopaminergic midbrain share a similar anatomical organization across species, and lesion, neuroimaging, and electrophysiological recording studies have demonstrated remarkable homologies between species across a range of functions ascribed to distinct striatal subregions (e.g., reward valuation, action selection, and motor habit formation; see Balleine & O'Doherty, 2010, and Liljeholm & O'Doherty, 2012, for review). Considered together, there is a strong body of evidence suggesting that rodents and primates employ homologous neural mechanisms that support cognitive and motivational processes relevant to decision making.

CROSS-SPECIES CONSIDERATIONS OF REINFORCERS

There are a number of potentially significant differences with respect to how decision making is assessed in rodents and humans that must be considered when making cross-species comparisons (Kalenscher & van Wingerden, 2011). One factor that tends to differ across decision-making assessments in rodents and humans is the nature of the reinforcers used. The two major dimensions across which reinforcers can differ in laboratory settings are whether they are (1) primary or secondary and (2) actual or hypothetical. Most assessments of decision making in animals employ primary reinforcers such as food and water, which are biologically relevant and require no learning for them to be reinforcing. In contrast, human subject research most often uses secondary reinforcers such as money, which are associated with primary reinforcers but have no intrinsic biological value for themselves. Exactly how the use of primary versus secondary reinforcers impacts decision making is still not fully understood; however, in the few instances in which they have been directly compared in humans, differences have been observed (e.g., see Jimura et al., 2011). These findings caution that apparent cross-species differences in decision making may be in part attributable to the different reinforcer types used and indicate that more studies directly comparing primary and secondary reinforcers will be important for reconciling cross-species differences in decision making at advanced ages. Secondary reinforcers further differ from the reinforcers used in animal studies in that they are sometimes hypothetical (i.e., subjects are asked to make choices "as if" they would actually receive the rewards). In contrast, animal studies always employ actual rewards delivered in real time. Notably, when compared directly, results obtained using hypothetical rewards often mirror those found in "real-life" decision making, suggesting that the actual/hypothetical distinction is not likely to significantly contribute to cross-species differences in choice behavior (Green & Myerson, 2013; Jimura et al., 2011; Sescousse, Caldu, Segura, & Dreher, 2013).

INTERTEMPORAL DECISION MAKING

Across both humans and rodent models, intertemporal choice is the form of cost–benefit decision making that has been most extensively studied in both young and aged subjects. We begin our review by considering behavioral findings, and then turn to data describing underlying neural mechanisms. Intertemporal decision making involves choices between reward options that differ in both magnitude and the time of their arrival (e.g., choices between small, immediate, and large, delayed rewards). All other things being equal, both rodents and humans strongly prefer large over small rewards. However, in both species, imposing a delay before delivery reduces or "discounts" the value of the larger reward, and thus reliably shifts choice preference toward smaller but more immediate rewards. This phenomenon, known as delay discounting, has been studied extensively and its governing principles are remarkably consistent across species, despite the fact that the delays employed in most human studies range from days to years, whereas those in animal studies are rarely greater than 120 s (Freeman, Green, Myerson, & Woolverton, 2009; Mazur, 2001; Smits, Stein, Johnson, Odum, & Madden, 2013; Stein, Pinkston, Brewer, Francisco, & Madden, 2012).

Several task designs have been used to assess intertemporal choice in rodents. Some intertemporal choice tasks employ so-called "adjusting" procedures, in which either the magnitude of, or delays to, reward delivery are changed on the basis of an animal's choices (e.g., repeated choices of the large, delayed reward would result in an increase in the delay or a decrease in the reward magnitude associated with this choice; see Dallery & Locey, 2005; Mazur, 1987; Richards, Mitchell, de Wit, & Seiden, 1997). There are disadvantages to these designs for rodent aging studies, however, including the need for many weeks or even months of testing to achieve stable performance. Other task designs employ so-called "fixed-delay" procedures, in which the large and small reward magnitudes are held constant, but the delays (usually to the large reward) are varied, either between sessions or within individual test sessions (Adriani & Laviola, 2003; Cardinal, Pennicott, Sugathapala, Robbins, & Everitt, 2001; Evenden & Ryan, 1996). Both young and aged rats tend to acquire these fixed-delay designs readily.

Our laboratory used a within-session, fixed-delay design to assess the effects of aging on intertemporal choice in rats (Simon et al., 2010). In this study, fully mature young adult (6 mo) and aged (24 mo) male Fischer 344 rats were tested in an operant test chamber, in which they made discrete-trial choices between two response levers. A press on one lever yielded a small reward (one food pellet) delivered immediately. A press on the other lever yielded a larger reward (four food pellets) delivered after a delay period, the duration of which changed in blocks of trials across each test session (0, 10, 20, 40, 60 s; see Figure 2) (Evenden & Ryan, 1996). Young and aged rats chose the large reward with equal frequency (nearly 100% of the time) when there was no delay to its delivery. However, as the delay to large reward delivery increased, young adult rats shifted their choice to the small but immediately available reward (i.e., the delays discounted the value of the large reward; Figure 2(B)). In contrast, aged rats as a group maintained their preference for the large delayed reward even at the longest delay examined (60 s), indicating that aging can result in robustly attenuated discounting of delayed rewards.

This age difference was not attributable to gross alterations in detecting or responding to the different reward magnitudes and delays employed in the task. A series of control experiments in the same rats showed equivalent preference for large over small rewards in the absence of delays and equivalent preference for immediate over delayed rewards when magnitudes were made equal. Moreover, both young and aged rats showed similar break points on high-ratio schedules of lever pressing for the food

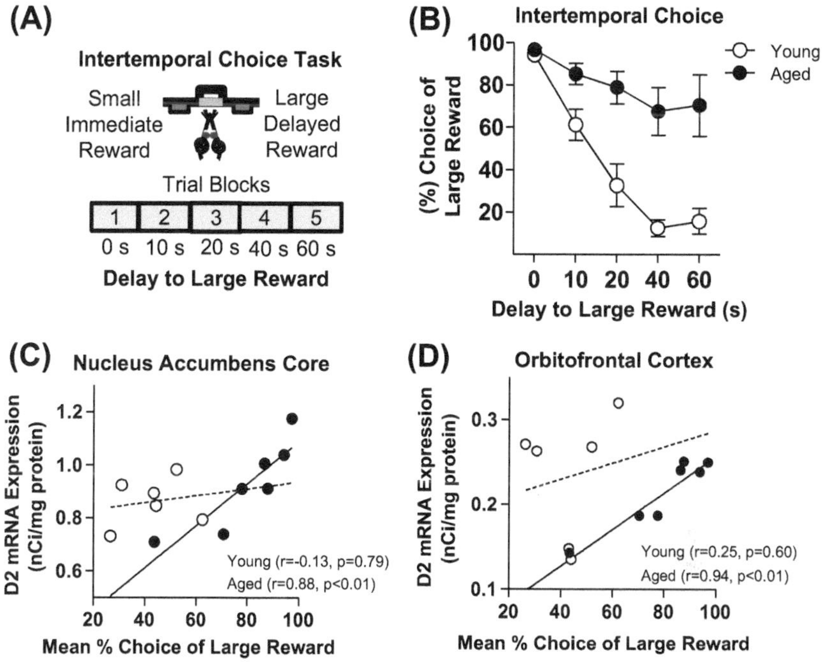

FIGURE 2 (A) Schematic diagram of the intertemporal choice task, which is conducted in standard operant chambers. Rats make discrete-trial choices between two levers, one yielding a small food reward delivered immediately and the other a large food reward delivered after a delay. Each session consists of five blocks of trials across which the delay to the large reward systematically increases from 0 to 60 s. Each trial block begins with forced-choice trials during which a single lever is presented, and which serve as reminders of the delay contingencies in effect for that block. These are followed by 10 free-choice trials, in which both levers are presented and rats are free to choose between the two. Percent choice of the large reward on these free-choice trials is the primary measure of interest. (B) Attenuated delay discounting in aged rats. All rats decreased choice of the large reward as the delay increased; however, aged rats showed significantly greater choice of the large delayed reward compared to young rats. (*Figure adapted from Simon et al., 2010; Neurobiology of Aging.*) (C), (D) D2 dopamine receptor mRNA expression (as assessed with *in situ* hybridization) in the nucleus accumbens core (C) and orbitofrontal cortex (D) in the young (open circles) and aged (closed circles) rats used in the intertemporal choice study shown in panel B. Among aged rats, D2 receptor mRNA expression in both the nucleus accumbens core and orbitofrontal cortex was strongly associated with mean percent choice of large reward, averaged across all blocks of trials. Specifically, among aged rats, greater D2 receptor mRNA expression in these regions predicted greater choice of the delayed large reward. Note that no relationship was observed between D2 receptor mRNA expression in the nucleus accumbens core or orbitofrontal cortex and mean percent choice of the large reward in young rats.

rewards used in the choice tasks, demonstrating that both age groups were equally motivated to perform the behavior necessary to obtain the food rewards. Finally, the maintained choice of delayed rewards in aged rats was likely not due solely to compromised behavioral flexibility, which we and others have reported in aged rats (Barense et al., 2002; Beas et al., 2013; Schoenbaum, Nugent, Saddoris, & Gallagher, 2002; Schoenbaum, Setlow, Saddoris, & Gallagher, 2006) and which could have impaired aged rats' ability to shift choice behavior across successive blocks of trials as the delay contingencies changed (Figure 2(A)). Aged rats showed the same pattern of choice behavior (greater choice of large, delayed rewards) even when the order in which the delays were presented was reversed (i.e., 60, 40, 20, 10, 0 s). These data agree with experimental research in humans, which shows that aged subjects are more likely to choose larger, delayed rewards over smaller, more immediate rewards compared to young adult cohorts (Eppinger, Nystrom, & Cohen, 2012; Green, Fry, & Myerson, 1994; Löckenhoff, O'Donoghue, & Dunning, 2011). Moreover, the fact that environmental conditions are identical across the life span in young and aged rats suggests that experiential factors do not fully account for age-related differences in intertemporal choice in humans.

More recently, Roesch and colleagues (Roesch, Bryden, Cerri, Haney, & Schoenbaum, 2012) used a different task design to evaluate the effects of age on choices involving delayed rewards. In this work, young adult (3 mo) and aged (22–24 mo) Long Evans rats sampled different olfactory cues that indicated the availability of either large versus small, or immediate versus delayed, sucrose solution rewards. Both young and aged rats similarly preferred the large- over the small-magnitude reward. Compared to young rats, however, aged rats showed a small but reliable increase in preference for delayed over immediate rewards. Together with the findings from Simon et al. (2010), these data indicate that aging results in an increased tolerance of time delays in rats. It is important to note, however, that unlike the design employed in Simon et al. (2010), reward magnitude and delay were varied independently in Roesch et al. (2012), and thus the design did not directly assess the effects of age on the integration of reward magnitude and delay. Indeed, in the Simon et al. (2010) study, we failed to observe age differences in preference for delayed over immediate rewards when the reward magnitudes were identical. It is possible that the shorter delays employed by Roesch et al. (1–7 s compared to 10–60 s in Simon et al., 2010) afforded enhanced sensitivity for detecting age-related differences in preference for delayed rewards. It will be important in future work to differentiate at shorter delay intervals between the influences of age on time valuation and time perception. Studies employing peak interval procedures show that age can influence the subjective passage of time in rodents such that perceived delays are shorter than the actual delays (Lejeune, Ferrara, Soffie, Bronchart, & Wearden, 1998; Meck, Church, & Wenk, 1986), and time perception has the potential to alter the degree to which such delays reduce reward value (Galtress, Garcia, & Kirkpatrick, 2012; Wittmann & Paulus, 2008).

An important contribution of the work by Roesch et al. (2012) is that it represents the first neurobiological investigation of decision making involving delayed reward in aged rodents. Previous work in young rats showed that OFC damage results in attenuated discounting of the large reward in an intertemporal choice task (Winstanley, Theobald, Cardinal, & Robbins, 2004; although see Mobini et al., 2002). In Roesch et al. (2012), single-unit neural activity was recorded from OFC in young and aged rats while they performed the olfactory-guided choice task described earlier. Using these procedures, the authors identified one population of neurons that exhibited preferential firing to immediate compared to delayed rewards, whereas another population of neurons exhibited the opposite pattern and fired preferentially to delayed rewards. In young rats, neurons with preferential firing to immediate rewards were predominant, consistent with young rats' greater preference for immediate over delayed rewards (Roesch, Taylor, & Schoenbaum, 2006). In contrast to young rats, neurons with a preference for delayed rewards were over-represented in aged rats, as might be expected given the aged rats' increased preference for delayed rewards (Roesch et al., 2012). A similar age by delay interaction has been observed in the human ventral striatum using functional MRI (discussed later).

In both humans and rodents, distinct aspects of information processing regarding intertemporal choice have been ascribed to discrete subregions of the OFC. Lateral OFC activation in humans predicts choices of delayed rewards (Boettiger et al., 2007; McClure, Laibson, Loewenstein, & Cohen, 2004) and negatively correlates with relative preference for small immediate rewards on an intertemporal choice task (Hariri et al., 2006). Consistent with these human data, a study in rats showed that lesions of the lateral OFC increased preference for small, immediate over large, delayed rewards (Mar, Walker, Theobald, Eagle, & Robbins, 2011). This increase in delay discounting may be attributable to the role of this OFC subregion in self-control and specifically in suppressing responses associated with immediate rewards (Elliott, Dolan, & Frith, 2000; Man, Clarke, & Roberts, 2009; Schoenbaum, Nugent, Saddoris, & Setlow, 2002). In contrast, activation of the medial OFC in humans is associated with choice of immediate relative to delayed rewards (McClure, York, & Montague, 2004), and positively correlates with relative preference for small immediate rewards in an intertemporal choice task (Hariri et al., 2006). Consistent with these findings, Mar et al. (2011) also found that medial OFC lesions in rats decreased the choice of small, immediate over large, delayed rewards (attenuated delay discounting). Thus, subregional differences in OFC contributions to intertemporal choice reveal strong parallels between rodents and humans, and it will be important to differentiate the effects of advanced age on the medial and lateral OFC to better understand age-related changes in intertemporal choice across species.

Like the OFC, the ventral striatum (particularly the core subregion of the nucleus accumbens) has also been strongly implicated in the representation of time-discounted value during intertemporal choice (Cardinal et al., 2001; Galtress et al., 2012; McClure, Laibson, et al., 2004; although see also Kable & Glimcher, 2007). Recent fMRI studies in humans have examined age differences in the role of the ventral striatum during intertemporal decision making. Reward-related neural activation in the ventral striatum was reduced by temporal delay in younger but not older adults; ventral striatal signal increased in response to both short and long delays in older adults (Eppinger, Schuck, Nystrom, & Cohen, 2013; Samanez-Larkin et al., 2011). A larger age group difference in neural signal was reported in the Eppinger et al. study and is consistent with the larger behavioral difference reported by this group. In particular, the young adults were relatively more impatient in the Eppinger et al. study compared to the Samanez-Larkin et al. study, and this was reflected in the larger magnitude of the ventral striatal signal difference. Importantly, the age by delay interaction in ventral striatal activity found by these authors in human subjects is strikingly similar to the findings from OFC recordings of neural activity in aged rats (Roesch et al., 2012). These data suggest that greater equivalence in prefrontal corticostriatal activity in response to immediate and delayed rewards may reflect a reduction in the value placed on reward immediacy, with a resulting relative increase in the value of delayed rewards.

The neurotransmitter dopamine strongly modulates the activity of the OFC and striatal systems described above, and has been heavily implicated in a range of cognitive functions including intertemporal choice (Bayer & Glimcher, 2005; Floresco, 2013; Robbins & Arnsten, 2009). In addition, aging is associated with attenuated dopamine signaling, suggesting that age-related alterations in intertemporal choice could stem at least in part from changes in PFC–striatal dopamine signaling (Backman, Lindenberger, Li, & Nyberg, 2010; Kaasinen & Rinne, 2002; Li et al., 2013; Volkow et al., 1998; Wong et al., 1984; Zhang & Roth, 1997). A large body of work has shown that phasic dopamine signaling encodes information regarding the anticipated value of expected outcomes, as well as the difference between expected and actual outcomes (Schultz, 2010; Sugam, Day, Wightman, & Carelli, 2012). Such anticipatory and feedback signals are thought to be critical for integrating behavioral outcomes with previously acquired information in order to modify subsequent behavior. While it remains unclear how phasic dopamine signals contribute to ongoing choice behavior when subjects must decide among multiple options, pharmacological manipulations in rodents have provided some insight regarding how tonic changes in dopamine signaling can impact intertemporal decisions. Systemic administration of dopamine agonists tends to increase choice of large, delayed rewards, consistent with the clinical effects of such drugs in reducing impulsive behavior in individuals with attention-deficit hyperactivity disorder. Notably, these effects may depend in part on baseline levels of delay discounting as well as the specific task parameters employed (Cardinal, Robbins, & Everitt, 2000; de Wit, Enggasser, & Richards, 2002; Zeeb, Floresco, & Winstanley, 2010). The results of studies using specific dopaminergic manipulations within prefrontal corticostriatal circuits generally agree with those employing systemic agonists. For example, manipulations that decrease dopamine signaling, such as intra-OFC administration of D2-like dopamine receptor antagonists and viral-mediated overexpression of the dopamine transporter protein in the ventral striatum, increase the choice of small, immediate over large, delayed rewards (Adriani et al., 2009; Pardey, Kumar, Goodchild, & Cornish, 2013; Zeeb et al., 2010). Conversely, administration of the indirect dopamine agonist amphetamine into the ventral striatum decreases the choice of small, immediate over large, delayed rewards (Mitchell, Shimp, Ouimet, McLaurin, & Setlow, 2013).

To better understand relationships between age-related alterations in intertemporal choice and dopamine signaling, our laboratory employed *in situ* hybridization procedures to evaluate dopamine receptor mRNA expression in the brains of the young and aged rats characterized in the intertemporal choice task described above (Simon et al., 2010; Figure 2(A) and (B)). *In situ* hybridization is a procedure that localizes the expression of specific mRNA sequences (in this case, the sequences encoding dopamine receptor proteins) in brain tissue. This method can be used to evaluate dopamine receptor expression in a regionally specific manner and offers a degree of receptor specificity not attainable with currently available dopamine receptor ligands employed in PET imaging and/or receptor autoradiography studies (Bizon, Lauterborn, Isackson, & Gall, 1996; Simon et al., 2011). Pertinent to the dopamine receptor mRNA analysis, it is important to note that although as a group, aged rats showed a strong preference for large delayed rewards relative to young rats, there was significant individual variability in choice performance among aged rats, with some aged rats discounting delayed rewards to a much larger degree than others (see Figure 2(B)). Among the aged rats, D2 dopamine receptor mRNA expression in both the core subregion of the nucleus accumbens and in the OFC strongly predicted preference for the large, delayed reward (Figure 2(C) and (D), closed circles). Although the number of subjects available for this analysis was small, it is notable that these relationships were not evident in young rats (Figure 2(C) and (D), open circles), nor with D1 dopamine receptor mRNA expression evaluated in adjacent brain sections (not shown). These data are consistent with findings from studies in which dopamine signaling was directly manipulated in these structures (detailed above), and suggest that variability in OFC and ventral striatal dopamine signaling in aging contributes to some aspects of individual differences in intertemporal choice.

Notably, D2 receptor mRNA expression changes do not easily account for the striking differences in choice behavior between young and aged rats, as D2 mRNA expression did not significantly vary as a function of chronological age. As findings from PET imaging and autoradiography studies in both humans and rodents indicate that translational and/or posttranslational aspects of D2 receptor signaling *do* change with age, additional studies that assess these other aspects of D2 receptor signaling in relation to intertemporal choice are still needed. Nevertheless, the data generated from the *in situ* hybridization study serve to illustrate the general approach of integrating molecular and behavioral methodologies in rodent subjects.

In summary, the behavioral data from older humans and rodents performing intertemporal choice tasks strongly parallel one another. Moreover, there are converging data from human and rodent studies to support that dopaminergic signaling within corticostriatal circuits is a critical mediator of intertemporal choice in both species, and that altered dopaminergic signaling contributes to age-related variability in intertemporal choice. Neuroimaging approaches, including PET imaging to evaluate regional changes in brain neurochemistry across species, could provide additional links between rodents and humans. Such data would lend further confidence in shared neural mechanisms of decision making across species, and would support future studies in rodent models directed at investigation of molecular and cellular mechanisms that mediate age-related changes in intertemporal choice using methodologies that are at the current time infeasible in human subjects.

PROBABILISTIC (RISKY) DECISION MAKING

Probabilistic, or risky, decision making refers to choices among options that differ in the probabilities with which the outcomes of those options (either positive or negative in valence) are delivered. Numerous behavioral task designs have been used to assess risky decision making in human subjects, and more specifically to compare performance of young and aged adults. Despite this body of work, the influence of age on risky decision making is less clear than in the case of intertemporal choice. For example, some studies have shown that aged individuals are more risk averse compared to young (Deakin, Aitken, Robbins, & Sahakian, 2004; Kumar, 2007), consistent with reports of decreased impulsivity and sensation seeking in the elderly (Roalf, Mitchell, Harbaugh, & Janowsky, 2011). In contrast, other findings show no age-related changes in risk-based decisions, or even that aged individuals are more likely than the young to select high-risk options under some conditions (Deakin et al., 2004; Denburg, Tranel, & Bechara, 2005; Henninger, Madden, & Huettel, 2010; Kumar, 2007).

As is the case with intertemporal choice, risky decision making can be modeled in animal subjects. There are a number of task designs in which preference for certain versus risky outcomes can be assessed in animal models (Chen, Lakshminarayanan, & Santos, 2006; Platt & Huettel, 2008; Rosati & Hare, 2011). Figure 3(A) shows one version of such a task that is commonly used in rodents (Cardinal & Howes, 2005; St Onge & Floresco, 2010). In this task, which follows the same design as the intertemporal choice task in Figure 2(A), rats make discrete-trial choices between two levers: one that yields a small certain reward and another that yields a large but probabilistically delivered reward. As in the intertemporal choice task, the probability with which the large reward is omitted (the "cost") changes in blocks of trials over the course of each test session (Figure 3(A)), allowing assessment of the degree to which different probabilities of omission discount the value of the large reward.

In our laboratories, we used this task to compare risky decision making in young and aged rats (Gilbert et al., 2012). Unlike the results of animal studies of intertemporal choice, there were no group differences between young and aged rats' choices of the large probabilistic versus small certain reward. However, much like the findings from the human literature that support both increased and decreased risk taking in the elderly, there was significantly greater individual variability among aged compared to young rats. The vast majority of young rats showed a typical "optimal" pattern of choice behavior, with increasing probabilities of large reward omission systematically shifting choice toward the small, certain reward (i.e., probability of omission discounted the value of the large reward; Figure 3(B)); however, only a small subset of aged rats showed this pattern of performance. Instead, many aged rats showed little to no discounting associated with increased probability of reward omission, whereas others showed steeper discounting compared to young cohorts (Figure 3(C)). Importantly, these data agree with findings from humans that find little relationship between patterns of performance in aged subjects on tasks that assess risk-based decision making versus intertemporal choice (Samanez-Larkin & Knutson, 2014).

Findings from both humans and rodents suggest that individual differences in cognitive abilities may account for individual differences in risky decision making. The past several decades of human research were reviewed in a meta-analysis that focused on gambling tasks and risky investment choices. This analysis found no evidence for systematic adult age differences in risk preferences (Hertwig & Gigerenzer, 2011; Mata, Josef, Samanez-Larkin, & Hertwig, 2011), but instead identified a subset of tasks in which older adults choose to avoid risk, and other tasks in which older adults choose to seek risk more often than younger adults (Mata et al., 2011). Notably, in many of these tasks, the expression of this "risk preference" is opposite of the reward-maximizing strategy.

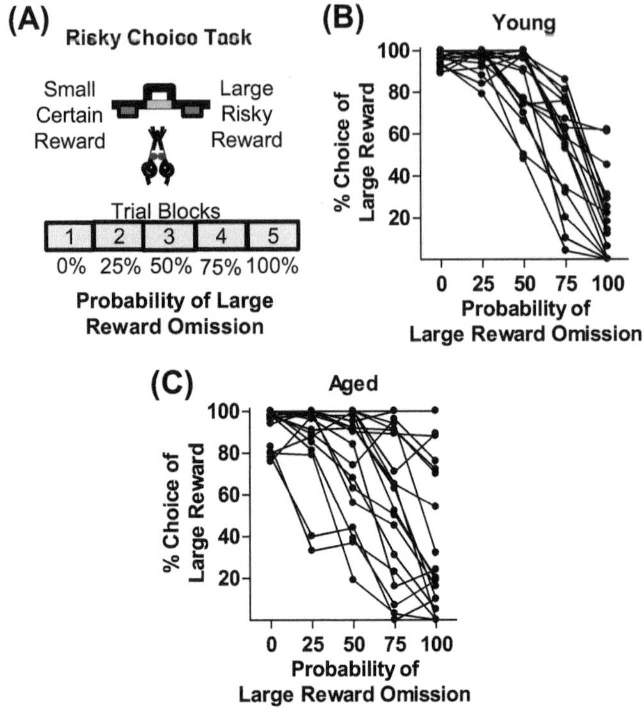

FIGURE 3 (A) Schematic diagram of the risky choice task, which is conducted in standard operant chambers and uses a design similar to that used to assess intertemporal choice (Figure 2). Rats make discrete-trial choices between two levers, one yielding a small, guaranteed food reward and the other a large food reward that is delivered with varying probabilities. Each session consists of five blocks of trials, across which the probability of large reward omission systematically increases from 0% to 100%. Each block of trials begins with forced-choice trials (on which only a single lever is presented), which serve as a reminder of the contingencies in effect for that block. These are followed by free-choice trials on which both levers are presented and the rats are free to choose between the two. Percent choice of the large reward on these free-choice trials is the primary measure of interest. (B), (C) Individual performance of young and aged Fischer 344 rats on the risky choice task. Each line represents data from a single rat (averaged across five consecutive sessions of task performance). Note that the majority of young rats displayed an "optimal" pattern of choice behavior, choosing the large reward when there was a low probability of omission but shifting their preference to the small, certain reward as the probability of reward omission increased. Significantly greater individual variability in performance was observed among aged rats, with only a subset of aged rats showing the same pattern of discounting observed in young rats. Some aged rats showed significantly attenuated choice of the small, certain reward and maintained preference for the large uncertain reward, even when this choice was clearly disadvantageous (i.e., when it was associated with 100% probability of omission). Other aged rats showed elevated choice of the small, certain reward, even under conditions in which there was a low probability of omission of the large reward. (*Adapted from Gilbert et al.* (2012); *Frontiers in Neuroscience.*)

Thus, in these tasks, apparent age differences in risk preferences may instead result from cognitive limitations (Henninger et al., 2010). Consistent with this account, tasks that require subjects to learn from recent experience show larger age differences in performance than do tasks in which performance does not depend on learning (Green, Myerson, Lichtman, Rosen, & Fry, 1996; Mata et al., 2011; Mather, 2006). In rodents, a study by St Onge and Floresco (2010) showed that inactivation of the medial PFC, a region important for behavioral flexibility and updating decision-reward contingencies, increased choice of the large, probabilistic reward, even when these choices resulted in overall less food delivery. Hence, one interpretation of the varied pattern of probabilistic decision making in aging is that it reflects the presence or magnitude of PFC-mediated cognitive deficits. With respect to this point, it is notable that recent work from our laboratory has identified multiple behavioral manifestations of PFC dysfunction among aged rats (Beas et al., 2013). As described in more detail below important avenues of future work will involve determining the extent to which PFC- or hippocampal-mediated cognitive deficits that accompany normal aging account for individual differences observed in risk-based decision making.

THE ROLE OF AGE-RELATED MEMORY IMPAIRMENT IN DECISION MAKING

Memory dysfunction associated with hippocampus and medial temporal lobe structures accompanies aging across species and has the potential to contribute to altered decision making (Buckner, 2004; Burke et al., 2012; Gallagher et al., 1993; Glisky, 2007). Specifically, while young subjects can readily learn and remember reward–cost contingencies when making decisions, impaired memory for previously learned reward–cost relationships might force aged subjects to employ less integrative strategies such as deciding solely on the basis of reward magnitude. In the context of intertemporal choice, age-related memory impairment might thus contribute to the increased preference for large, delayed rewards (Simon et al., 2010). While it should be acknowledged that hippocampal damage actually enhances preference for small, immediate over large, delayed rewards (Abela & Chudasama, 2013; Mariano et al., 2009), outright lesions do not accurately mimic the effects of age on the hippocampus and related structures. Indeed, despite ample evidence for impaired hippocampal function in aging across species, the number of hippocampal neurons does not change as a function of age or cognitive abilities (Keuker, Luiten, & Fuchs, 2003; Rapp & Gallagher, 1996; Rasmussen, Schliemann, Sorensen, Zimmer, & West, 1996). With this in mind, neurochemical changes that have been linked to hippocampal memory dysfunction are likely more relevant for understanding the contributions of age-related changes in hippocampal function to decision making. For example, recent work from our laboratories showed that lower levels of hippocampal $\alpha 4\beta 2$ nicotinic receptor binding in young rats predict greater choice of the large, delayed reward in an intertemporal choice task (Mendez, Damborsky, Winzer-Serhan, Bizon, & Setlow, 2013). Marked reductions in nicotinic receptor expression are well described in the aged rat hippocampus and have been linked to mnemonic dysfunction (Aubert, Rowe, Meaney, Gauthier, & Quirion, 1995; Bartus, Dean, Beer, & Lippa, 1982; Perry, Martin-Ruiz, & Court, 2001). Extending such findings to the context of decision making may help elucidate the neural mechanisms that govern intertemporal choice in aged subjects.

In contrast to findings indicating a role for medial temporal lobe structures in intertemporal choice, findings from rodent studies do not support a critical role for the hippocampus in risky decision making. In our own work, we observed no relationship between hippocampal-dependent spatial memory impairment and risky choice task performance among the aged rat population shown in Figure 3 (Gilbert et al., 2012). These data are consistent with the findings of Abela and Chudasama (2013), who showed that hippocampal lesions in young rats had no effect on risky choice. Indeed, amnestic patients with hippocampal damage perform similarly to controls on probabilistic learning tasks, suggesting that processing of probabilistic information can occur independent of medial temporal lobe memory systems (Knowlton, Mangels, & Squire, 1996).

In contrast to hippocampal-mediated episodic memory, deficits in PFC-mediated working memory might be expected to impair the ability to maintain long-term decision strategies that require integration of reward value and the outcomes of one's choices over successive experiences. In other words, individuals with impaired working memory might be more readily influenced by event-specific, moment-to-moment fluctuations in decision outcomes. In the context of a risky choice task, subjects with intact working memory would be unlikely to be derailed by an occasional trial in which reward is omitted, whereas subjects with impaired working memory might be more likely to immediately shift toward a less costly option upon encountering a negative consequence (resulting in overall greater discounting of probabilistic rewards). In the context of intertemporal choice, better working memory is associated with less discounting of delayed rewards in young adult subjects (Shamosh et al., 2008; Shimp, Mitchell, Beas, Bizon, & Setlow, 2014), and cognitive training to enhance working memory in chronic stimulant users reduces discounting of delayed monetary rewards in subsequent assessments (Bickel, Yi, Landes, Hill, & Baxter, 2011). The relationships between working memory and delay discounting in young subjects tend to contradict findings from aged population-based studies, however, in which both impaired working memory and attenuated delay discounting have been reported. These findings suggest that the cognitive strategies used to govern intertemporal choice may become decoupled from working memory in aged individuals. To date, explicit comparisons have not been made between working memory and cost–benefit decision making in aged rats; however, animal models should be useful for dissecting the cognitive and neurobiological mechanisms that support age-related changes in these relationships.

CONCLUSION

Rodent models have been invaluable to our understanding of the neurobehavioral underpinnings of human cognition and behavior under both normal and pathological conditions. Rats and mice are capable of performing complex cognitive tasks, and decades of research show that performance on such tasks is mediated by anatomically and functionally homologous brain systems in rodents and primates (including humans). Rodents also lend themselves to molecular, cellular, genetic, and environmental manipulations that are often infeasible in primates. This combination of factors renders rodents excellent subjects for addressing a range of questions concerning age-related alterations in cognitive function, including cost–benefit decision making.

The data described in this chapter show convergence in the effects of age on intertemporal and risky choice in rodents and humans, and reveal novel findings regarding the mechanisms of these age-related alterations. As in humans, aged rats tested in intertemporal choice tasks show increased tolerance for delayed rewards (less discounting) compared to their young counterparts, as well as corresponding alterations in the same neural systems implicated in intertemporal choice in humans (e.g., orbitofrontal cortex, dopamine signaling in the ventral striatum). Risky choice behavior has been less well studied in aged rodent models, but available data indicate the presence of significant variability in risk preference in aging, which may be linked to variability in PFC-mediated executive functions (Beas et al., 2013).

Considered together, these findings provide initial validation for the use of rodents to investigate the influence of aging on cost–benefit decision making, and suggest possible avenues for future research in human subjects (e.g., medial temporal lobe and cholinergic contributions to age-related changes in decision making). Importantly, rodent models should be useful for further defining critical neurobiological underpinnings of altered decision making in aging, as well as for evaluating the emergence and evolution of such alterations. In particular, the restricted life span of rodents provides a unique opportunity to evaluate the impact of isolated environmental and biological factors on decision quality, in a longitudinal manner across the full life span. Finally, experiments in aged rodents to date have been conducted in models of "normal" cognitive aging in which frank neurodegeneration and pathology associated with many age-related neurodegenerative diseases are absent; however, these same approaches could be applied to disease-relevant animal models. Despite the fact that impaired decision making can be a significant contributor to disease burden and reduced quality of life, there has been little investigation of decision making using models that recapitulate aspects of age-related neurodegenerative conditions such as Alzheimer's or Parkinson's disease (Gleichgerrcht, Ibanez, Roca, Torralva, & Manes, 2010; Rokosik & Napier, 2012). Such work will be important for understanding and improving cognitive outcomes across the full spectrum of human aging.

References

Abela, A. R., & Chudasama, Y. (2013). Dissociable contributions of the ventral hippocampus and orbitofrontal cortex to decision-making with a delayed or uncertain outcome. *European Journal of Neuroscience*, *37*(4), 640–647.

Adriani, W., Boyer, F., Gioiosa, L., Macri, S., Dreyer, J. L., & Laviola, G. (2009). Increased impulsive behavior and risk proneness following lentivirus-mediated dopamine transporter over-expression in rats' nucleus accumbens. *Neuroscience*, *159*(1), 47–58.

Adriani, W., & Laviola, G. (2003). Elevated levels of impulsivity and reduced place conditioning with d-amphetamine: Two behavioral features of adolescence in mice. *Behavioral Neuroscience*, *117*(4), 695–703.

Alexander, G. E., Ryan, L., Bowers, D., Foster, T. C., Bizon, J. L., Geldmacher, D. S., et al. (2012). Characterizing cognitive aging in humans with links to animal models. *Frontiers in Aging Neuroscience*, *4*, 21.

Aubert, I., Rowe, W., Meaney, M. J., Gauthier, S., & Quirion, R. (1995). Cholinergic markers in aged cognitively impaired Long-Evans rats. *Neuroscience*, *67*(2), 277–292.

Backman, L., Lindenberger, U., Li, S. C., & Nyberg, L. (2010). Linking cognitive aging to alterations in dopamine neurotransmitter functioning: Recent data and future avenues. *Neuroscience and Biobehavioral Reviews*, *34*(5), 670–677.

Balleine, B. W., & O'Doherty, J. P. (2010). Human and rodent homologies in action control: Corticostriatal determinants of goal-directed and habitual action. *Neuropsychopharmacology*, *35*(1), 48–69.

Banuelos, C., LaSarge, C. L., McQuail, J. A., Hartman, J. J., Gilbert, R. J., Ormerod, B. K., et al. (2013). Age-related changes in rostral basal forebrain cholinergic and GABAergic projection neurons: Relationship with spatial impairment. *Neurobiology of Aging*, *34*(3), 845–862.

Barense, M. D., Fox, M. T., & Baxter, M. G. (2002). Aged rats are impaired on an attentional set-shifting task sensitive to medial frontal cortex damage in young rats. *Learning & Memory*, *9*(4), 191–201.

Bartus, R. T., Dean, R. L., 3rd, Beer, B., & Lippa, A. S. (1982). The cholinergic hypothesis of geriatric memory dysfunction. *Science*, *217*(4558), 408–414.

Baxter, M. G., Parker, A., Lindner, C. C., Izquierdo, A. D., & Murray, E. A. (2000). Control of response selection by reinforcer value requires interaction of amygdala and orbital prefrontal cortex. *The Journal of Neuroscience : The Official Journal of the Society for Neuroscience*, *20*(11), 4311–4319.

Bayer, H. M., & Glimcher, P. W. (2005). Midbrain dopamine neurons encode a quantitative reward prediction error signal. *Neuron*, *47*(1), 129–141.

Beas, B. S., Setlow, B., & Bizon, J. L. (2013). Distinct manifestations of executive dysfunction in aged rats. *Neurobiology of Aging*, *34*(9), 2164–2174.

Bechara, A., & Van Der Linden, M. (2005). Decision-making and impulse control after frontal lobe injuries. *Current Opinion in Neurology*, *18*(6), 734–739.

Bickel, W. K., Yi, R., Landes, R. D., Hill, P. F., & Baxter, C. (2011). Remember the future: Working memory training decreases delay discounting among stimulant addicts. *Biological Psychiatry*, *69*(3), 260–265.

Birrell, J. M., & Brown, V. J. (2000). Medial frontal cortex mediates perceptual attentional set shifting in the rat. *The Journal of Neuroscience: The Official Journal of the Society for Neuroscience*, *20*(11), 4320–4324.

Bizon, J. L., Foster, T. C., Alexander, G. E., & Glisky, E. L. (2012). Characterizing cognitive aging of working memory and executive function in animal models. *Frontiers in Aging Neuroscience*, *4*, 19.

Bizon, J. L., Helm, K. A., Han, J. S., Chun, H. J., Pucilowska, J., Lund, P. K., et al. (2001). Hypothalamic–pituitary–adrenal axis function and corticosterone receptor expression in behaviourally characterized young and aged Long-Evans rats. *The European Journal of Neuroscience*, *14*(10), 1739–1751.

Bizon, J. L., LaSarge, C. L., Montgomery, K. S., McDermott, A. N., Setlow, B., & Griffith, W. H. (2009). Spatial reference and working memory across the lifespan of male Fischer 344 rats. *Neurobiology of Aging*, *30*(4), 646–655.

Bizon, J. L., Lauterborn, J. C., Isackson, P. J., & Gall, C. M. (1996). Acidic fibroblast growth factor mRNA is expressed by basal forebrain and striatal cholinergic neurons. *The Journal of Comparative Neurology*, *366*(3), 379–389.

Boettiger, C. A., Mitchell, J. M., Tavares, V. C., Robertson, M., Joslyn, G., D'Esposito, M., et al. (2007). Immediate reward bias in humans: Fronto-parietal networks and a role for the catechol-O-methyltransferase 158(Val/Val) genotype. *Journal of Neuroscience*, *27*(52), 14383–14391.

Brown, V. J., & Bowman, E. M. (2002). Rodent models of prefrontal cortical function. *Trends in Neurosciences*, *25*(7), 340–343.

Buckner, R. L. (2004). Memory and executive function in aging and AD: Multiple factors that cause decline and reserve factors that compensate. *Neuron*, *44*(1), 195–208.

Burke, S. N., Ryan, L., & Barnes, C. A. (2012). Characterizing cognitive aging of recognition memory and related processes in animal models and in humans. *Frontiers in Aging Neuroscience*, *4*, 15.

Cardinal, R. N., & Howes, N. J. (2005). Effects of lesions of the nucleus accumbens core on choice between small certain rewards and large uncertain rewards in rats. *BMC Neuroscience*, *6*, 37.

Cardinal, R. N., Pennicott, D. R., Sugathapala, C. L., Robbins, T. W., & Everitt, B. J. (2001). Impulsive choice induced in rats by lesions of the nucleus accumbens core. *Science*, *292*(5526), 2499–2501.

Cardinal, R. N., Robbins, T. W., & Everitt, B. J. (2000). The effects of d-amphetamine, chlordiazepoxide, alpha-flupenthixol and behavioural manipulations on choice of signalled and unsignalled delayed reinforcement in rats. *Psychopharmacology*, *152*(4), 362–375.

Chen, M. K., Lakshminarayanan, V., & Santos, L. R. (2006). How basic are behavioral biases? Evidence from capuchin monkey trading behavior. *Journal of Political Economy*, *114*(3), 517–537.

Dallery, J., & Locey, M. L. (2005). Effects of acute and chronic nicotine on impulsive choice in rats. *Behavioural Pharmacology*, *16*(1), 15–23.

Deakin, J., Aitken, M., Robbins, T., & Sahakian, B. J. (2004). Risk taking during decision-making in normal volunteers changes with age. *Journal of the International Neuropsychological Society: JINS*, *10*(4), 590–598.

Denburg, N. L., Tranel, D., & Bechara, A. (2005). The ability to decide advantageously declines prematurely in some normal older persons. *Neuropsychologia*, *43*(7), 1099–1106.

de Wit, H., Enggasser, J. L., & Richards, J. B. (2002). Acute administration of d-amphetamine decreases impulsivity in healthy volunteers. *Neuropsychopharmacology*, *27*(5), 813–825.

Dias, R., Robbins, T. W., & Roberts, A. C. (1996). Dissociation in prefrontal cortex of affective and attentional shifts. *Nature*, *380*(6569), 69–72.

Elliott, R., Dolan, R. J., & Frith, C. D. (2000). Dissociable functions in the medial and lateral orbitofrontal cortex: Evidence from human neuroimaging studies. *Cerebral Cortex*, *10*(3), 308–317.

Eppinger, B., Nystrom, L. E., & Cohen, J. D. (2012). Reduced sensitivity to immediate reward during decision-making in older than younger adults. *PloS One*, *7*(5), e36953.

Eppinger, B., Schuck, N. W., Nystrom, L. E., & Cohen, J. D. (2013). Reduced striatal responses to reward prediction errors in older compared with younger adults. *Journal of Neuroscience*, *33*(24), 9905–9912.

Evenden, J. L., & Ryan, C. N. (1996). The pharmacology of impulsive behaviour in rats: The effects of drugs on response choice with varying delays of reinforcement. *Psychopharmacology*, *128*(2), 161–170.

Floresco, S. B. (2013). Prefrontal dopamine and behavioral flexibility: Shifting from an "inverted-U" toward a family of functions. *Frontiers in Neuroscience*, *7*, 62.

Floresco, S. B., St Onge, J. R., Ghods-Sharifi, S., & Winstanley, C. A. (2008). Cortico-limbic-striatal circuits subserving different forms of cost-benefit decision making. *Cognitive, Affective, & Behavioral Neuroscience*, *8*(4), 375–389.

Foster, T. C., Defazio, R. A., & Bizon, J. L. (2012). Characterizing cognitive aging of spatial and contextual memory in animal models. *Frontiers in Aging Neuroscience*, *4*, 12.

Freeman, K. B., Green, L., Myerson, J., & Woolverton, W. L. (2009). Delay discounting of saccharin in rhesus monkeys. *Behavioural Processes*, *82*(2), 214–218.

Gallagher, M., Burwell, R., & Burchinal, M. (1993). Severity of spatial learning impairment in aging: Development of a learning index for performance in the Morris water maze. *Behavioral Neuroscience*, *107*(4), 618–626.

Gallagher, M., McMahan, R. W., & Schoenbaum, G. (1999). Orbitofrontal cortex and representation of incentive value in associative learning. *Journal of Neuroscience: The Official Journal of the Society for Neuroscience*, *19*(15), 6610–6614.

Galtress, T., Garcia, A., & Kirkpatrick, K. (2012). Individual differences in impulsive choice and timing in rats. *Journal of the Experimental Analysis of Behavior*, *98*(1), 65–87.

Gaykema, R. P., van Weeghel, R., Hersh, L. B., & Luiten, P. G. (1991). Prefrontal cortical projections to the cholinergic neurons in the basal forebrain. *Journal of Comparative Neurology*, *303*(4), 563–583.

Gilbert, R. J., Mitchell, M. R., Simon, N. W., Banuelos, C., Setlow, B., & Bizon, J. L. (2012). Risk, reward, and decision-making in a rodent model of cognitive aging. *Frontiers in Neuroscience*, *5*, 144.

Gleichgerrcht, E., Ibanez, A., Roca, M., Torralva, T., & Manes, F. (2010). Decision-making cognition in neurodegenerative diseases. *Nature Reviews Neurology*, *6*(11), 611–623.

Glisky, E. L. (2007). Changes in cognitive function in human aging. In D. R. Riddle (Ed.), *Brain aging: Models, methods, and mechanisms* CRC Press Boca Raton (FL).

Green, L., Fry, A. F., & Myerson, J. (1994). Discounting of delayed rewards - a life-span comparison. *Psychological Science*, *5*(1), 33–36.

Green, L., & Myerson, J. (2013). How many impulsivities? A discounting perspective. *Journal of the Experimental Analysis of Behavior*, *99*(1), 3–13.

Green, L., Myerson, J., Lichtman, D., Rosen, S., & Fry, A. (1996). Temporal discounting in choice between delayed rewards: the role of age and income. *Psychology and Aging*, *11*(1), 79–84.

Haberman, R. P., Colantuoni, C., Stocker, A. M., Schmidt, A. C., Pedersen, J. T., & Gallagher, M. (2011). Prominent hippocampal CA3 gene expression profile in neurocognitive aging. *Neurobiology of Aging*, *32*(9), 1678–1692.

Hariri, A. R., Brown, S. M., Williamson, D. E., Flory, J. D., de Wit, H., & Manuck, S. B. (2006). Preference for immediate over delayed rewards is associated with magnitude of ventral striatal activity. *Journal of Neuroscience: The Official Journal of the Society for Neuroscience, 26*(51), 13213–13217.

Henninger, D. E., Madden, D. J., & Huettel, S. A. (2010). Processing speed and memory mediate age-related differences in decision making. *Psychology and Aging, 25*(2), 262–270.

Hertwig, R., & Gigerenzer, G. (2011). Behavioral inconsistencies do not imply inconsistent strategies. *Frontiers in Psychology, 2*, 292.

Jimura, K., Myerson, J., Hilgard, J., Keighley, J., Braver, T. S., & Green, L. (2011). Domain independence and stability in young and older adults' discounting of delayed rewards. *Behavioural Processes, 87*(3), 253–259.

Jones, J. L., Esber, G. R., McDannald, M. A., Gruber, A. J., Hernandez, A., Mirenzi, A., et al. (2012). Orbitofrontal cortex supports behavior and learning using inferred but not cached values. *Science, 338*(6109), 953–956.

Kaasinen, V., & Rinne, J. O. (2002). Functional imaging studies of dopamine system and cognition in normal aging and Parkinson's disease. *Neuroscience & Biobehavioral Reviews, 26*(7), 785–793.

Kable, J. W., & Glimcher, P. W. (2007). The neural correlates of subjective value during intertemporal choice. *Nature Neuroscience, 10*(12), 1625–1633.

Kable, J. W., & Glimcher, P. W. (2009). The neurobiology of decision: Consensus and controversy. *Neuron, 63*(6), 733–745.

Kalenscher, T., & van Wingerden, M. (2011). Why we should use animals to study economic decision making—a perspective. *Frontiers in Neuroscience, 5*, 82.

Kesner, R. P., & Churchwell, J. C. (2011). An analysis of rat prefrontal cortex in mediating executive function. *Neurobiology of Learning and Memory, 96*(3), 417–431.

Keuker, J. I., Luiten, P. G., & Fuchs, E. (2003). Preservation of hippocampal neuron numbers in aged rhesus monkeys. *Neurobiology of Aging, 24*(1), 157–165.

Knowlton, B. J., Mangels, J. A., & Squire, L. R. (1996). A neostriatal habit learning system in humans. *Science, 273*(5280), 1399–1402.

Kumar, A. (2007). *Who gambles in the stock market?* Austin: McCombs School of Business, University of Texas at Austin.

Kumar, A., & Foster, T. C. (2013). Linking redox regulation of NMDAR synaptic function to cognitive decline during aging. *Journal of Neuroscience: The Official Journal of the Society for Neuroscience, 33*(40), 15710–15715.

Lejeune, H., Ferrara, A., Soffie, M., Bronchart, M., & Wearden, J. H. (1998). Peak procedure performance in young adult and aged rats: Acquisition and adaptation to a changing temporal criterion. *Quarterly Journal of Experimental Psychology, 51*(3), 193–217.

Levy, D. J., & Glimcher, P. W. (2012). The root of all value: A neural common currency for choice. *Current Opinion in Neurobiology, 22*(6), 1027–1038.

Li, S. C., Papenberg, G., Nagel, I. E., Preuschhof, C., Schroder, J., Nietfeld, W., et al. (2013). Aging magnifies the effects of dopamine transporter and D2 receptor genes on backward serial memory. *Neurobiology of Aging, 34*(1), 358, e351–310.

Liljeholm, M., & O'Doherty, J. P. (2012). Contributions of the striatum to learning, motivation, and performance: An associative account. *Trends in Cognitive Sciences, 16*(9), 467–475.

Löckenhoff, C. E., O'Donoghue, T., & Dunning, D. (2011). Age differences in temporal discounting: the role of dispositional affect and anticipated emotions. *Psychology and Aging, 26*(2), 274–284.

Man, M. S., Clarke, H. F., & Roberts, A. C. (2009). The role of the orbitofrontal cortex and medial striatum in the regulation of prepotent responses to food rewards. *Cerebral Cortex, 19*(4), 899–906.

Mar, A. C., Walker, A. L., Theobald, D. E., Eagle, D. M., & Robbins, T. W. (2011). Dissociable effects of lesions to orbitofrontal cortex subregions on impulsive choice in the rat. *Journal of Neuroscience: The Official Journal of the Society for Neuroscience, 31*(17), 6398–6404.

Mariano, T. Y., Bannerman, D. M., McHugh, S. B., Preston, T. J., Rudebeck, P. H., Rudebeck, S. R., et al. (2009). Impulsive choice in hippocampal but not orbitofrontal cortex-lesioned rats on a nonspatial decision-making maze task. *European Journal of Neuroscience, 30*(3), 472–484.

Mata, R., Josef, A. K., Samanez-Larkin, G. R., & Hertwig, R. (2011). Age differences in risky choice: A meta-analysis. *Annals of the New York Academy, 1235*, 18–29.

Mather, M. (2006). A review of decision-making processes: Weighing the risks and benefits of aging. In L. L. Carstensen, & C. R. Hartel (Eds.), *When I'm 64*. Washington, DC: The National Academies Press.

Mazur, J. E. (1987). An adjusting procedure for studying delayed reinforcement. In M. L. Commons, J. E. Mazur, J. A. Nevin, & H. Rachlin (Eds.), *Quantitative analysis of behavior*. Hillsdale: Erlbaum.

Mazur, J. E. (2001). Hyperbolic value addition and general models of animal choice. *Psychological Review, 108*(1), 96–112.

McClure, S. M., Laibson, D. I., Loewenstein, G., & Cohen, J. D. (2004a). Separate neural systems value immediate and delayed monetary rewards. *Science, 306*(5695), 503–507.

McClure, S. M., York, M. K., & Montague, P. R. (2004b). The neural substrates of reward processing in humans: The modern role of FMRI. *Neuroscientist, 10*(3), 260–268.

Meck, W. H., Church, R. M., & Wenk, G. L. (1986). Arginine vasopressin innoculates against age-related increases in sodium-dependent high affinity choline uptake and discrepancies in the content of temporal memory. *European Journal of Pharmacology, 130*(3), 327–331.

Mendez, I. A., Damborsky, J. C., Winzer-Serhan, U. H., Bizon, J. L., & Setlow, B. (2013). a4b2 and a7 nicotinic acetylcholine receptor binding predicts choice preference in two cost benefit decision making tasks. *Neuroscience, 230*, 121–131.

Miller, E. K., & Cohen, J. D. (2001). An integrative theory of prefrontal cortex function. *Annual Review of Neuroscience, 24*, 167–202.

Mitchell, M. R., Shimp, K. G., Ouimet, D. J., McLaurin, B. I., & Setlow, B. (2013). Acute administration of d-amphetamine into nucleus accumbens decreases impulsive choice. *Abstract Annual Meeting Society for Neuroscience*, program number: 855.06.

Mobini, S., Body, S., Ho, M. Y., Bradshaw, C. M., Szabadi, E., Deakin, J. F., et al. (2002). Effects of lesions of the orbitofrontal cortex on sensitivity to delayed and probabilistic reinforcement. *Psychopharmacology (Berl), 160*(3), 290–298.

Morrison, J. H., & Baxter, M. G. (2012). The ageing cortical synapse: hallmarks and implications for cognitive decline. *Nature Reviews Neuroscience, 13*(4), 240–250.

Pardey, M. C., Kumar, N. N., Goodchild, A. K., & Cornish, J. L. (2013). Catecholamine receptors differentially mediate impulsive choice in the medial prefrontal and orbitofrontal cortex. *Journal of Psychopharmacology, 27*(2), 203–212.

Perry, E. K., Martin-Ruiz, C. M., & Court, J. A. (2001). Nicotinic receptor subtypes in human brain related to aging and dementia. *Alcohol, 24*(2), 63–68.

Paxinos G., & Watson C (1998). The Rat Brain in Stereotaxic Coordinates. 4th ed., San Diego: Academic Press, p. 237.

Peters, J., & Buchel, C. (2011). The neural mechanisms of inter-temporal decision-making: understanding variability. *Trends in Cognitive Sciences, 15*(5), 227–239.

Platt, M. L., & Huettel, S. A. (2008). Risky business: the neuroeconomics of decision making under uncertainty. *Nature Neuroscience, 11*(4), 398–403.

Rapp, P. R., & Gallagher, M. (1996). Preserved neuron number in the hippocampus of aged rats with spatial learning deficits. *Proceedings of the National Academy of Sciences of the United States of America, 93*(18), 9926–9930.

Rasmussen, T., Schliemann, T., Sorensen, J. C., Zimmer, J., & West, M. J. (1996). Memory impaired aged rats: No loss of principal hippocampal and subicular neurons. *Neurobiology of Aging, 17*(1), 143–147.

Richards, J. B., Mitchell, S. H., de Wit, H., & Seiden, L. S. (1997). Determination of discount functions in rats with an adjusting-amount procedure. *Journal of the Experimental Analysis of Behavior*, *67*(3), 353–366.

Roalf, D. R., Mitchell, S. H., Harbaugh, W. T., & Janowsky, J. S. (2011). Risk, reward, and economic decision making in aging. *The Journals of Gerontology. Series B, Psychological Sciences and Social Sciences*, *67*(3), 289–298.

Robbins, T. W., & Arnsten, A. F. T. (2009). The neuropsychopharmacology of fronto-executive function: Monoaminergic modulation. *Annual Review of Neuroscience*, *32*, 267–287.

Roberson, E. D., Defazio, R. A., Barnes, C. A., Alexander, G. E., Bizon, J. L., Bowers, D., et al. (2012). Challenges and opportunities for characterizing cognitive aging across species. *Frontiers in Aging Neuroscience*, *4*, 6.

Roesch, M. R., Bryden, D. W., Cerri, D. H., Haney, Z. R., & Schoenbaum, G. (2012). Willingness to wait and altered encoding of time-discounted reward in the orbitofrontal cortex with normal aging. *Journal of Neuroscience: The Official Journal of the Society for Neuroscience*, *32*(16), 5525–5533.

Roesch, M. R., Taylor, A. R., & Schoenbaum, G. (2006). Encoding of time-discounted rewards in orbitofrontal cortex is independent of value representation. *Neuron*, *51*(4), 509–520.

Rokosik, S. L., & Napier, T. C. (2012). Pramipexole-induced increased probabilistic discounting: Comparison between a rodent model of Parkinson's disease and controls. *Neuropsychopharmacology*, *37*(6), 1397–1408.

Rosati, A. G., & Hare, B. (2011). Chimpanzees and bonobos distinguish between risk and ambiguity. *Biology Letters*, *7*(1), 15–18.

Rose, J. E., & Woolsey, C. N. (1948). The orbitofrontal cortex and its connections with the mediodorsal nucleus in rabbit, sheep and cat. *Research Publications—Association for Research in Nervous and Mental Disease*, *27*(1 vol.), 210–232.

Rudebeck, P. H., & Murray, E. A. (2011). Dissociable effects of subtotal lesions within the macaque orbital prefrontal cortex on reward-guided behavior. *Journal of Neuroscience: The Official Journal of the Society for Neuroscience*, *31*(29), 10569–10578.

Samanez-Larkin, G. R., & Knutson, B. (2014). Reward processing and risky decision making in the aging brain. In V. Reyna, & V. Zayas (Eds.), *The neuroscience of risky decision making* (pp. 123–142). Washington DC: American Psychological Association.

Samanez-Larkin, G. R., Mata, R., Radu, P. T., Ballard, I. C., Carstensen, L. L., & McClure, S. M. (2011). Age differences in striatal delay sensitivity during intertemporal choice in healthy adults. *Frontiers in Neuroscience*, *5*, 126.

Schoenbaum, G., Nugent, S., Saddoris, M. P., & Gallagher, M. (2002b). Teaching old rats new tricks: Age-related impairments in olfactory reversal learning. *Neurobiology of Aging*, *23*(4), 555–564.

Schoenbaum, G., Nugent, S. L., Saddoris, M. P., & Setlow, B. (2002a). Orbitofrontal lesions in rats impair reversal but not acquisition of go, no-go odor discriminations. *Neuroreport*, *13*(6), 885–890.

Schoenbaum, G., Setlow, B., Saddoris, M. P., & Gallagher, M. (2006). Encoding changes in orbitofrontal cortex in reversal-impaired aged rats. *Journal of Neurophysiology*, *95*(3), 1509–1517.

Schultz, W. (2010). Dopamine signals for reward value and risk: Basic and recent data. *Behavioral and Brain Functions*, *6*, 24.

Sescousse, G., Caldu, X., Segura, B., & Dreher, J. C. (2013). Processing of primary and secondary rewards: A quantitative meta-analysis and review of human functional neuroimaging studies. *Neuroscience & Biobehavioral Reviews*, *37*(4), 681–696.

Shamosh, N. A., Deyoung, C. G., Green, A. E., Reis, D. L., Johnson, M. R., Conway, A. R., et al. (2008). Individual differences in delay discounting: Relation to intelligence, working memory, and anterior prefrontal cortex. *Psychological Science*, *19*(9), 904–911.

Shimp, K. G., Mitchell, M. R., Beas, B. S., Bizon, J. L., & Setlow, B. (in press). Affective and cognitive mechanisms of risky decision making. *Neurobiology of Learning and Memory*.

Simon, N. W., LaSarge, C. L., Montgomery, K. S., Williams, M. T., Mendez, I. A., Setlow, B., et al. (2010). Good things come to those who wait: Attenuated discounting of delayed rewards in aged Fischer 344 rats. *Neurobiol Aging*, *31*(5), 853–862.

Simon, N. W., Montgomery, K. S., Beas, B. S., Mitchell, M. R., LaSarge, C. L., Mendez, I. A., et al. (2011). Dopaminergic modulation of risky decision-making. *Journal of Neuroscience*, *31*(48), 17460–17470.

Smits, R. R., Stein, J. S., Johnson, P. S., Odum, A. L., & Madden, G. J. (2013). Test-retest reliability and construct validity of the experiential discounting task. *Experimental and Clinical Psychopharmacology*, *21*(2), 155–163.

St Onge, J. R., & Floresco, S. B. (2010). Prefrontal cortical contribution to risk-based decision making. *Cerebral Cortex*, *20*(8), 1816–1828.

Stein, J. S., Pinkston, J. W., Brewer, A. T., Francisco, M. T., & Madden, G. J. (2012). Delay discounting in Lewis and Fischer 344 rats: Steady-state and rapid-determination adjusting-amount procedures. *Journal of the Experimental Analysis of Behavior*, *97*(3), 305–321.

Sugam, J. A., Day, J. J., Wightman, R. M., & Carelli, R. M. (2012). Phasic nucleus accumbens dopamine encodes risk-based decision-making behavior. *Biological Psychiatry*, *71*(3), 199–205.

Uylings, H. B., Groenewegen, H. J., & Kolb, B. (2003). Do rats have a prefrontal cortex? *Behavioural Brain Research*, *146*(1–2), 3–17.

Volkow, N. D., Gur, R. C., Wang, G. J., Fowler, J. S., Moberg, P. J., Ding, Y. S., et al. (1998). Association between decline in brain dopamine activity with age and cognitive and motor impairment in healthy individuals. *The American Journal of Psychiatry*, *155*(3), 344–349.

Winstanley, C. A., Theobald, D. E., Cardinal, R. N., & Robbins, T. W. (2004). Contrasting roles of basolateral amygdala and orbitofrontal cortex in impulsive choice. *Journal of Neuroscience: The Official Journal of the Society for Neuroscience*, *24*(20), 4718–4722.

Wittmann, M., & Paulus, M. P. (2008). Decision making, impulsivity and time perception. *Trends in Cognitive Sciences*, *12*(1), 7–12.

Wong, D. F., Wagner, H. N., Jr., Dannals, R. F., Links, J. M., Frost, J. J., Ravert, H. T., et al. (1984). Effects of age on dopamine and serotonin receptors measured by positron tomography in the living human brain. *Science*, *226*(4681), 1393–1396.

Zeeb, F. D., Floresco, S. B., & Winstanley, C. A. (2010). Contributions of the orbitofrontal cortex to impulsive choice: Interactions with basal levels of impulsivity, dopamine signalling, and reward-related cues. *Psychopharmacology (Berl)*, *211*(1), 87–98.

Zhang, L., & Roth, G. S. (1997). The effect of aging on rat striatal D1 receptor mRNA-containing neurons. *Neurobiology of Aging*, *18*(2), 251–255.

Zhang, H. Y., Watson, M. L., Gallagher, M., & Nicolle, M. M. (2007). Muscarinic receptor-mediated GTP-Eu binding in the hippocampus and prefrontal cortex is correlated with spatial memory impairment in aged rats. *Neurobiology of Aging*, *28*(4), 619–626.

CHAPTER

3

Decision Neuroscience and Aging

Gregory R. Samanez-Larkin

Department of Psychology, Yale University, New Haven, CT, USA

Until recently we have known little about how core decision processes change with age and how aging may impact the structure and function of corresponding ventromedial frontostriatal neural systems (Samanez-Larkin & Knutson, 2014). The chapter begins by briefly orienting the reader to frontostriatal brain networks, and then reviews age differences in a series of reward-related decision-making contexts. A range of decision-related processes are covered, from adult age differences in basic sensitivity to gains and losses to areas of decision making that require increasing integration of information, and from the qualification of potential benefits with associated costs (such as temporal delays or risk) to the rapid computation and updating of reward signals during feedback-driven learning. Each of the sections that follow first briefly reviews the behavioral evidence, and then reviews the often very limited initial evidence for age differences in neural structure and function associated with the behavioral differences in reward processing and decision making. The studies reviewed focus almost exclusively on monetary incentives, although reference will be made to the few existing studies that examine age differences in other types of rewards. A closing discussion covers how the findings might be organized within emerging frameworks and theories and provides direction for future research.

OVERVIEW OF FRONTOSTRIATAL NEURAL CIRCUITRY

The neural circuitry underlying reward processing and decision making includes a distributed, interconnected network of cortical and subcortical brain regions. Many of these areas, such as the striatum—a set

http://dx.doi.org/10.1016/B978-0-12-417148-0.00003-0

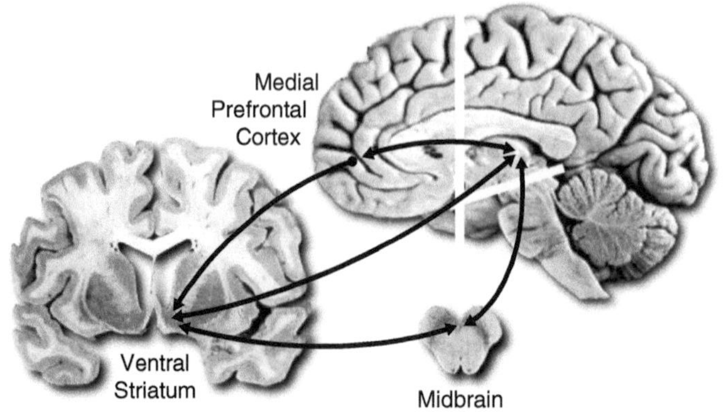

FIGURE 1 A ventromedial frontostriatal brain circuit. The four nodes in the network (connected with lines and arrows) are the ventral tegmental area in the midbrain (lower right), the nucleus accumbens in the ventral striatum (lower left), the medial prefrontal cortex (upper center), and the dorsomedial nucleus of the thalamus (unlabeled in the upper right). The sagittal view in the upper right includes a vertical white bar indicating the approximate location of the coronal slice in the lower left and includes an angled horizontal white bar indicating the approximate location of the axial slice of the midbrain in the lower right. *Underlay brain images adapted from Williams and Jew (1997).*

of gray matter nuclei deep in the brain that includes the caudate, putamen, and nucleus accumbens—and the medial and lateral prefrontal cortex, are rich in dopamine receptors and receive direct input from midbrain dopamine neurons (see Figure 1). Early evidence suggesting that dopamine is released during the subjective experience of reward and administration of many drugs of abuse, for which people have strong cravings and are highly motivated to seek, led to the hypothesis that dopamine is the "pleasure chemical" (Wise, 1980). However, subsequent research over the past several decades has clarified that although dopamine plays a primary role in motivation and learning (Wise, 2004), it is not the neurochemical source of feelings of pleasure (Berridge, 2012). Although dopamine release in the striatum and medial frontal cortex has been shown to increase during both the anticipation and receipt of rewards, this dopamine signal is better characterized as a reward prediction error rather than a simple reward signal (Glimcher, 2011). Prediction errors signal the difference in magnitude between an expected reward and an actual reward, and they serve to update expectations of reward when encountering a stimulus or performing an action in the future. In summary, dopamine release in this network of brain regions plays an important role in learning to make future predictions of reward based on recent feedback.

However, dopamine is not the only important neurochemical signal in this interconnected network of frontal and striatal brain regions.

These regions also communicate through the release of GABA and glutamate (Alexander, Crutcher, & DeLong, 1990; Alexander, DeLong, & Strick, 1986). The connectivity of this circuit is depicted in Figure 1. Although age differences in dopamine have received a great deal of attention in cognitive aging research (e.g., Braver & Barch, 2002; Li, Lindenberger, & Bäckman, 2010), very little research has focused on interactions between neurochemicals, which all decline to some extent with age (Mora, Segovia, & Del Arco, 2007). Connections between the prefrontal cortex and striatum play an important role not only in the representation, computation, and updating of reward-related signals, but also in cognitive control and the integration of reward signals with other information relevant to making decisions (e.g., potential costs of obtaining a reward such as temporal delays or risk; Haber & Knutson, 2010; Haber, 2003). Unfortunately, almost none of the studies reviewed here (or elsewhere, e.g., Eppinger & Bruckner, this volume) include direct measures of the dopamine system or of any other neurochemical yet many of these studies speculate on the potential contribution of age differences in dopamine. In contrast, these studies rarely consider contributions from other neurotransmitters. A hope is that research will catch up in the coming years.

Rather than focusing on neurochemistry, this chapter instead focuses on examining structural and functional age differences across adulthood in brain regions such as the striatum and medial prefrontal cortex and how these differences may be associated with age differences in decision making. Although cross-sectional and longitudinal data document structural atrophy across adulthood within each of these regions (Raz, 2005; Raz, Rodrigue, & Haacke, 2007), only recently have studies begun to explore age differences in function within regions and structural connectivity between regions. The majority of studies reviewed here use functional magnetic resonance imaging to measure neural activity in individual brain regions while engaged in a task. Functional magnetic resonance imaging datasets are four dimensional (three dimensions of space plus time), with measures of activity across the brain collected approximately every 2 s. Other studies use diffusion tensor imaging to assess the structural integrity of white matter pathways that connect regions. Diffusion tensor images are also collected in a magnetic resonance imaging scanner but they produce a single three-dimensional dataset and not a time-varying estimate of changes in connectivity. To foreshadow our conclusions, we will argue that the majority of documented age-related deficits in decision making are due to age-related declines in the ability to integrate novel information over time and that these integration deficits are associated with a relative disconnection of communication across frontostriatal networks in old age.

GAINS AND LOSSES

Do individuals become more or less excited about winning or losing money in old age? Initial behavioral research revealed that although younger and older adults do not differ in their self-reported feelings of positive arousal/activation during the anticipation or receipt of monetary gains, older adults report lower levels of negative arousal/activation during the anticipation of monetary losses (Nielsen, Knutson, & Carstensen, 2008; Samanez-Larkin et al., 2007). This asymmetry in gain and loss anticipation as a function of age is consistent with a large body of behavioral research demonstrating an age-related positivity effect (Carstensen & Mikels, 2005; Mather & Carstensen, 2005).

Functional magnetic resonance imaging studies that have examined adult age differences in the basic function of the reward system are consistent with the behavioral effects reported above; neural activity in the striatum during anticipation shows similar modulation by reward magnitude in younger and older adults (Samanez-Larkin et al., 2007) and receipt of monetary gains (Cox, Aizenstein, & Fiez, 2008; Samanez-Larkin et al., 2007; Samanez-Larkin, Kuhnen, Yoo, & Knutson, 2010; Schott et al., 2007). These studies provide initial evidence that basic neural responses to the anticipation and receipt of monetary gains are relatively preserved from young adulthood to old age.

However, a different pattern emerges for anticipatory responses to monetary losses. Older compared to younger adults show reduced reactivity in the caudate (within the striatum) and the anterior insula (a deep cortical region between the frontal and temporal lobes) during anticipation of monetary loss (Samanez-Larkin et al., 2007). This asymmetry in anticipatory neural activity was replicated in an independent sample (Wu, Samanez-Larkin, Katovich, & Knutson, 2014). Interestingly, these age differences do not extend to loss *outcomes*. When older adults lose money, they are as reactive to those losses as younger adults (Samanez-Larkin et al., 2007). As will be discussed later in the chapter in the "Learning" section, this anticipatory (but not consummatory) valence effect does not account for many of the observed age differences in decision making.

Further, the vast majority of decisions encountered in daily life require not only the simple processing of potential gains and losses but also the integration of these signals with each other and with other relevant information. In the next two sections we will review recent findings on decisions that require the integration of information about potential outcomes (e.g., monetary gains and losses of different sizes) and information about associated costs of obtaining a reward (e.g., temporal delays or risk).

INTERTEMPORAL DECISION MAKING

Intertemporal choices are decisions in everyday life that involve selecting between outcomes available at different times in the future. Making an intertemporal decision requires deciding whether the additional money offered at a later date is worth waiting the extra time delay required to receive the larger reward (relative to a smaller reward available sooner). It requires the integration of information about reward size and time delay, but is otherwise a fairly simple decision, at least computationally (i.e., resisting an impulse for immediate satisfaction may create demand for cognitive control but computing the subjective value of an option by scaling the outcome according to the subjective cost of the delay is fairly simple). The time delays and outcomes in intertemporal choice tasks are certain; that is, if you choose $5 now over $10 in 2 weeks you will receive $5 now with 100% certainty. If you choose $10 in 2 weeks, you will receive $10 in 2 weeks with 100% certainty. Individual differences in temporal discounting, or the reduction in the subjective value of a particular reward due to the time delay until delivery, are common (Peters & Büchel, 2011). Although discounting behavior is highly variable in humans, the majority of studies that have examined age differences in temporal discounting report an increasing willingness to wait in older age, which corresponds to a lower discount rate for time (Löckenhoff, 2011). This behavioral effect has been observed in both humans and rats (Simon et al., 2010b; Beas, Setlow, Samanez-Larkin, & Bizon, this volume). Intertemporal choice may be viewed as an area where decision making improves with age. Older adults make quantitatively better decisions with respect to maximizing absolute units of reward; they more often choose larger, later rewards over sooner, smaller rewards compared to younger adults.

Recent functional neuroimaging studies have examined age differences in intertemporal choice. Parallel to the behavioral findings, the studies find that neural activation in the ventral striatum is reduced when the reward can only be obtained after a significant temporal delay in younger but not older adults (Eppinger, Nystrom, & Cohen, 2012; Samanez-Larkin et al., 2011a). Ventral striatal signal increases to both short and long delays in healthy older adults, which is not the case for younger adults. In general, the age group differences across the existing studies are strikingly similar (see Figure 2(A) and (B)). In addition, evidence of an age by delay interaction similar to that identified in the human ventral striatum has been recently observed in the orbitofrontal cortex of rodents (Roesch, Bryden, Cerri, Haney, & Schoenbaum, 2012a) (see Figure 2(C)).

There are at least two opposing accounts of these data. The findings could be viewed as evidence for age-related decline or improvement. It is possible that the age differences in temporal discounting are a serendipitous result of neural decline with age (Eppinger et al., 2012).

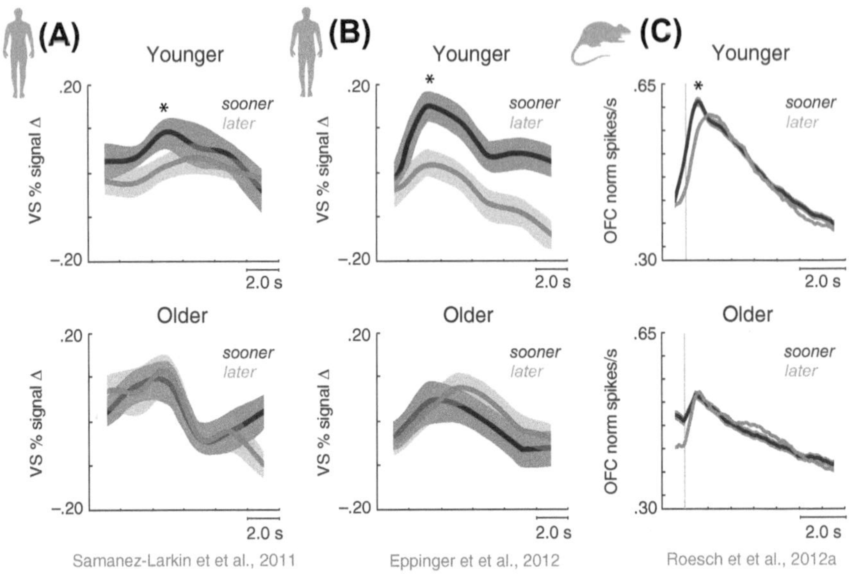

FIGURE 2 (A, B) Young adults show reduced activation of the ventral striatum (VS) for rewards available at longer (gray line) compared to shorter (black line) time delays, whereas this oversensitivity to immediacy is not present in older adults. Older adults show equivalent activation of the VS for short and long delays. y-axis is percentage change in the blood-oxygen-level-dependent signal. (C) Similarly, in younger rats, reward-responsive neurons in the orbitofrontal cortex (OFC) fire less strongly to delayed rewards with lower firing rates for long (gray line) compared to short (black line) time delays. For older adult rats, reward-responsive neurons in the OFC show similar firing rates to both long (gray line) and short (black line) time delays. The vertical gray line indicates reward delivery. y-axis is normalized spikes per second. Figure panels adapted from (A) Samanez-Larkin et al. (2011a), (B) Eppinger et al. (2012), and (C) Roesch et al. (2012a). In all plots, shaded error bars are s.e.m.

This decline account posits that structural or neurochemical reductions (e.g., lower tonic dopamine) in old age reduce sensitivity to immediacy and associated impulsivity, which may contribute to quantitatively "better" decisions. However, evidence that dopamine depletion in animals most often increases instead of decreases discount rates (Phillips, Walton, & Jhou, 2006) is inconsistent with a model attributing age differences in time discounting to dopamine decline with age. Although this assumption is often made, evidence for neural signal differences between age groups is not definitive evidence for age-related neurobiological deterioration (even in an animal model).

An alternate account is that these behavioral and neural effects are evidence for improvement over the life span (Samanez-Larkin et al., 2011a). Although there is some level of neurobiological decline in these regions with age, relatively similar responses to both short and long delays are observed in older adults. Others have speculated that this age-related improvement may be related to increased experience with the realization of delayed reward over an individual's lifetime (Li, Baldassi, Johnson, & Weber, 2013). Responses to delayed rewards in older adults may be the result of experience-based tuning of reward signals (Samanez-Larkin et al., 2011a) reducing the demand for new integration of novel information. This latter interpretation suggests that it is as if the older adults know that $20 is going to be just as good in 2 weeks as it is today. In contrast, the younger adults have not had the opportunity to realize interest rates over decades and appreciate the long-term rewards of waiting.

An important qualification to the improvement account is the evidence that similar behavioral and neural effects are observed in younger and older rodents (Roesch et al., 2012a, 2012b; Simon et al., 2010b) who have been reared in well-controlled environments with ad libitum access to food and water. Before starting the experiments the younger and older animals had the same lack of experience with delayed rewards. This leaves open several possibilities: (1) the same behavioral and neural age differences in humans and rodents occur for different reasons, (2) there is a neurobiological aging process not associated with experience that is in common in both species, or (3) some combination of both of these possibilities is at work. Future research should examine how this increased willingness to wait may be related to other cognitive processes underlying decision making that are likely to change with age similarly across species (Gilbert et al., 2011). Additionally, an age-related increase in the willingness to wait may have positive or negative consequences in other domains. More generally, the extent to which these changes with age prove advantageous or disadvantageous for decision making in the real world depends on the context (Mata et al., 2012).

RISKY DECISION MAKING

In contrast to the certain benefits and certain delays offered in the intertemporal choices described above, many decisions encountered in everyday life are associated with uncertain rewards. Before reviewing the existing findings on risky decision making, it is important to clarify some terminology. Uncertainty increases as the probability of obtaining a reward moves away from 0 (certainly not receiving the reward) or 1 (certainly receiving the reward) and is maximal at 0.5 (where there is an equal chance of receiving or not receiving the reward). Uncertainty is not the same as risk. Although psychologists and medical researchers and professionals often use the term "risk" to indicate that there is a non zero probability of something bad happening, we use the term "risk" here as it is used in finance and statistics—as the variance of potential outcomes regardless of whether they are gains or losses. Here we review studies on risky decision making that compare safe (no variance) options or less risky (lower variance) options with more risky (higher variance) options. While intertemporal decisions require the integration of potential benefits with the associated costs of waiting, risky decisions require the integration of potential benefits with the associated costs of uncertainty and risk. Risky decisions arguably require a higher level of integration than intertemporal decisions because the decision maker has to consider the *many* possible outcomes of each individual option when making a choice.

Recent studies have begun to examine adult age differences in choice among risky and safe options. There are strong societal stereotypes of older adults as being more risk averse than middle-aged or younger adults. However, stereotypes of risk aversion with age are not supported by results from well-controlled experimental tasks (Mather, 2006). Focusing on gambling tasks and risky investment decisions, a meta-analysis found no evidence for systematic adult age differences in risk taking (Mata, Josef, Samanez-Larkin, & Hertwig, 2011). Rather, the meta-analysis identified a subset of tasks in which older adults are more risk averse and other tasks in which older adults are more risk seeking than younger adults (Mata et al., 2011). It is important to note that in many of these tasks the expression of this "risk preference" is simply a deviation from the reward maximizing strategy in the task. That is, for many of the tasks, the reward maximizing strategy is either to be relatively risk seeking or relatively risk averse (and not risk neutral). Therefore, it is possible that what appear to be age differences in risk preferences are instead due to cognitive limitations (Henninger, Madden, & Huettel, 2010) in performing these tasks that require a higher level of information integration.

Very few brain imaging studies involving choices between low- and high-risk options have compared younger and older adults (Hosseini et al., 2010; Lee, Leung, Fox, Gao, & Chan, 2008; Samanez-Larkin et al., 2010). One study used an investment task that was designed to mimic financial decisions in everyday life by including a series of choices between small-stakes investments in risky stocks and safe bonds (Kuhnen & Knutson, 2005). To maximize earnings in the task, individuals need to learn from feedback on previous trials which assets are the most profitable. The task quantifies both mistakes choosing (risky) stocks and mistakes choosing (safe) bonds. In an adult life-span sample of young, middle-aged, and older adults, researchers found no age differences in risk aversion, but observed age differences in choosing risky stock options (Samanez-Larkin et al., 2010). The age differences were not due to excessive bond choices (which might indicate excessive risk aversion) but were due to both choosing stocks too early in a block or choosing suboptimal stock late in a block (see Figure 3). A parsimonious interpretation of these effects is that older adults are having more difficulty learning rapidly from feedback in this

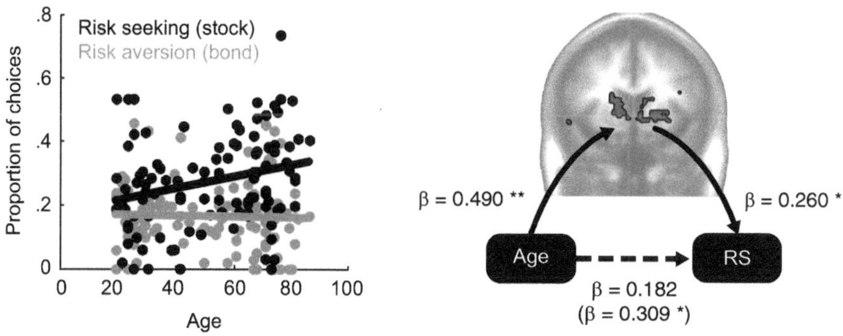

FIGURE 3 In a risky-decision task, older adults make more mistakes when choosing assets that are associated with risky rewards (selection of stocks), but do not differ from younger adults in risk aversion (selection of bonds). The behavioral age differences were associated with increased neural variability with age in the striatum (outlined gray areas overlaid on the brain are all voxels that exceeded $p < 0.0001$, uncorrected) and this neural measure of variability mediated the associations between age and risky stock (RS) mistakes. *Figure adapted from Samanez-Larkin et al. (2010).*

novel situation. This pattern of behavior replicated in two independent samples (Samanez-Larkin, Wagner, & Knutson, 2011b; Samanez-Larkin et al., 2010).

Consistent with neurocomputational theory suggesting that neuromodulatory cell-firing gets noisier with age (Li & Sikström, 2002; Li, Naveh-Benjamin, & Lindenberger, 2005), this age-related performance effect was mediated by a neural measure of functional variability in the ventral striatum (Samanez-Larkin et al., 2010) (see Figure 3). Neural activity variability increased with age in the midbrain and striatum, and the age effects in these two regions replicated in an independent study using a completely unrelated task that did not involve reward (Garrett, Kovacevic, McIntosh, & Grady, 2010). Note that the vast majority of functional brain imaging studies compare mean signal between task conditions of interest. Variability of the neural signal may be an important, overlooked individual difference measure relevant to understanding age differences in brain function (Garrett et al., 2013).

This research suggests that variability in forming representations of reward value that require integration of information in a novel environment may increase with age. Consistent with this, related evidence suggests that older adults have more difficulty estimating the value of ambiguous stimuli during reward-learning tasks (Eppinger & Kray, 2011) and are less sensitive to expected value (i.e., the mathematical product of potential outcome size and probability) when making risky decisions compared to younger adults (Weller, Levin, & Denburg, 2011). In sum, these findings suggest that what may appear to be age differences in risk preference may instead be differences in cognitive ability. In support of this conclusion, neuroimaging studies of risky decisions that are not dependent on rapid learning from recent experience show similar neural activation of prefrontal regions in younger and older adults (Hosseini et al., 2010). More recent studies, reviewed in the next section, have focused specifically on age differences in rapid learning-based decisions.

LEARNING

Learning to integrate prior feedback is often crucial for making optimal decisions. In contrast to the studies of basic reward processing, which suggest relative consistency across adulthood into old age, the literature on reward learning reveals consistent age-related declines in performance (Eppinger, Hämmerer, & Li, 2011). In many cases older adults learn more slowly than younger adults, although with enough experience they often reach the same performance asymptotes as younger adults (Hämmerer, Li, Müller, & Lindenberger, 2011; Samanez-Larkin, Worthy, Mata, McClure, & Knutson, 2014).

There has been a great deal of debate about age differences in sensitivity to positive and negative feedback in reward learning—so-called "valence effects." Some evidence suggests that older adults are more sensitive to positive than negative feedback compared to younger adults during learning (Denburg, Recknor, Bechara, & Tranel, 2006; Wood, Busemeyer, Koling, Cox, & Davis, 2005). Others have suggested the opposite—that older adults are relatively more sensitive to negative than positive feedback (Eppinger, Schuck, Nystrom, & Cohen, 2013; Hämmerer et al., 2011; Simon, Howard, & Howard, 2010a). If there is this shift toward negative-feedback sensitivity, it likely happens later in old age (Frank & Kong, 2008; Simon et al., 2010a). Yet other studies do not find evidence for age differences in valence effects during learning (Lighthall, Gorlick, Schoeke, Frank, & Mather, 2012; Samanez-Larkin et al., 2007, 2014). Across reward-learning tasks, the average effect reported is a main effect of age without an age by valence interaction (Eppinger et al., 2011). This is consistent with a meta-analysis showing the same lack of a consistent age difference in valence effects on decision tasks that are not learning dependent (Mata et al., 2011) in spite of limited findings and theory suggesting that there should be an age-related valence difference (Depping & Freund, 2011). Overall, age differences in reward-learning and decision-making tasks do not appear to be specifically due to the differential processing of gains or losses but are instead due to older adults' general difficulty with learning.

Neuroimaging studies have revealed that older adults compared to younger adults show reduced ventral striatal activation, especially during the early stages of learning (Mell et al., 2009), and reduced sensitivity of frontal cortical regions throughout learning (Eppinger, Kray, Mock, & Mecklinger, 2008; Eppinger et al., 2011; Hämmerer et al., 2011). Recent studies have extended these findings to show that these age differences may be due to older adults' difficulty with dynamically computing prediction errors in novel environments (Chowdhury et al., 2013; Eppinger et al., 2013). Supporting a dissociation between basic reward sensitivity and reward-based learning, striatal regions are similarly activated in younger and older adults during simple reward-based tasks that do not require novel learning, but these same regions in the same subjects show increased neural activity variability (Samanez-Larkin et al., 2010) and reduced representation of prediction errors (Samanez-Larkin et al., 2014) during tasks that require learning. How is it possible that the same striatal regions that seem to be functionally as active across late adulthood when processing basic rewards or making intertemporal choices also show functional irregularities in risky decision-making and learning tasks? One explanation may be that a broader neural network (as detailed in the opening summary of brain circuitry) is required for rapid, novel integration of information and lies at the source of the age differences during learning-based decision making.

A study explored this possibility by examining the structural connectivity of the frontostriatal circuit depicted in Figure 1 using diffusion tensor imaging in a group of younger, middle-aged, and older adults who had previously completed a probabilistic reward-learning task (Samanez-Larkin, Levens, Perry, Dougherty, & Knutson, 2012). Participants had to integrate recent feedback after each choice to learn which option would yield higher earnings. The results revealed that the structural integrity of pathways through the prefrontal cortex declined with age and was associated with individual differences in reward learning such that higher structural integrity was associated with better learning (Samanez-Larkin et al., 2012) (see Figure 4). The findings suggest

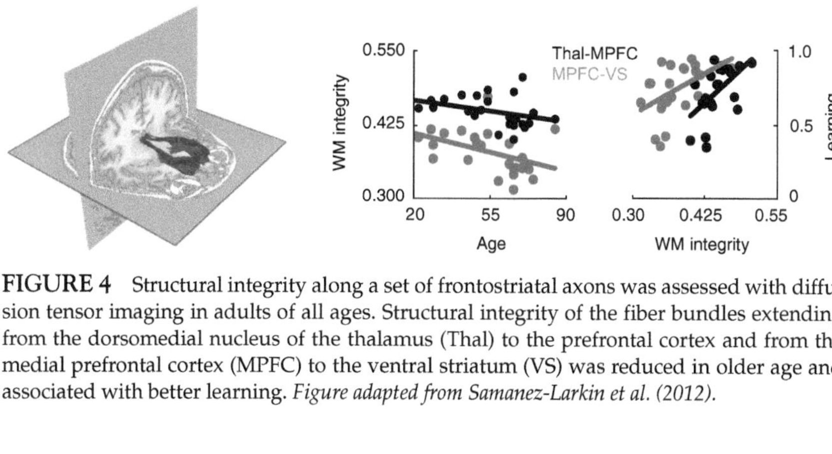

FIGURE 4 Structural integrity along a set of frontostriatal axons was assessed with diffusion tensor imaging in adults of all ages. Structural integrity of the fiber bundles extending from the dorsomedial nucleus of the thalamus (Thal) to the prefrontal cortex and from the medial prefrontal cortex (MPFC) to the ventral striatum (VS) was reduced in older age and associated with better learning. *Figure adapted from Samanez-Larkin et al. (2012).*

that the source of age-related striatal functional variability in the striatum observed in risky decision making (Samanez-Larkin et al., 2010) or the reduced representation of prediction errors in the medial prefrontal cortex and striatum (Chowdhury et al., 2013; Eppinger et al., 2013; Samanez-Larkin et al., 2014) may be the result of structural changes affecting communication across regions supporting reward learning. Interestingly, these pathways are very likely glutamatergic rather than dopaminergic.

Only two studies of which we are aware have examined adult age differences in functional connectivity between frontal and striatal regions during reward-based tasks. One study found no differences between healthy younger and older adults in functional connectivity between the midbrain and ventral striatum, midbrain and medial prefrontal cortex, or ventral striatum and medial prefrontal cortex, during a simple reward-processing task (Schott et al., 2007). Another study using a learning-based risky-decision task found reduced functional connectivity between the ventral striatum and medial prefrontal cortex in older age, but functional connectivity between these regions was not related to decision performance controlling for age (Samanez-Larkin et al., 2010). In the same study, higher functional connectivity between the ventral striatum and regions of the insula and ventrolateral prefrontal cortex were associated with better decision making but were not associated with age (Samanez-Larkin et al., 2010). Future studies should directly examine associations between structural and functional measures of connectivity and how each are related to reward processing and decision performance to clarify the effects of structural change on function across this network.

In summary, many of the age differences in decision making reviewed throughout this chapter may be closely related to age differences in learning (both over short and long histories of experiences). Arguably, most decisions made in everyday life are driven by predictions of reward based on previous experiences with a particular stimulus or action. Older adults may become more tolerant of delays when making intertemporal decisions partially due to accumulated experience with realizing rewards after delays—a result of a lifetime of learning that may have crystallized representations of delayed reward over time. In contrast, the increase in risky decision mistakes described above is likely due to the demands of the task that require rapid learning and integration of information in a novel environment—in which previous experience with risky rewards outside of the task does not confer any benefit. In both cases, understanding age differences in learning-based integration of information is critical. Future research should more directly assess the extent to which learning accounts for age differences in decision making (e.g., Eppinger & Bruckner, this volume).

CONCLUSIONS

Although some have claimed that basic motivational function may decline with age (Eppinger et al., 2012), this claim is inconsistent with decades of behavioral research on the psychology of aging (Carstensen, 2006; Carstensen, Mikels, & Mather, 2005; Charles & Carstensen, 2010) and a number of neuroscientific studies (Samanez-Larkin & Carstensen, 2011; Samanez-Larkin, 2011). As reviewed in this chapter, basic motivational processes (e.g., reward sensitivity) and associated brain function appear to remain relatively intact across much of adulthood and into old age (Samanez-Larkin & Carstensen, 2011; Samanez-Larkin, 2010). When decisions require the integration of information about benefits with costs, older adults are more tolerant of time delays in intertemporal decision tasks but make more mistakes in risky-decision tasks. Both of these diverging effects have been associated with age differences in striatal and prefrontal neural activity. Subcortical regions like the ventral striatum that appear functionally intact or even enhanced for reward tasks with relatively low cognitive demands show irregularities in decision tasks with higher cognitive demands for integration. Studies of network structure suggest that these specific decision impairments are related to broader circuit dysfunction in frontostriatal systems (Samanez-Larkin et al., 2012) that potentially extend beyond dopamine loss alone. When reward signals that are already well established are elicited (e.g., by the cueing of a potential $5 reward or a delayed reward), older adults perform better. When there is a demand for new learning about rewards that requires broader network interaction (e.g., in novel, learning-based risky decisions), older adults are impaired.

Overall, research on decision neuroscience and aging is still very much in its infancy and there are many unexplored topics. All of the primary studies reviewed here use secondary reinforcers, money or points, as the reward, and there are almost no studies examining age differences in other types of rewards (Jimura et al., 2011; Rademacher, Salama, Gründer, & Spreckelmeyer, 2014). Emerging studies suggest that there are overlooked age differences across reward types. For example, one study has recently shown that ventral striatal activity in older adults may be more sensitive to social rather than monetary rewards in older compared to younger adults (Rademacher et al., 2014). Emerging evidence also suggests that age differences in self-reported risk tolerance are highly variable across recreational, health, social, and financial domains (Rolison, Hanoch, Wood, & Liu, 2013). In addition to exploring reward type and domain generality or specificity, it would also be interesting to examine whether age differences in different types of decisions are related. For example, we are not aware of any published brain imaging studies that have compared decisions in the same subjects to examine whether, for example, tolerance of intertemporal delays is associated with tolerance of risk in old age, although some initial studies have been published with only younger adults (Peters & Büchel, 2009).

Relatedly, although many assumptions are made about the role of dopamine in age differences in decision making, almost no studies have collected direct measures of the dopamine system (or any other neurochemical system, for that matter). To fully test these hypotheses, positron emission tomography could be used to assess multiple aspects of neuromodulatory systems including receptors, transporters, and presynaptic markers and combined with functional magnetic resonance imaging to establish whether age differences observed in neural function are related to specific neurochemical change (Dreher, Meyer-Lindenberg, Kohn, & Berman, 2008). This work might help resolve competing hypotheses about whether the majority of age differences in decision making are due to simple loss of dopamine or broader changes in neurochemical systems across a wider network of brain regions.

Related to this last point, cognitive aging research has historically focused overwhelmingly on age-related declines in attention, memory, and cognitive control and corresponding lateral cortical and medial temporal brain systems (Buckner, 2004; Grady, 2008, 2012; Hedden & Gabrieli, 2004; West, 1996) rather than on the ventromedial frontostriatal systems reviewed here. Now that a number of studies have begun to characterize age differences in frontostriatal circuits as well, the next step will be to examine how changes in frontostriatal and fronto-medial-temporal networks might interact. Although one study suggests that working memory deficits may *not* be the primary source of age-related differences in learning and risky decision making (Samanez-Larkin et al., 2011b), this does not rule out other possible contributions from lateral cortical or medial temporal systems. For example, the age-related difficulty with information integration when making novel decisions suggests that the computation of new reward representations may be less distinct in older age (Li & Sikström, 2002), perhaps partially due to a difficulty with pattern separation in the hippocampus (Bizon & Gallagher, 2005; Clelland et al., 2009). Although not depicted in Figure 1, there are also prominent connections between the regions displayed and regions of lateral frontal cortex and the medial temporal lobes including the hippocampus (Haber & Knutson, 2010; Haber, 2003).

A final, important direction for future research will be to better establish links between performance on laboratory tasks and decision behavior in everyday life. Many assumptions are made because the tasks mimic everyday decisions and involve real (albeit quite small) monetary incentives, but almost no research has focused on validating these tasks. Nevertheless, there are some promising initial findings linking performance on some of the laboratory tasks reviewed above to measures of financial well-being in everyday life such as accumulated assets, avoidance of debt, debt-to-assets ratio, and credit scores (Knutson, Samanez-Larkin, & Kuhnen, 2011; Kuhnen, Samanez-Larkin, & Knutson, 2013; Samanez-Larkin et al., 2010). In general, though, there are currently very few studies that have directly examined adult age differences in monetary decision making in the real world (Agarwal, Driscoll, Gabaix, & Laibson, 2009; Korniotis & Kumar, 2011; Mata & Nunes, 2010). Future work should attempt to integrate laboratory measures, including brain imaging, with real world measures of decision making not only to better characterize changes in decision making across adulthood but also to facilitate translation from the laboratory to everyday life.

Acknowledgments

G.R.S.L. is supported by a Pathway to Independence Award (R00-AG042596) from the National Institute on Aging and was partially supported during the preparation of this chapter by the Scientific Research Network on Decision Neuroscience and Aging (R24-AG039350). Portions of this chapter were adapted from Samanez-Larkin, G.R. (2013) Financial Decision Making and the Aging Brain. *Observer* 26 (5), 30–33 and Samanez-Larkin, G.R., Knutson, B. (2014) Reward processing and risky decision making in the aging brain. In V. Reyna & V. Zayas (Eds.) *The Neuroscience of Risky Decision Making*. Washington DC: American Psychological Association, pp. 123–142. Thanks to Jennifer Bizon, Joseph McQuail, Todd Hagen, Daniel Weiner, and Eric Johnson for conversations and suggestions that helped shape this chapter.

References

Agarwal, S., Driscoll, J. C., Gabaix, X., & Laibson, D. I. (2009). The age of reason: financial decisions over the life-cycle with implications for regulation. *Brookings Papers on Economic Activity, 40*(2), 51–117.

Alexander, G. E., Crutcher, M. D., & DeLong, M. R. (1990). Basal ganglia-thalamocortical circuits: parallel substrates for motor, oculomotor, "prefrontal" and "limbic" functions. *Progress in Brain Research, 85*, 119–146.

Alexander, G. E., DeLong, M. R., & Strick, P. L. (1986). Parallel organization of functionally segregated circuits linking basal ganglia and cortex. *Annual Review of Neuroscience, 9*, 357–381. http://dx.doi.org/10.1146/annurev.ne.09.030186.002041.

Berridge, K. C. (2012). From prediction error to incentive salience: mesolimbic computation of reward motivation. *The European Journal of Neuroscience, 35*(7), 1124–1143. http://dx.doi.org/10.1111/j.1460-9568.2012.07990.x.

Bizon, J. L., & Gallagher, M. (2005). More is less: neurogenesis and age-related cognitive decline in Long-Evans rats. *Science of Aging Knowledge Environment: SAGE KE, 2005*(7), re2. http://dx.doi.org/10.1126/sageke.2005.7.re2.

Braver, T. S., & Barch, D. M. (2002). A theory of cognitive control, aging cognition, and neuromodulation. *Neuroscience and Biobehavioral Reviews, 26*(7), 809–817.

Buckner, R. L. (2004). Memory and executive function in aging and AD: multiple factors that cause decline and reserve factors that compensate. *Neuron, 44*(1), 195–208. http://dx.doi.org/10.1016/j.neuron.2004.09.006.

Carstensen, L. L. (2006). The influence of a sense of time on human development. *Science, 312*(5782), 1913–1915. http://dx.doi.org/10.1126/science.1127488.

Carstensen, L. L., & Mikels, J. A. (2005). At the intersection of emotion and cognition: aging and the positivity effect. *Current Directions in Psychological Science, 14*(3), 117–121.

Carstensen, L. L., Mikels, J. A., & Mather, M. (2005). Aging and the intersection of cognition, motivation and emotion. In J. E. Birren & K. W. Schaie (Eds.), *Handbook of the psychology of aging* (6th ed.). Academic Press.

Carstensen, L. L., Pasupathi, M., Mayr, U., & Nesselroade, J. R. (2000). Emotional experience in everyday life across the adult life span. *Journal of Personality and Social Psychology, 79*(4), 644–655.

Charles, S. T., & Carstensen, L. L. (2010). Social and emotional aging. *Annual Review of Psychology, 61*, 383–409. http://dx.doi.org/10.1146/annurev.psych.093008.100448.

Chowdhury, R., Guitart-Masip, M., Lambert, C., Dayan, P., Huys, Q., Düzel, E., et al. (2013). Dopamine restores reward prediction errors in old age. *Nature Neuroscience, 16*(5), 648–653. http://dx.doi.org/10.1038/nn.3364.

Clelland, C. D., Choi, M., Romberg, C., Clemenson, G. D., Fragniere, A., Tyers, P., et al. (2009). A functional role for adult hippocampal neurogenesis in spatial pattern separation. *Science, 325*(5937), 210–213. http://dx.doi.org/10.1126/science.1173215.

Cox, K. M., Aizenstein, H. J., & Fiez, J. A. (2008). Striatal outcome processing in healthy aging. *Cognitive, Affective, & Behavioral Neuroscience, 8*(3), 304–317.

Denburg, N. L., Recknor, E. C., Bechara, A., & Tranel, D. (2006). Psychophysiological anticipation of positive outcomes promotes advantageous decision-making in normal older persons. *International Journal of Psychophysiology, 61*(1), 19–25. http://dx.doi.org/10.1016/j.ijpsycho.2005.10.021.

Depping, M. K., & Freund, A. M. (2011). Normal aging and decision making: The role of motivation. *Human Development, 54*(6), 349–367. http://dx.doi.org/10.1159/000334396.

Dreher, J.-C., Meyer-Lindenberg, A., Kohn, P., & Berman, K. F. (2008). Age-related changes in midbrain dopaminergic regulation of the human reward system. *Proceedings of the National Academy of Sciences of the United States of America, 105*(39), 15106–15111. http://dx.doi.org/10.1073/pnas.0802127105.

Eppinger, B., Hämmerer, D., & Li, S.-C. (2011). Neuromodulation of reward-based learning and decision making in human aging. *Annals of the New York Academy of Sciences, 1235*(1), 1–17. http://dx.doi.org/10.1111/j.1749-6632.2011.06230.x.

Eppinger, B., & Kray, J. (2011). To choose or to avoid: age differences in learning from positive and negative feedback. *Journal of Cognitive Neuroscience, 23*(1), 41–52. http://dx.doi.org/10.1162/jocn.2009.21364.

Eppinger, B., Kray, J., Mock, B., & Mecklinger, A. (2008). Better or worse than expected? Aging, learning, and the ERN. *Neuropsychologia, 46*(2), 521–539. http://dx.doi.org/10.1016/j.neuropsychologia.2007.09.001.

Eppinger, B., Nystrom, L. E., & Cohen, J. D. (2012). Reduced sensitivity to immediate reward during decision-making in older than younger adults. *PloS One, 7*(5), e36953. http://dx.doi.org/10.1371/journal.pone.0036953.g005.

Eppinger, B., Schuck, N. W., Nystrom, L. E., & Cohen, J. D. (2013). Reduced striatal responses to reward prediction errors in older compared with younger adults. *The Journal of Neuroscience, 33*(24), 9905–9912. http://dx.doi.org/10.1523/JNEUROSCI.2942-12.2013.

Frank, M. J., & Kong, L. (2008). Learning to avoid in older age. *Psychology and Aging, 23*(2), 392–398. http://dx.doi.org/10.1037/0882-7974.23.2.392.

Garrett, D. D., Kovacevic, N., McIntosh, A. R., & Grady, C. L. (2010). Blood oxygen level-dependent signal variability is more than just noise. *The Journal of Neuroscience, 30*(14), 4914–4921. http://dx.doi.org/10.1523/JNEUROSCI.5166-09.2010.

Garrett, D. D., Samanez-Larkin, G. R., MacDonald, S. W. S., Lindenberger, U., McIntosh, A. R., & Grady, C. L. (2013). Moment-to-moment brain signal variability: a next frontier in human brain mapping? *Neuroscience and Biobehavioral Reviews, 37*(4), 610–624. http://dx.doi.org/10.1016/j.neubiorev.2013.02.015.

Gilbert, R. J., Mitchell, M. R., Simon, N. W., Bañuelos, C., Setlow, B., & Bizon, J. L. (2011). Risk, reward, and decision-making in a rodent model of cognitive aging. *Frontiers in Neuroscience, 5*, 144. http://dx.doi.org/10.3389/fnins.2011.00144.

Glimcher, P. W. (2011). Understanding dopamine and reinforcement learning: The dopamine reward prediction error hypothesis. *Proceedings of the National Academy of Sciences of the United States of America, 108*(Suppl. 3), 15647–15654. http://dx.doi.org/10.1073/pnas.1014269108.

Grady, C. (2012). The cognitive neuroscience of ageing. *Nature Reviews Neuroscience, 13*(7), 491–505. http://dx.doi.org/10.1038/nrn3256.

Grady, C. L. (2008). Cognitive neuroscience of aging. *Annals of the New York Academy of Sciences, 1124*, 127–144. http://dx.doi.org/10.1196/annals.1440.009.

Haber, S. N. (2003). The primate basal ganglia: Parallel and integrative networks. *Journal of Chemical Neuroanatomy, 26*(4), 317–330.

Haber, S. N., & Knutson, B. (2010). The reward circuit: linking primate anatomy and human imaging. *Neuropsychopharmacology: Official Publication of the American College of Neuropsychopharmacology, 35*(1), 4–26. http://dx.doi.org/10.1038/npp.2009.129.

Hämmerer, D., Li, S.-C., Müller, V., & Lindenberger, U. (2011). Life span differences in electrophysiological correlates of monitoring gains and losses during probabilistic reinforcement learning. *Journal of Cognitive Neuroscience, 23*(3), 579–592. http://dx.doi.org/10.1162/jocn.2010.21475.

Hedden, T., & Gabrieli, J. D. E. (2004). Insights into the ageing mind: A view from cognitive neuroscience. *Nature Reviews Neuroscience, 5*(2), 87–96. http://dx.doi.org/10.1038/nrn1323.

Henninger, D. E., Madden, D. J., & Huettel, S. A. (2010). Processing speed and memory mediate age-related differences in decision making. *Psychology and Aging, 25*(2), 262–270. http://dx.doi.org/10.1037/a0019096.

Hosseini, S. M. H., Rostami, M., Yomogida, Y., Takahashi, M., Tsukiura, T., & Kawashima, R. (2010). Aging and decision making under uncertainty: behavioral and neural evidence for the preservation of decision making in the absence of learning in old age. *NeuroImage, 52*(4), 1514–1520. http://dx.doi.org/10.1016/j.neuroimage.2010.05.008.

Jimura, K., Myerson, J., Hilgard, J., Keighley, J., Braver, T. S., & Green, L. (2011). Domain independence and stability in young and older adults' discounting of delayed rewards. *Behavioural Processes, 87*(3), 253–259. http://dx.doi.org/10.1016/j.beproc.2011.04.006.

Knutson, B., Adams, C. M., Fong, G. W., & Hommer, D. (2001). Anticipation of increasing monetary reward selectively recruits nucleus accumbens. *The Journal of Neuroscience, 21*(RC159), 1–5.

Knutson, B., Samanez-Larkin, G. R., & Kuhnen, C. M. (2011). Gain and loss learning differentially contribute to life financial outcomes. *PloS One, 6*(9), e24390. http://dx.doi.org/10.1371/journal.pone.0024390.

Korniotis, G. M., & Kumar, A. (2011). Do older investors make better investment decisions? *The Review of Economics and Statistics, 93*(1), 244–265. http://dx.doi.org/10.1162/REST_a_00053.

Kuhnen, C. M., & Knutson, B. (2005). The neural basis of financial risk taking. *Neuron, 47*(5), 763–770. http://dx.doi.org/10.1016/j.neuron.2005.08.008.

Kuhnen, C. M., Samanez-Larkin, G. R., & Knutson, B. (2013). Serotonergic genotypes, neuroticism, and financial choices. *PloS One, 8*(1), e54632. http://dx.doi.org/10.1371/journal.pone.0054632.

Lee, T. M. C., Leung, A. W. S., Fox, P. T., Gao, J.-H., & Chan, C. C. H. (2008). Age-related differences in neural activities during risk taking as revealed by functional MRI. *Social Cognitive and Affective Neuroscience, 3*(1), 7–15. http://dx.doi.org/10.1093/scan/nsm033.

Li, S.-C., & Sikström, S. (2002). Integrative neurocomputational perspectives on cognitive aging, neuromodulation, and representation. *Neuroscience and Biobehavioral Reviews, 26*(7), 795–808.

Li, S.-C., Lindenberger, U., & Bäckman, L. (2010). Dopaminergic modulation of cognition across the life span. *Neuroscience and Biobehavioral Reviews*, *34*(5), 625–630. http://dx.doi.org/10.1016/j.neubiorev.2010.02.003.

Li, S.-C., Naveh-Benjamin, M., & Lindenberger, U. (2005). Aging neuromodulation impairs associative binding: A neurocomputational account. *Psychological Science*, *16*(6), 445–450. http://dx.doi.org/10.1111/j.0956-7976.2005.01555.x.

Li, Y., Baldassi, M., Johnson, E. J., & Weber, E. U. (2013). Complementary cognitive capabilities, economic decision making, and aging. *Psychology and Aging*, *28*(3), 595–613. http://dx.doi.org/10.1037/a0034172.

Lighthall, N. R., Gorlick, M. A., Schoeke, A., Frank, M. J., & Mather, M. (2012). Stress modulates reinforcement learning in younger and older adults. *Psychology and Aging*, *28*(1), 35–46. http://dx.doi.org/10.1037/a0029823.

Löckenhoff, C. E. (2011). Age, time, and decision making: From processing speed to global time horizons. *Annals of the New York Academy of Sciences*, *1235*(1), 44–56. http://dx.doi.org/10.1111/j.1749-6632.2011.06209.x.

Mata, R., Josef, A. K., Samanez-Larkin, G. R., & Hertwig, R. (2011). Age differences in risky choice: A meta-analysis. *Annals of the New York Academy of Sciences*, *1235*(1), 18–29. http://dx.doi.org/10.1111/j.1749-6632.2011.06200.x.

Mata, R., & Nunes, L. (2010). When less is enough: Cognitive aging, information search, and decision quality in consumer choice. *Psychology and Aging*, *25*(2), 289–298. http://dx.doi.org/10.1037/a0017927.

Mata, R., Pachur, T., Helversen, von, B., Hertwig, R., Rieskamp, J., & Schooler, L. (2012). Ecological rationality: A framework for understanding and aiding the aging decision maker. *Frontiers in Neuroscience*, *6*, 19. http://dx.doi.org/10.3389/fnins.2012.00019.

Mather, M. (2006). A review of decision-making processes: Weighing the risks and benefits of aging. *When I'm 64*, 145–173.

Mather, M., & Carstensen, L. L. (2005). Aging and motivated cognition: The positivity effect in attention and memory. *Trends in Cognitive Sciences*, *9*(10), 496–502. http://dx.doi.org/10.1016/j.tics.2005.08.005.

Mell, T., Wartenburger, I., Marschner, A., Villringer, A., Reischies, F. M., & Heekeren, H. R. (2009). Altered function of ventral striatum during reward-based decision making in old age. *Frontiers in Human Neuroscience*, *3*, 34. http://dx.doi.org/10.3389/neuro.09.034.2009.

Mora, F., Segovia, G., & Del Arco, A. (2007). Glutamate-dopamine-GABA interactions in the aging basal ganglia. *Brain Research Reviews*, *58*(2), 340–353. http://dx.doi.org/10.1016/j.brainresrev.2007.10.006.

Nielsen, L., Knutson, B., & Carstensen, L. L. (2008). Affect dynamics, affective forecasting, and aging. *Emotion*, *8*(3), 318–330. http://dx.doi.org/10.1037/1528-3542.8.3.318.

Peters, J., & Büchel, C. (2009). Overlapping and distinct neural systems code for subjective value during intertemporal and risky decision making. *The Journal of Neuroscience*, *29*(50), 15727–15734. http://dx.doi.org/10.1523/JNEUROSCI.3489-09.2009.

Peters, J., & Büchel, C. (2011). The neural mechanisms of inter-temporal decision-making: Understanding variability. *Trends in Cognitive Sciences*, *15*(5), 227–239. http://dx.doi.org/10.1016/j.tics.2011.03.002.

Phillips, P. E. M., Walton, M. E., & Jhou, T. C. (2006). Calculating utility: Preclinical evidence for cost–benefit analysis by mesolimbic dopamine. *Psychopharmacology*, *191*(3), 483–495. http://dx.doi.org/10.1007/s00213-006-0626-6.

Rademacher, L., Salama, A., Gründer, G., & Spreckelmeyer, K. N. (2014). Differential patterns of nucleus accumbens activation during anticipation of monetary and social reward in young and older adults. *Social Cognitive and Affective Neuroscience*, *9*(6), 825–831. http://dx.doi.org/10.1093/scan/nst047.

Raz, N. (2005). The aging brain observed in vivo: Differential changes and their modifiers. In R. Cabeza, L. Nyberg, & D. Park (Eds.), *Cognitive neuroscience of aging: Linking cognitive and cerebral aging* (pp. 19–57). New York, NY: Oxford University Press.

Raz, N., Rodrigue, K. M., & Haacke, E. M. (2007). Brain aging and its modifiers: Insights from in vivo neuromorphometry and susceptibility weighted imaging. *Annals of the New York Academy of Sciences, 1097*, 84–93. http://dx.doi.org/10.1196/annals.1379.018.

Roesch, M. R., Bryden, D. W., Cerri, D. H., Haney, Z. R., & Schoenbaum, G. (2012a). Willingness to wait and altered encoding of time-discounted reward in the orbitofrontal cortex with normal aging. *The Journal of Neuroscience, 32*(16), 5525–5533. http://dx.doi.org/10.1523/JNEUROSCI.0586-12.2012.

Roesch, M. R., Esber, G. R., Bryden, D. W., Cerri, D. H., Haney, Z. R., & Schoenbaum, G. (2012b). Normal aging alters learning and attention-related teaching signals in basolateral amygdala. *The Journal of Neuroscience, 32*(38), 13137–13144. http://dx.doi.org/10.1523/JNEUROSCI.2393-12.2012.

Rolison, J. J., Hanoch, Y., Wood, S., & Liu, P.-J. (2013). Risk-taking differences across the adult life span: A question of age and domain. *The Journals of Gerontology Series B: Psychological Sciences and Social Sciences, 69*(6), 870–880. http://dx.doi.org/10.1093/geronb/gbt081.

Samanez-Larkin, G. R. (April 22, 2010). In B. Knutson & L. L. Carstensen (Eds.), *Incentive processing in the aging brain*. Stanford University. Retrieved from http://purl.stanford.edu/vy834vv5149.

Samanez-Larkin, G. R. (2011). *Decision making over the life span*. New York: Wiley-Blackwell.

Samanez-Larkin, G. R., & Carstensen, L. L. (2011). Socioemotional functioning and the aging brain. In J. Decety & J. T. Cacioppo (Eds.), *The handbook of social neuroscience* (pp. 507–521). New York: Oxford University Press.

Samanez-Larkin, G. R., & Knutson, B. (2014). Reward processing and risky decision making in the aging brain. In V. F. Reyna & V. Zayas (Eds.), *The neuroscience of risky decision making* (pp. 123–142). Washington DC: American Psychological Association.

Samanez-Larkin, G. R., Wagner, A. D., & Knutson, B. (2011b). Expected value information improves financial risk taking across the adult life span. *Social Cognitive and Affective Neuroscience, 6*(2), 207–217. http://dx.doi.org/10.1093/scan/nsq043.

Samanez-Larkin, G. R., Gibbs, S. E. B., Khanna, K., Nielsen, L., Carstensen, L. L., & Knutson, B. (2007). Anticipation of monetary gain but not loss in healthy older adults. *Nature Neuroscience, 10*(6), 787–791. http://dx.doi.org/10.1038/nn1894.

Samanez-Larkin, G. R., Kuhnen, C. M., Yoo, D. J., & Knutson, B. (2010). Variability in nucleus accumbens activity mediates age-related suboptimal financial risk taking. *The Journal of Neuroscience, 30*(4), 1426–1434. http://dx.doi.org/10.1523/JNEUROSCI.4902-09.2010.

Samanez-Larkin, G. R., Mata, R., Radu, P. T., Ballard, I. C., Carstensen, L. L., & McClure, S. M. (2011a). Age differences in striatal delay sensitivity during intertemporal choice in healthy adults. *Frontiers in Neuroscience, 5*, 126. http://dx.doi.org/10.3389/fnins.2011.00126.

Samanez-Larkin, G. R., Levens, S. M., Perry, L. M., Dougherty, R. F., & Knutson, B. (2012). Frontostriatal white matter integrity mediates adult age differences in probabilistic reward learning. *The Journal of Neuroscience, 32*(15), 5333–5337. http://dx.doi.org/10.1523/JNEUROSCI.5756-11.2012.

Samanez-Larkin, G. R., Worthy, D. A., Mata, R., McClure, S. M., & Knutson, B. (2014). Adult age differences in frontostriatal representation of prediction error but not reward outcome. *Cognitive, Affective, & Behavioral Neuroscience, 14*(2), 672–682. http://dx.doi.org/10.3758/s13415-014-0297-4.

Schott, B. H., Niehaus, L., Wittmann, B. C., Schütze, H., Seidenbecher, C. I., Heinze, H.-J., et al. (2007). Ageing and early-stage Parkinson's disease affect separable neural mechanisms of mesolimbic reward processing. *Brain, 130*(Pt 9), 2412–2424. http://dx.doi.org/10.1093/brain/awm147.

Simon, J. R., Howard, J. H., & Howard, D. V. (2010a). Adult age differences in learning from positive and negative probabilistic feedback. *Neuropsychology, 24*(4), 534–541. http://dx.doi.org/10.1037/a0018652.

Simon, N. W., Lasarge, C. L., Montgomery, K. S., Williams, M. T., Mendez, I. A., Setlow, B., et al. (2010b). Good things come to those who wait: Attenuated discounting of delayed rewards in aged Fischer 344 rats. *Neurobiology of Aging*, *31*(5), 853–862. http://dx.doi.org/10.1016/j.neurobiolaging.2008.06.004.

Weller, J. A., Levin, I. P., & Denburg, N. L. (2011). Trajectory of risky decision making for potential gains and losses from ages 5 to 85. *Journal of Behavioral Decision Making*, *24*(4), 331–344. http://dx.doi.org/10.1002/bdm.690.

West, R. L. (1996). An application of prefrontal cortex function theory to cognitive aging. *Psychological Bulletin*, *120*(2), 272–292.

Williams, T. H., & Jew, J. Y. (1997). *The human brain*. Retrieved from http://web.archive.org/web/20050401051631/http://www.vh.org/adult/provider/anatomy/BrainAnatomy/BrainAnatomy.html.

Wise, R. A. (1980). The dopamine synapse and the notion of "pleasure centers" in the brain. *Trends in Neurosciences*, *3*(4), 91–95. http://dx.doi.org/10.1016/0166-2236(80)90035-1.

Wise, R. A. (2004). Dopamine, learning and motivation. *Nature Reviews Neuroscience*, *5*(6), 483–494. http://dx.doi.org/10.1038/nrn1406.

Wood, S., Busemeyer, J., Koling, A., Cox, C. R., & Davis, H. (2005). Older adults as adaptive decision makers: Evidence from the Iowa gambling task. *Psychology and Aging*, *20*(2), 220–225. http://dx.doi.org/10.1037/0882-7974.20.2.220.

Wu, C. C., Samanez-Larkin, G. R., Katovich, K., & Knutson, B. (2014). Affective traits link to reliable neural markers of incentive anticipation. *NeuroImage*, *84*(1), 279–289. http://dx.doi.org/10.1016/j.neuroimage.2013.08.055.

CHAPTER

4

Towards a Mechanistic Understanding of Age-Related Changes in Learning and Decision Making: A Neuro-Computational Approach

Ben Eppinger[1], *Rasmus Bruckner*[2]

[1]Department of Psychology, Technische Universität Dresden, Germany; [2]Department of Psychology, Humboldt-Universität zu Berlin, Germany

Many of our decisions involve uncertainty about the potential outcomes of choices. In some of these situations the probabilities of outcomes are known (or approximated), such as in medical decisions about treatment options (e.g., cancer therapy). In other situations outcome probabilities are unknown and we have to learn about the likelihood with which a certain action leads to a desired outcome. Such situations may involve high-level financial decisions such as investments in stocks or bonds, but they also apply to decisions during grocery shopping when having to choose between different varieties of apples.

Stereotypes about older adults suggest that they might be more risk avoidant and conservative decision makers than younger adults (for a review see Mather, 2006; Mather et al., 2012). Such behavior might be adaptive in situations in which the decision context favors risk-avoidant choices, but may lead to suboptimal decisions in situations that favor risky choice. Recent theoretical ideas suggest that decision making deficits may become obvious once age-related decline in fluid cognitive functions (e.g., processing speed or reasoning abilities) offsets relative increase or stability in more crystalized abilities (learned or acculturated knowledge) (Agarwal, Driscoll, Gabaix, & Laibson, 2009; Samanez-Larkin, 2013).

http://dx.doi.org/10.1016/B978-0-12-417148-0.00004-2

Results from empirical studies on age differences in decision making under uncertainty show mixed results regarding age-related changes in risky-choice behavior. Some studies report age-related deficits in decision making, whereas others found no significant differences between younger and older adults (Mata, Josef, Samanez-Larkin, & Hertwig, 2011; Mather et al., 2012). Current meta-analytic data point to a dissociation between studies that focus on explicitly stated probabilities and studies in which the outcome of an option has to be learned (Mata et al., 2011). That is, the current literature suggests that age-related deficits in decision making under uncertainty are primarily due to impairments in learning probabilistic reward structures.

Building on this dissociation, in the current chapter we will concentrate on the psychological and neurophysiological underpinnings of age-related deficits in decision making tasks in which the expected value of choice options has to be learned. We will outline the relationship between age-related changes in the dopamine (DA) system as well as functional changes in subcortical and prefrontal networks involved in making decisions from experience. Furthermore, we will focus on potential links between neuro-computational theories of reinforcement learning and age-related deficits in experience-driven decision making. Finally, we will conclude with a summary of the current research, identify gaps that need to be filled in the future, and provide evidence for potential targets for interventions that aim at improving learning and decision making abilities in old age.

AGE-RELATED DECLINE IN THE DOPAMINE SYSTEM

We start the chapter with a brief review of age-related changes in the dopamine system and their impact on learning and decision making functions in older adults. Age-related changes in the dopamine system have been observed across various areas in the brain. For example, positron emission tomography (PET) and single-photon emission computed tomography studies suggest that aging is associated with a decline in pre- and postsynaptic markers of DA D1, and D2 receptor density is reduced in older compared to younger adults. Age-related reductions in D1 receptor density (about 7% per decade) have been reported in the basal ganglia (caudate nucleus and putamen) (Bäckman et al., 2009; MacDonald, Karlsson, Rieckmann, Nyberg, & Bäckmann, 2012; Wang et al., 1998). Similar findings have been reported for D2 receptor density in the striatum (Volkow et al., 2000; Volkow, Wang, et al., 1998) and the prefrontal cortex (Volkow et al., 2000). Moreover, there is evidence for an association between age-related decline in D2 receptors in the prefrontal cortex and metabolism in the prefrontal and cingulate cortex as well as correlations between D2 receptor decline and performance deficits in the measures of executive control (the Wisconsin Card Sort Test) (Volkow, Gur, et al., 1998; Volkow et al., 2000). Presynaptic markers of DA function also show substantial decline with age. The binding potential for the DA transporter in the striatum is significantly lower in older than younger adults (Erixon-Lindroth et al., 2005; Troiano et al., 2010; Wong, Müller, Kuwabara, Studenski, & Bohnen, 2012). Although these results point to a substantial negative relationship between age and DA function, it should be noted that so far, there are no longitudinal assessments of age-related changes in DA neurotransmission. Therefore, we lack precise estimates and a detailed understanding of age-related change in pre- and postsynaptic measures of the DA system as well as the relation between baseline DA levels, age-related change, and individual differences in cognitive performance. Furthermore, so far it has not been established whether different aspects of the DA system are differentially affected by age.

Effects of Age-Related Dopamine Decline on Cognitive Function

Age-related decline in DA function has been associated with deficits in various cognitive abilities (Braver & Barch, 2002; Bäckman, Lindenberger, Li, & Nyberg, 2010; Li, Lindenberger, & Sikström, 2001). In particular, studies point to an association between decline in D1 receptor density in the striatum and working memory (WM) (Braskie et al., 2008; Bäckman et al., 2009). This finding is consistent with theoretical ideas that suggest that deficits in the updating of WM representations in older adults are due to reduced phasic DA responses that are projected to the prefrontal cortex (Braver & Barch, 2002; Braver et al., 2001). The so-called gating theory suggests that midbrain DA signals regulate the access of new information to WM (Braver & Cohen, 2000). More specifically, the theory holds that DA prediction error (Pe) signals are used to learn when the WM gate should be opened in order to allow new information to access WM and to guide behavior. Consistent with the theory, results of a behavioral study point to specific deficits in older adults when they have to update WM context representations (Braver et al., 2001). These deficits may result from reduced dopaminergic Pe signaling during WM gating in the dorsolateral prefrontal cortex. Results from a PET study on WM training in younger adults show that WM updating training induces transient DA release in the striatum, which seems in line with the predictions of the gating theory (Bäckman et al., 2011). To summarize, based on these findings it is tempting to assume that reductions in DA phasic signaling with age lead to a deficient updating of WM representations and by this affect multiple cognitive operations in older adults that rely on short-term storage and updating of information.

Effects of Age-Related Dopamine Decline on Learning and Decision Making from Experience

Compared to associations between DA and cognitive measures, relationships between age differences in motivational functions such as reward-based learning and decision making and DA are less well established. This is somewhat surprising, given the rapid progress of research on the involvement of the DA system in reward processing, reinforcement learning, and decision making in younger adults. Moreover, in contrast to cognitive functions, there are relatively detailed mechanistic models of the role of DA (and other neurotransmitters such as norepinephrine) in reinforcement learning and decision making (Aston-Jones & Cohen, 2005; Montague, Hyman, & Cohen, 2004). One advantage of these neuro-computational theories is that they allow us to be more specific regarding age-related changes in the underlying neural mechanisms. For example, reductions in phasic dopaminergic learning signals from the ventral tegmental area should lead to deficits in the updating of reward value representations and to behavioral impairments in reinforcement learning (Eppinger, Haemmerer, & Li, 2011; Nieuwenhuis et al., 2002). Empirical findings support these results, showing age-related behavioral deficits in reinforcement learning, reduced learning effects in reward-related evoked potential (ERP) components in older adults, reduced prediction error signals in the ventral striatum in the elderly as well as alterations in the structural integrity of the midbrain (Chowdhury, Guitart-Masip, Lambert, Dolan, & Düzel, 2013; Chowdury et al., 2013; Eppinger, Kray, Mock, & Mecklinger, 2008; Eppinger, Schuck, Nystrom, & Cohen, 2013; Samanez-Larkin, Levens, Perry, Dougherty, & Knutson, 2012; Schott et al., 2007). Moreover, a combined PET and neuroimaging (fMRI) study in younger and older adults showed age-related changes in the relationship between midbrain DA synthesis and reward-related fMRI activity (Dreher, Meyer-Lindenberg, Kohn, & Berman, 2008).

Work on the direct relationship between age-related changes in DA neuromodulation and age differences in decision making is scarce. However, findings in younger adults revealed an association between reduced DA D2 autoreceptor availability in the midbrain, increased stimulated DA release in the ventral striatum, and enhanced trait impulsivity (Buckholtz et al., 2010). That is, these findings suggest that in younger adults, enhanced DA release in the ventral striatum (as induced by amphetamine) is associated with greater impulsivity. Based on these findings it could be argued that reduced DA release in the ventral striatum in older adults may result in less impulsive behavior (Eppinger, Nystrom, & Cohen, 2012).

There are many open questions in this emerging field of research. For example, it is unclear how aging affects tonic versus phasic activity modes of DA (and their interaction) and what the implications of these effects are for learning and decision making. Another issue that merits further research is the relationship between age-related changes in variability of DA activity and age-related deficits in learning and decision making (Garrett et al., 2013). For example, findings by Samanez-Larkin and colleagues (2010) indicate that suboptimal financial decision making in older adults is associated with increases in variability of fMRI activity in the ventral striatum. A more general question that emerges from this work is whether aging may lead to greater decision noise, that is, unstructured variance in choices and preferences in older adults, and whether these effects are reflected in increased intra-individual variability of neurophysiological measures (Li et al., 2001).

Taken together, there is strong evidence for age-related changes in different aspects of the DA system. These age differences in DA neuromodulation seem to have profound effects on many cognitive and motivational functions. The ubiquity of these effects has lead to some degree of frustration among researchers, and to the notion that DA may be involved in almost every cognitive and motivational function. However, it should be noted that many previous approaches lacked a precise theory of the mechanism by which DA affects specific cognitive or motivational processes. Recent progress in computational approaches and combinations of modeling and neuroimaging techniques will allow us to move on and develop mechanistic rather than descriptive theories of age-related changes in cognitive and motivational functions.

AGE DIFFERENCES IN LEARNING FROM EXPERIENCE

As outlined nicely by Mata et al. (2011), age-related impairments in decisions from experience might result from an underlying deficit in learning the expected value of decision options. The purpose of the following paragraphs is to provide a link between age differences in decisions from experience and age-related changes in neurophysiological mechanisms of reinforcement learning. For the purpose of this chapter we will primarily focus on age differences in learning from uncertain (probabilistic) reward information as well as age-related changes in the neural systems involved in learning from experience. We will also visit the field of computational neuroscience to examine mechanistic ideas about age-related changes in learning and decision making from experience.

Findings from electrophysiological ERP studies suggest that older adults are impaired in learning from uncertain (probabilistic) reward, whereas age-related learning impairments are less pronounced when reward is deterministic (reward information is always reliable) (Eppinger et al., 2008; Pietschmann, Endrass, Czerwon, & Kathmann, 2011). Learning impairments in older adults are associated with deficits in error detection, as indicated by a reduced error-related negativity, an ERP component that is elicited by erroneous responses (Eppinger & Kray, 2011; Eppinger et al., 2008; Herbert, Eppinger, & Kray, 2011; Pietschmann et al., 2011). Furthermore, older adults show less differentiated ERP responses to positive and negative feedback during learning, indicating that they have difficulties in representing valence information (Eppinger et al., 2008; Herbert et al., 2011). Taken together, these findings suggest that older adults may have deficits in learning the expected value of reward if contingencies between states, actions, and rewards are probabilistic (Eppinger et al., 2011; Hämmerer & Eppinger, 2012).

Recent findings from fMRI studies show that these learning impairments might be due to age differences in dopaminergic teaching signals that are projected from the midbrain (ventral tegmental area and substantia nigra) to the ventral striatum and ventromedial prefrontal cortex (vmPFC) (Chowdury et al., 2013; Eppinger, Schuck, et al., 2013; Samanez-Larkin, Worthy, Mata, McClure, & Knutson, 2014). These learning signals reflect discrepancies between actual and expected outcomes (prediction errors) and can be captured using reinforcement learning models (Niv & Schoenbaum, 2008). In environments that involve a continuous updating of predictions about the expected value of a stimulus or action, these models use the temporal difference (TD) learning algorithm to formalize learning (Sutton & Barto, 1998).

Temporal Difference Learning

The core idea of TD learning is that, during learning, the expected value of a stimulus or state is continuously updated as a function of the difference between the sum of the current reward and the future value prediction minus the current value prediction (see Figure 1 and Eqn (1)). For example during grocery shopping one might encounter a new product (for example, a new variety of apples). Before eating the apple, the prediction regarding the taste might be neutral or slightly positive (otherwise one would not have bought it). Assume that the apple tastes extraordinarily good. That is, the taste is better than predicted. This should be reflected in a strong positive Pe (see Figure 1). However, one moment later you might realize that the apple is not an

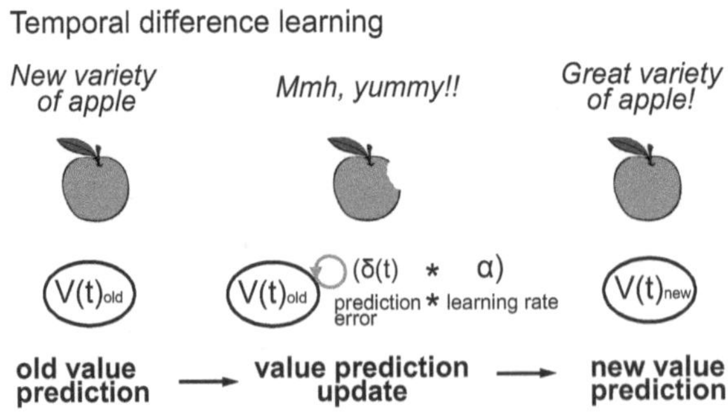

FIGURE 1 Illustration and schematic picture of the temporal difference reinforcement learning algorithm.

organic product (as you might have preferred). This would induce a negative Pe and reduce the expected value of the apple. According to reinforcement learning theory, the prediction error is used to continuously update value predictions. After repeated experience with the same variety of apples (that is, with learning), the value prediction gets more and more accurate.

More formally, according to the TD algorithm the prediction error $\delta(t)$ is defined as the immediate reward $R(t)$ plus the predicted future value $V(t+1)$ minus the current value prediction $V(t)$ (Eqn (1)):

$$\delta(t) = R(t) + \gamma \cdot V(t+1) - V(t)$$

The Pe $\delta(t)$ is used to update the old value prediction (Eqn (2)):

$$V(t)\,\text{new} = Vt\,(\text{old}) + \alpha \cdot \delta(t)$$

The (exponential) discount factor $0<\gamma<1$ in Eqn (1) accounts for the fact that humans (and other animals) tend to discount the value of future reward. That is, more distant reward is perceived as less valuable (high discount rate) than more immediate reward. In the apples example above, assume that you would have to buy an apple today but can consume it only 2 days from now. The expected value of this apple (apart from being less fresh than today) is presumably lower than the value of an apple that could be consumed right away.

The learning rate $0<\alpha<1$ in Eqn (2) determines how much a specific event affects future value predictions. A learning rate close to 1 would suggest that the most recent outcome has a strong effect on the value prediction, whereas a small learning rate indicates that much experience has to accumulate to affect value predictions. In the apple example, a low learning rate in subject A would mean that new information (such as where the apple comes from or where it was bought) does not have much impact on the value prediction (e.g., because subject A does not care about this information). In contrast, a high learning rate in subject B would mean that this information has a strong impact on value predictions (e.g., because subject B does care about the origin of the apple).

To summarize, a core feature of reinforcement learning theory is that reward prediction errors are used to learn (update) the expected future value associated with stimuli (states) and/or actions. Deficits in DA phasic Pe signaling may lead to less differentiated reward representation in the vmPFC and therefore to impairments in reinforcement learning (Eppinger et al., 2011). In a recent study we used reinforcement learning modeling in combination with fMRI to investigate the effects of aging on approach and avoidance learning (Eppinger, Schuck, et al., 2013). Behavioral findings showed that older adults are impaired in learning from reward (when they have to choose actions that lead to reward), but not in avoidance learning (when they have to learn to avoid stimuli that lead to negative outcomes) (see Eppinger, Schuck, et al., 2013). To examine whether we can explain age-related deficits in learning from reward based on the association between model parameters and neural activity, we examined correlations between Pe estimates and the blood oxygenation level-dependent (BOLD) signal. Results of this analysis showed that impairments in learning from reward in older adults were associated with reduced Pe signaling in two areas that receive strong projections from the dopamine system, the ventral striatum and the vmPFC. In contrast, as in the behavioral results, we found no evidence for age differences in the correlations between prediction errors and BOLD activity during learning from negative feedback.

A study by Chowdury et al. (2013) revealed very similar results during probabilistic reinforcement learning. Moreover, using a pharmacological intervention with the dopamine precursor L-DOPA, these authors could show that the Pe signals in the ventral striatum in the elderly could be partially restored by enhancing DA levels. That is, the results by Chowdury et al. (2013) point to a potential pharmacological intervention to improve learning and decision making abilities in old age. Taken together, these findings are nicely consistent with the idea that reduced dopaminergic signaling from the midbrain may lead to less differentiated reward representations in the vmPFC and to behavioral impairments in learning.

However, although these interpretations are consistent with several previous theoretical accounts and empirical findings (Eppinger et al., 2011; Hämmerer & Eppinger, 2012; Nieuwenhuis et al., 2002), it should be noted that the interactions between the midbrain DA system and the prefrontal cortex might be more complex than currently suggested. For example, electrophysiological data in monkeys indicate that the ventral striatum prediction error signal critically depends on intact projections from the vmPFC (Takahashi et al., 2011). That is, it could be that reduced Pe signals in the ventral striatum in older adults are not due to diminished DA projections, but rather due to deficits in vmPFC representations in the elderly. Support for this view comes from a study by Samanez-Larkin et al. (2012), which indicates that the diminished integrity of white matter pathways from the medial prefrontal cortex to the ventral striatum partially mediates the association between age and reduced learning performance in older adults.

Age Differences in Different Types of Reinforcement Learning

As stated above, our definition of decisions from experience refers to decision making tasks in which participants have to learn about the probability of outcomes in order to make optimal decisions that incorporate risk. It should be noted that this definition is agnostic with respect to learning mechanisms involved. So far we have mostly addressed situations in which younger and older adults learn to choose actions based on past experience. This type of reinforcement learning is sometimes referred to as model-free learning, because it is purely experience driven and does not rely on a forward model of the environment. Model-free learning is powerful and computationally robust. However, it also has its limitations, because it relies on multiple repetitions of associations and tends to be inflexible and slow (Doll, Simon, & Daw, 2012; Gershman, Markman, & Otto, 2013). Thus, model-free learning and decision making mechanisms may fail in more complex situations in which contingencies in the world change and we have to rapidly adjust behavior.

For these situations we need adaptive decision mechanisms that allow us to anticipate the consequences of future actions and to choose the sequence of future actions that has the highest probability to lead to the desired goal (Doll et al., 2012). Current decision making theories refer to these mechanisms as model-based learning and decision making (Balleine & O'Doherty, 2010; Daw, Niv, & Dayan, 2005). The advantage of model-based mechanisms is that they allow us to rapidly and flexibly adjust behavior to changes in the environment (such as changes in outcome probabilities). The downside is that they are computationally expensive because they involve a complete representation of the decision space (all possible combinations of states, actions, and rewards in a given situation). In a recent behavioral study we investigated the interplay of model-based and model-free decision making mechanisms in younger and older adults using a two-stage Markov decision task (see Figure 2(A)). In the first stage of this task, participants have to choose between two options (the two airplanes in Figure 2(A)). Depending on their choice, they transition to either the second-stage options with light gray background (see Figure 2(A), right-hand side), or the second-stage options with dark gray background (see Figure 2(A), left-hand side). In the second stage, they have to make another decision between two options (the figures in the second stage). Subsequently, they receive feedback for their choice (either a reward of 10 Eurocents or no reward). Feedback for the second-stage options is probabilistic and changes over time (see Figure 2(A)). The idea of this task is that in order to reach a preferred (rewarded) state in the second stage, participants have to engage in a strategic decision in the first stage. That is, they have to integrate model-free information about the reward probabilities in the second stage of the task with a model-based representation of the transition structure in the first stage of the task (see Figure 2(A) and (B)). Intuitively this means that in the second stage of the task, participants have to continuously learn which is the currently best option (model-free learning). However, in order to get the currently preferred stimulus in the first stage, they have to make a model-based decision, that is, they have to incorporate the transition probabilities into their decision. Thus, in order to get to the lower-right figure with light gray background in Figure 2(A) (second stage) one has to choose the

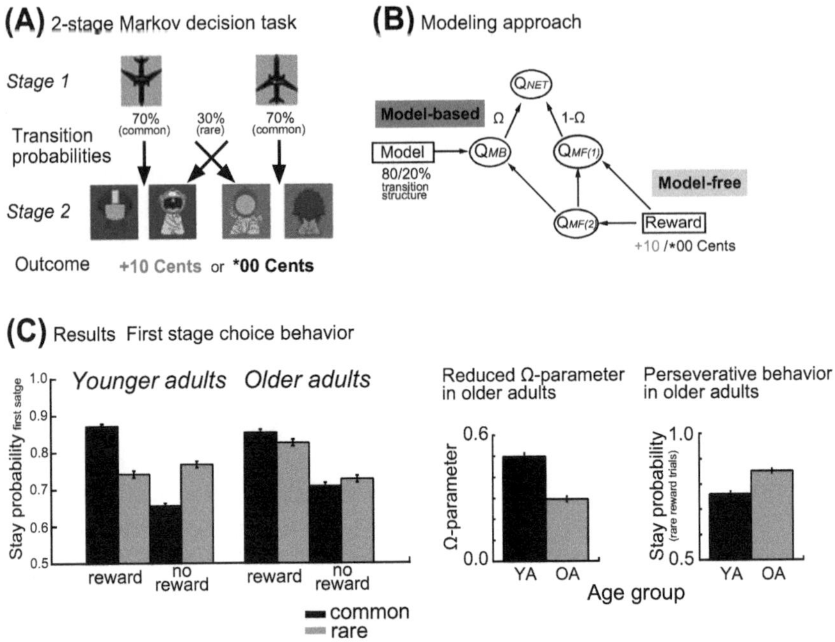

FIGURE 2 (A) Schematic picture of the two-stage Markov decision task. In the first stage of this task participants have to make a goal-directed decision that integrates knowledge of the transition structure with knowledge of the currently best option on the second stage. (B) A hybrid reinforcement learning algorithm is used to model choice behavior in the task. The model provides an estimate of the relative contribution of model-free and model-based decision mechanisms to behavior. (C) The behavioral results show a shift from model-based to model-free choice behavior in older compared to younger adults. *Figure adapted with permission from Eppinger, Walter, et al. (2013).*

upper-right option in the first stage. However, given the probabilistic nature of the transition structure, from time to time one will also end up at the other two states (figures with dark gray background in Figure 2(A)). The critical dependent variable in this task is the choice behavior in the first stage when participants have to integrate their knowledge of the transition structure with model-free information about the currently best option in the second stage. Choice behavior in the first stage of this task was fit using a hybrid reinforcement learning algorithm (Daw, Gershman, Seymour, Dayan, & Dolan, 2011; Eppinger, Walter, Heekeren, & Li, 2013; Wunderlich, Smittenaar, & Dolan, 2012) (for a schematic depiction see Figure 2(B)). This algorithm assumes that choices in the first stage of the task are driven by a weighted combination of model-based reinforcement learning (Q_{MB}), which accounts for the transition structure, and model-free SARSA (λ) TD learning ($Q_{MF(1)}$ and $Q_{MF(2)}$). The weighting of model-based versus model-free decision mechanisms is determined by the free parameter omega (Ω). If Ω approaches 0 behavior is model free, which is reflected in a main effect of reward. In contrast, an Ω value close to 1 indicates model-based choice behavior, which is reflected in an interaction between transition structure and reward on the previous trial. Results show substantial age-related deficits in model-based behavior in older compared to younger adults (Figure 2(C)). These deficits seem to be particularly pronounced in situations in which unexpected reward on the second stage indicates that the decision strategy on the first stage has to be adjusted. In these situations, older adults choose the suboptimal option, whereas younger adults engage in a strategic exploration of the decision space using their knowledge of the task transition structure. The neurophysiological mechanisms that lead to these deficits in model-based behavior in older adults are not yet clear. Work in younger adults suggests that fronto-partial areas may play a critical role in learning model-based representations (Gläscher, Daw, Dayan, & O'Doherty, 2010; Lee, Shimojo, & O'Doherty, 2014). Consistent with these findings, recent results from our group suggest that deficits in the learning of task transition structures (that is, learning how to navigate in a task in order to reach a goal) are associated with a reduced recruitment of the lateral prefrontal cortex (Eppinger, Heekeren, & Li, 2013b). Taken together, the current data point to substantial deficits of older adults in model-based learning and decision making. These deficits may affect choice behavior in experiential decision making tasks, particularly in environments that involve nonstationary reward and transition structures.

CONCLUSIONS

We conclude with a brief summary of the psychological and neurobiological processes underlying learning and decision making deficits and with a description of potential interventions to improve learning and decision making in older adults.

Most of our everyday decisions involve uncertainty about the potential outcomes. To reduce uncertainty we have to sample different options and associated rewards (different types of apples or different stocks or bonds for investment). Therefore, in decisions from experience we have to learn the outcome probability of an option. In this chapter we explored the psychological and neurophysiological underpinnings of learning impairments, which are relevant for the understanding of age-related changes in decisions from experience. In particular, we focused on age-related changes in the neurocomputational mechanisms of reinforcement learning. Recent results in this emerging field of research suggest that age-related impairments in learning of the expected utility of options might be due to a reduced updating of reward value representations in the vmPFC (Eppinger et al., 2011; Hämmerer & Eppinger, 2012). Whether these effects are due to reduced dopaminergic projections from the midbrain to the ventral striatum or whether they result from a diminished representational capacity of the vmPFC in older adults (or both) is currently unclear (Eppinger, Schuck, et al., 2013). Thus, based on the current data it seems straightforward to link age-related deficits in decisions from experience to these impairments in model-free reinforcement learning. However, model-free reinforcement learning tends to be relatively slow and inflexible, due to the large number of repetitions that needs to approximate the value of options. Therefore, it seems reasonable to assume that decisions from experience also involve faster and more flexible learning mechanisms that allow the decision maker to rapidly adjust behavior to changes in the environment, such as changes in reward probabilities. Current decision theories assume that these learning mechanisms involve the representation of a forward model of the decision space that includes all possible combinations of states, actions, and outcomes (Balleine & O'Doherty, 2010; Daw et al., 2005). The decision maker uses this model representation to choose the option that yields the highest long-term outcome in a given situation. Thus, these learning and decision making mechanisms provide the basis for flexible decisions. However, they also come at the cost of being computationally demanding and effortful (Otto, Gershman, Markman, & Daw, 2013). Recent behavioral and fMRI data suggest that model-based learning and decision making is impaired in older adults (Eppinger, Heekeren, & Li, 2012; Eppinger, Walter, et al., 2013). These impairments seem to be associated with a substantial under-recruitment of the lateral prefrontal cortex during the learning of higher-order contingencies in the decision space. Certainly, more research is needed to define and understand age-related changes in model-free and model-based decision mechanisms as well as their interactions and boundary conditions (Lee et al., 2014).

Most of the studies that directly targeted the dopamine system using PET have focused on age differences in WM updating and executive control, but more or less ignored motivational functions (Bäckman, Nyberg, Lindenberger, Li, & Farde, 2006). This is surprising, given the well-established role of DA for motivation and the fact that we seem to have a much better mechanistic understanding of reward-based learning and decision processes than WM or executive control. Future studies should fill this gap, ideally by combining neurocomputational approaches with functional neuroimaging. Ultimately, the goal of this research should be to link results back to everyday life situations that involve decisions from experience, to allow not only to learn about the involved mechanisms but also to learn how to improve decision making under uncertainty across the life span.

Potential Interventions to Ameliorate Learning Deficits in Older Adults

Naturally, findings on age-related deficits in DA function and their consequences for behavior raise the question about pharmacological interventions in old age that might ameliorate cognitive deficits. Data from a recent study suggest that the DA precursor L-DOPA, which is commonly used to treat later-stage Parkinson's disease, partially restores striatal Pe signaling in older adults (Chowdury et al., 2013). However, in this study older adults did not seem to benefit from this treatment in terms of performance, which raises questions about the usefulness of an intervention using L-DOPA. Furthermore, it should be noted that L-DOPA may induce negative side effects such as nausea, arrhythmia, and extreme emotional states, and the consequences of longer-term use of such medications are unclear. Additionally, the outcome of pharmacological studies using dopamine agonists is less straightforward than one would wish. Another study that used an L-DOPA manipulation in combination with a task that taxes interference control showed a negative effect in younger adults (possibly due to excessive DA levels) and no effect on performance in older adults (Onur, Piefke, Lie, Thiel, & Fink, 2011). Similar to these results, a study using DA agonists and antagonists during memory encoding in older adults did not show significant differences in drug effects on memory when compared to younger adults (Morcom et al., 2010). Thus, the results of studies using pharmacological interventions in combination with cognitive tasks are mixed, and the effects are generally weak. One apparent problem with most of the pharmacological interventions is that the mechanisms by which these drugs interact with the neuromodulatory system are very complex and probably not specific to a certain cognitive function. Furthermore, the drug effects may depend on individual difference in baseline DA levels as well as genetic predispositions. These factors add another level of complexity to the development of potential pharmacological interventions. Drugs that are assumed to enhance cognitive function but are less specifically associated with dopamine, such as Modafinil, have, to our knowledge, not been systematically investigated in age-comparative studies.

Another way to interact with the DA system is to provide primary and secondary reinforcers in the context of cognitive or motivational tasks to support performance. Recent work in younger adults suggests that performance-dependent reward incentives support executive control abilities (such as the ability to switch between tasks or to perform two tasks in parallel) (Savine & Braver, 2013). Similar effects were obtained with respect to episodic memory performance for rewarded, as compared to non-rewarded, information (Adcock, Thangavel, Withfield-Gabrieli, Knutson, & Gabrieli, 2006; Wittmann et al., 2005). An age-comparative ERP study (Eppinger et al., 2010) showed that reward during learning enhances subsequent memory performance to a similar degree in younger and older adults. Similar findings were obtained by Mather and Schoeke (2011). Work by Anguera and colleagues (2013) suggests that training using a video game enhances cognitive control abilities and improves prefrontal brain function. These effects may partially be due to the rewarding properties of the computer game. Taken together, these results seem to support a seemingly trivial conclusion, namely, that younger as well as older adults seem to learn and perform better in situations that involve incentives. The boundary conditions of these effects as well as the underlying neurophysiological mechanisms, however, are not yet determined.

To summarize, in this chapter we provided a link between age-related impairments in decisions from experience and age-related deficits in different types of reinforcement learning. Moreover, we showed that computational approaches in combination with neuroimaging can provide an important tool to advance our mechanistic understanding of age differences in decision making. Accumulating evidence suggests that age differences in Pe signaling may be one of the mechanisms underlying age-related impairments in model-free reinforcement learning (Chowdury et al., 2013; Eppinger, Schuck, et al., 2013; Samanez-Larkin et al., 2014). These effects are most likely due to age differences in dopaminergic neuromodulation. In contrast, age deficits in more complex types of learning, such as the learning of task structures or state spaces, seem to be associated with a reduced recruitment of prefrontal areas (Eppinger, Heekeren, & Li, under review). Both learning deficits may contribute to age-related changes in decisions from experience, particularly in uncertain and ambiguous decision situations. Given the ubiquity of these situations in our daily life, future research should try to improve decision making abilities in older adults by supporting learning mechanisms.

References

Adcock, R. A., Thangavel, A., Withfield-Gabrieli, S., Knutson, B., & Gabrieli, J. D. E. (2006). Reward-motivated learning: mesolimbic activation precedes memory formation. *Neuron, 50*, 507–517.

Agarwal, S., Driscoll, J., Gabaix, X., & Laibson, D. (2009). The age of reason: Financial decisions over the lifecycle with implications for regulation. Brookings Papers on Economic Activity, Fall, 51–117.

Anguera, J. A., Boccanfuso, J., Rintoul, J. L., Al-Hashimi, O., Faraji, F., Janowich, J., et al. (2013). Video game training enhances cognitive control in older adults. *Nature, 50*, 97–103.

Aston-Jones, G., & Cohen, J. D. (2005). An integrative theory of locus coeruleus-norepinephrine function: adaptive gain and optimal performance. *Annual Review of Neuroscience, 28*, 403–450.

Bäckman, L., Karlsson, S., Fischer, H., Karlsson, P., Brehmer, Y., Rieckmann, A., et al. (2009). Dopamine D(1) receptors and age differences in brain activation during working memory. *Neurobiology of Aging, 32*, 1849–1856.

Bäckman, L., Lindenberger, U., Li, S.-C., & Nyberg, L. (2010). Linking cognitive aging to alterations in dopamine neurotransmitter functioning: recent data and future avenues. *Neuroscience and Biobehavioral Reviews, 34*, 670–677.

Bäckman, L., Nyberg, L., Lindenberger, U., Li, S.-C., & Farde, L. (2006). The correlative triade among aging, dopamine, and cognition. *Neuroscience and Biobehavioral Reviews, 30*(6), 791–807.

Bäckman, L., Nyberg, L., Soveri, A., Johansson, J., Andersson, M., Dahlin, E., et al. (2011). Effects of working-memory training on striatal dopamine release. *Science, 333*, 718.

Balleine, B. W., & O'Doherty, J. P. (2010). Human and rodent homologies in action control: Cortico-striatal determinants of goal-directed and habitual action. *Neuropsychopharmacology, 35*, 48–69.

Braskie, M. N., Wilcox, C. E., Landau, S. M., O'Neil, J. P., Baker, S. L., Madison, C. M., et al. (2008). Relationship of striatal dopamine synthesis capacity to age and cognition. *Journal of Neuroscience, 28*, 14320–14328.

Braver, T. S., & Barch, D. M. (2002). A theory of cognitive control, aging cognition, and neuromodulation. *Neuroscience and Biobehavioral Reviews, 26*, 809–817.

Braver, T. S., Barch, D. M., Keys, B. A., Carter, C. S., Cohen, J. D., Kaye, J. A., et al. (2001). Context processing in older adults: Evidence for a theory relating cognitive control to neurobiology in healthy aging. *Journal of Experimental Psychology: General, 130*(4), 746–763.

Braver, T. S., & Cohen, J. (2000). On the control of control: the role of dopamine in regulating prefrontal function and working memory. In S. Monsell, & J. Driver (Eds.), *Attention & performance* (XVIII) (pp. 713–737). Cambridge, MA: MIT Press.

Buckholtz, J. W., Treadway, M. T., Cowan, R. L., Woodward, N. D., Li, R., Ansari, M. S., et al. (2010). Dopaminergic network differences in human impulsivity. *Science, 329*, 532.

Chowdhury, R., Guitart-Masip, M., Lambert, C., Dolan, R. J., & Düzel, E. (2013). Structural integrity of the substantia nigra and subthalamic nucleus predicts flexibility of instrumental learning in older-age individuals. *Neurobiology of Aging, 34*, 2261–2270.

Chowdury, R., Guitart-Masip, M., Lambert, C., Dayan, P., Huys, Q., Duezel, E., et al. (2013). Dopamine restores reward prediction errors in old age. *Nature Neuroscience, 16*, 648–653.

Daw, N. D., Gershman, S. J., Seymour, B., Dayan, P., & Dolan, R. J. (2011). Model-based influences on humans' choices and striatal prediction errors. *Neuron, 69*, 1204–1215.

Daw, N. D., Niv, Y., & Dayan, P. (2005). Human and rodent homologies in action control: Cortico-striatal determinants of goal-directed and habitual action. *Nature Neuroscience, 8*, 1704–1711.

Doll, B. B., Simon, D. A., & Daw, N. D. (2012). The ubiquity of model-based reinforcement learning. *Current Opinion in Neurobiology, 22*, 1075–1081.

Dreher, J.-C., Meyer-Lindenberg, A., Kohn, P., & Berman, K. F. (2008). Age-related changes in midbrain dopaminergic regulation of the human reward system. *Proceedings of the National Academy of Sciences, 105*, 15106–15111.

Eppinger, B., Haemmerer, D., & Li, S.-C. (2011). Neuromodulation of reward-based learning and decision making in human aging. *Annals of the New York Academy of Sciences, 1235*, 1–17.

Eppinger, B., Heekeren, H. R., & Li, S.-C. (2012). *When two birds in the bush are better than one in the hand: age-related impairments in learning to predict future rewards. Paper presented at the Annual Meeting of the Society for Neuroscience.* Lousiana: New Orleans.

Eppinger, B., Herbert, M., & Kray, J. (2010). We remember the good things. Age differences in learning and memory. *Neurobiology of Learning and Memory, 93*, 515–521.

Eppinger, B., & Kray, J. (2011). To choose or to avoid: Age differences in learning form positive and negative feedback. *Journal of Cognitive Neuroscience, 23*, 41–52.

Eppinger, B., Kray, J., Mock, B., & Mecklinger, A. (2008). Better or worse than expected? Aging, learning, and the ERN. *Neuropsychologia, 46*, 521–539.

Eppinger, B., Nystrom, L., & Cohen, J. D. (2012b). Reduced sensitivity to immediate reward during decision-making in older than younger adults. *PLoS ONE, 7*(5), 1–10.

Eppinger, B., Schuck, N. W., Nystrom, L. E., & Cohen, J. D. (2013a). Reduced striatal responses to reward prediction errors in older compared to younger adults. *Journal of Neuroscience, 33*, 9905–9912. http://dx.doi.org/10.1523/JNEUROSCI.2942-12.2013.

Eppinger, B., Walter, M., Heekeren, H. R., & Li, S.-C. (2013b). Of goals and habits: Age-related and individual differences in goal-directed decision-making. *Frontiers in Decision Neuroscience, 7*, 1–14.

Erixon-Lindroth, N., Farde, L., Robins Wahlin, T.-B., Sovago, J., Halldin, C., & Bäckman, L. (2005). The role of the striatal dopamine transporter in cognitive aging. *Psychiatry Research, 138*, 1–12.

Garrett, D. D., Samanez-Larkin, G. R., MacDonald, S. W. S., Lindenberger, U., McIntosh, A. R., & Grady, C. L. (2013). Moment-to-moment brain signal variability: A next frontier in human brain mapping. *Neuroscience and Biobehavioral Reviews, 37*, 610–624.

Gershman, S. J., Markman, A. B., & Otto, A. R. (2013). Retrospective revaluation in sequential decision making: A tale of two systems. *Journal of Experimental Psychology: General, 143*, 182–194.

Gläscher, J., Daw, N. D., Dayan, P., & O'Doherty, J. P. (2010). States versus rewards: Dissociable neural prediction error signals underlying model-based and model-free reinforcement learning. *Neuron, 66*, 585–595.

Hämmerer, D., & Eppinger, B. (2012). Dopaminergic and prefrontal contributions to reward-based learning and outcome monitoring during child development and aging. *Developmental Psychology, 48*, 862–874.

Herbert, M., Eppinger, B., & Kray, J. (2011). Younger but not older adults benefit from salient reward feedback during learning. *Frontiers in Cognition, 2*, 1–9.

Lee, S. W., Shimojo, S., & O'Doherty, J. P. (2014). Neural computations underlying arbitration between model-based and model-free learning. *Neuron, 81*, 687–699.

Li, S.-C., Lindenberger, U., & Sikström, S. (2001). Aging cognition: From neuromodulation to representation. *Trends in Cognitive Sciences, 5*(11), 479–486.

MacDonald, S. W., Karlsson, S., Rieckmann, A., Nyberg, L., & Bäckmann, L. (2012). Aging-related increases in behavioral variability: Relations to losses of dopamine D1 receptors. *Journal of Neuroscience, 32*, 8186–8191.

Mata, R., Josef, A. K., Samanez-Larkin, G. R., & Hertwig, R. (2011). Age differences in risky choice: A meta-analysis. *Annals of the New York Academy of Sciences, 1235*, 18–29.

Mather, M. (2006). A review of decision making processes: weighing the risks and benefits of aging. In L. L. Carstensen, & C. R. Hartel (Eds.), *When I'm 64* (pp. 145–173). Washington: The National Academies Press.

Mather, M., Mazar, N., Gorlick, M. A., Lighthall, N. R., Burgeno, J., Schoeke, A., et al. (2012). Risk preferences and aging: The "certainty effect" in older adults' decision making. *Psychology and Aging, 27*, 801–816.

Mather, M., & Schoeke, A. (2011). Positive outcomes enhance incidental learning for both younger and older adults. *Frontiers in Neuroscience, 5*, 1–10.

Montague, P. R., Hyman, S. E., & Cohen, J. D. (2004). Computational roles for dopamine in behavioral control. *Nature, 431*, 760–767.

Morcom, A. M., Bullmore, E. T., Huppert, F. A., Lennox, B., Praseedom, A., Linnington, H., et al. (2010). Memory encoding and dopamine in the aging brain: A psychopharmacological neuroimaging study. *Cerebral Cortex, 20*, 743–757.

Nieuwenhuis, S., Ridderinkhof, K. R., Talsma, D., Coles, M. G. H., Holroyd, C. B., Kok, A., et al. (2002). A computational account of altered error processing in older age: Dopamine and the error-related negativity. *Cognitive, Affective and Behavioral Neuroscience, 2*(1), 19–36.

Niv, Y., & Schoenbaum, G. (2008). Dialogues on prediction errors. *Trends in Cognitive Sciences, 12*, 265–272.

Onur, Ö. A., Piefke, M., Lie, C.-H., Thiel, C. M., & Fink, G. R. (2011). Modulatory effects of levodopa on cognitive control in young but not in older subjects: A pharmacological fMRI study. *Journal of Cognitive Neuroscience, 23*, 2797–2810.

Otto, A. R., Gershman, S. J., Markman, A. B., & Daw, N. D. (2013). The curse of planning: Dissecting multiple reinforcement learning systems by taxing the central executive. *Psychological Science, 24*, 751–761.

Pietschmann, M., Endrass, T., Czerwon, B., & Kathmann, N. (2011). Aging, probabilistic learning and performance monitoring. *Biological Psychology, 86*, 74–82.

Samanez-Larkin, G. R. (2013). Financial decision making and the aging brain. *APS Observer, 26*, 30–33.

Samanez-Larkin, G. R., Levens, S. M., Perry, L. M., Dougherty, R. F., & Knutson, B. (2012). Frontostriatal white matter integrity mediates adult age differences in probabilistic reward learning. *Journal of Neuroscience, 32*, 5333–5337.

Samanez-Larkin, G. R., Worthy, D. A., Mata, R., McClure, S. M., & Knutson, B. (2014). Adult age differences in frontostriatal representation of prediction error but not reward outcome. *Cognitive Affective and Behavioral Neuroscience, 14*, 672–682.

Samanez-Larkin, G. R., Kuhnen, C. M., Yoo, D. J., & Knutson, B. (2010). Variability in nucleus accumbens activity mediates age-related suboptimal financial risk taking. *Journal of Neuroscience, 27*, 1426–1434.

Savine, A. C., & Braver, T. S. (2013). Local and global effects of motivation on cognitive control. *Cognitive, Affective and Behavioral Neuroscience, 12*, 692–718.

Schott, B. H., Niehaus, L., Wittmann, B. C., Schuetze, H., Seidenbecher, C. I., Heintze, H.-J., et al. (2007). Ageing and early-stage Parkinsons's disease affect separable neural mechanisms of mesolimbic reward processing. *Brain, 130*, 2412–2424.

Sutton, R. S., & Barto, A. G. (1998). *Reinforcement learning: an introduction (adaptive computation and machine learning)*. Cambridge, MA: MIT Press.

Takahashi, Y. K., Roesch, M. R., Wilson, R. C., Toreson, K., O'Donnell, P., Niv, Y., et al. (2011). Expectancy-related changes in firing of dopamine neurons depend on orbitofrontal cortex. *Nature Neuroscience, 14*, 1590–1599.

Troiano, A. R., Schulzer, M., De La Fuente-Fernandez, R., Mak, E., McKenzie, J., Sossi, V., et al. (2010). Dopamine transporter PET in normal aging: Dopamine transporter decline and its possible role in preservation of motor function. *Synapse, 64*, 146–151.

Volkow, N. D., Gur, R. C., Wang, G.-J., Fowler, J. S., Mpberg, P. J., Ding, Y.-S., et al. (1998a). Association between decline in brain dopamine activity with age and cognitive and motor impairment in healthy individuals. *American Journal of Psychiatry, 155*(3), 344–349.

Volkow, N. D., Logan, J., Fowler, J. S., Wang, G.-J., Gur, R. C., Wong, C., et al. (2000). Association between age-related decline in brain dopamine activity and impairment in frontal and cingulate metabolism. *American Journal of Psychiatry, 157*(1), 75–80.

Volkow, N. D., Wang, G.-J., Fowler, J. S., Ding, Y.-S., Gur, R. C., Gatley, J., et al. (1998b). Parallel loss of presynaptic and postsynaptic dopamine markers in normal aging. *Annals of Neurology, 44*, 143–147.

Wang, Y., Chan, G. L. Y., Holden, J. E., Dobko, T., Mak, E., Schulzer, M., et al. (1998). Age-dependent decline of dopamine D1 receptors in human brain: a PET study. *Synapse, 30*, 56–61.

Wittmann, B. C., Schott, B. H., Guderian, S., Frey, J. U., Heinze, H.-J., & Duezel, E. (2005). Reward-related fMRI activation of dopaminergic midbrain is associated with hippocampus-dependent long-term memory formation. *Neuron, 45*, 459–467.

Wong, K. K., Müller, M. L. T.M., Kuwabara, H., Studenski, S., & Bohnen, N. I. (2012). Gender differences in nigrostriatal dopaminergic innervation are present at young-to-middle but not at older age in normal adults. *Journal of Clinical Neuroscience, 19*, 183–184.

Wunderlich, K., Smittenaar, P., & Dolan, R. J. (2012). Dopamine enhances model-based over model-free behavior. *Neuron, 75*, 418–424.

CHAPTER

5

Age-Associated Executive Dysfunction, the Prefrontal Cortex, and Complex Decision Making

Natalie L. Denburg[1,3], *William M. Hedgcock*[2,3]

[1]Department of Neurology, Carver College of Medicine, Iowa City, IA, USA; [2]Department of Marketing, Tippie College of Business, Iowa City, IA, USA; [3]Interdisciplinary Graduate Program in Neuroscience, Iowa City, IA, USA

Theories abound regarding how the "healthy" brain ages, and some of these go beyond conventional wisdom, which holds that aging is more or less synonymous with memory loss. Although memory does tend to decline with age, many older people experience far more dramatic declines in non-memory-related cognitive abilities, such as difficulties with concentration, problem-solving, and decision making. Unlike memory, which is strongly linked to the medial temporal region of the brain, these other abilities (referred to as "executive functions") are closely linked to the frontal lobes.

Older adulthood is a time of complex and critical decision making, in spite of age-related decline in frontal brain regions. To illustrate, older adults are faced with many complex and critical decisions regarding retirement, health care, finances, and living situations, and their ability to make such decisions successfully has a profound impact on the individual and society as a whole. Unfortunately, numerous neurologically and psychiatrically healthy older adults (i.e., persons not diagnosed with a neurologic or psychiatric disease, not suffering from Alzheimer's disease or any other of the "known" degenerative dementias) do not make advantageous decisions: they make poor financial choices, are taken advantage of by adult children, or get swindled.

http://dx.doi.org/10.1016/B978-0-12-417148-0.00005-4

We have proposed that the vulnerability of such older adults is caused, at least in part, by a specific neurobehavioral change: the prefrontal cortex of their brain is deteriorating and thereby affecting cognitive abilities referable to this brain region. New functional neuroimaging findings, along with results from behavioral, psychophysiological, and structural imaging studies of the brain, indicate that these seniors may be losing their ability to make complex choices that require effective emotional processing to analyze short-term and long-term considerations. Older adults in this category may fall prey to the promise of an immediate reward or a simple solution to a complicated problem. They may fail to detect the longer-range adverse consequences of their actions. Finally, they may assume long-term benefits in situations where there are none. We see these characteristics as direct consequences of neurological dysfunction in systems that are critical for bringing emotion-related signals to bear on decision making.

The decision-making problems mentioned set the groundwork for older adults to be obvious targets for fraud victimization. (However, the notion that older adults are disproportionately victimized has not gone unchallenged; see Ross, Grossmann, and Schryer, 2014, for a cautionary discussion of such data.) Deceiving the elderly is not a new problem, but it is one that has been growing in prevalence. To illustrate, financial abuse of elders aged 65 and older has risen from 8% in 1950 to an astounding 20% in 2010 (Infogroup/ORC, 2010; Kemp & Liao, 2006). These recent statistics may even underestimate the extent of the problem, with only 1 in 25 cases being reported (NCEA, 2005). In other words, money loss due to elderly fraud was 2.9 billion dollars as of 2011, an increase from 2.6 billion dollars in 2008 (MetLife, 2011). Sadly, these numbers do not take into account the devastation fraud can have on the elderly and their families, often wiping out entire savings and years of work in a single action, not to mention the psychological distress and loss of dignity that frequently ensues. Despite legislative emphasis on this issue (e.g., Death Planning Made Difficult, 2000), research efforts examining older consumers' real-world decision-making abilities are sorely lacking. The reasons why some elderly people are vulnerable to such schemes, and more generally prone to making poor decisions, are not well understood (Bruine de Bruin, Parker, & Fischhoff, 2012; Finucane et al., 2002; Moye & Marson, 2007; Samanez-Larkin, Wagner, & Knutson, 2011).

In this chapter, we will demonstrate how changes to the prefrontal cortex affect a wide range of decisions. We will review early examples from the neuroscience literature. We will then discuss age-related changes of the brain, specifically literature supporting the claim that the frontal lobes undergo disproportionate age-related changes. Next, implications of these changes for decision making across diverse tasks, such as the Iowa Gambling Task (IGT), will be discussed. We conclude with the assertion that these behavioral changes are due to a common cause that we term *age-associated executive dysfunction*, an impairment in emotion-related signals that are essential to decision making.

GUIDING OBSERVATIONS, THEORETICAL FRAMEWORKS, AND KEY EMPIRICAL TESTS

The following section reviews guiding observations, theoretical frameworks, and key empirical tests used in our decision-making work, including the famous case of Phineas Gage, the somatic marker hypothesis (SMH), the frontal aging hypothesis, and the creation of the IGT.

Phineas Gage

Phineas Gage's historical accident in 1848 provided crucial early clues about the importance of the prefrontal sector of the brain for reasoning and decision making, social behavior, and personality. Gage's work-related accident resulted in a tamping iron being driven through the front part of his head, entering just under the eye, piercing the frontal lobes of his brain, and exiting through the top front part of his head. Surprisingly, Gage survived and recovered from this notable accident, and exhibited normal intelligence, memory, speech, sensation, and movement. However, Gage displayed profound changes in abilities subsumed by the frontal lobes. Before the accident, he used good judgment, and had been responsible, socially well-adapted, and well-liked by peers and supervisors. Afterward, Gage exhibited impairments in many aspects of decision making, most notably poor judgment and social conduct. In addition, he demonstrated rather dramatic changes in personality involving irresponsibility, dishonesty, and unreliability. In short, he was "no longer Gage" (p. 340; Harlow, 1868).

The importance of the case of Phineas Gage can be more fully appreciated when one considers just how difficult it has been to unravel the cognitive and behavioral functions that are subserved by the prefrontal region of the human brain. The prefrontal sector, situated anterior to the motor/premotor cortices and superior to the Sylvian fissure, comprises an enormous expanse of the brain, forming nearly half of the entire cerebral mantle. In humans in particular, this region has expanded disproportionately. Throughout the history of neuropsychology, the psychological capacities associated with the prefrontal region have remained elusive and have been likened to a riddle (Teuber, 1964).

The Somatic Marker Hypothesis

The SMH is a neural theory of how emotions play a key role in decision making, and how this process depends on the ventromedial prefrontal cortex (VMPC) of the brain (Damasio, 1994); this theory was inspired by case studies of brain lesion patients such as Phineas Gage. The term somatic refers to body and brain-related signals, which we experience as emotions and feelings. According to the SMH, when faced with complex decisions, we make choices that are in our best interest only after properly weighing potential short-term and long-term outcomes. A key idea of this hypothesis is that when these outcomes are ambiguous or uncertain, then emotions, feelings, and the brain's ability to maintain an internal equilibrium are essential to making a decision. The VMPC is critical for triggering various bodily changes (somatic states) in response to stimuli such as cues for reward or punishment. As we make decisions under uncertainty, our assessment of their immediate and future potential consequences may trigger numerous responses that conflict with each other—a highly favorable potential consequence may trigger excitement and elation, while an aversive consequence may trigger pain and dread. The end result, though, is the emergence of an overall positive or negative signal—basically a "go" or "stop" signal (Damasio, 1994).

Damasio (1994) has proposed that numerous and conflicting signals may be triggered simultaneously, but sooner or later, stronger ones trump weaker ones. In this way, emotional processes are critical for decision making that is advantageous in the long run. However, people deprived of appropriate emotional signals—e.g., because of damage to the VMPC—may fail to perceive potential adverse long-term consequences (Bechara, Tranel, & Damasio, 2000). In this sense, too little emotion can be bad for advantageous decision making, just as too much emotion can be. In adapting the SMH, therefore, Denburg, Tranel, and Bechara (2005), Denburg, Recknor, Bechara, and Tranel (2006), and Denburg, Cole, et al. (2007) proposed that some ostensibly normal older people, who are free of obvious neurological or psychiatric disease, experience changes in reasoning and decision making because of dysfunction in a neural system that includes the brain's ventromedial prefrontal system. That is, they are losing their ability to make complex choices that depend critically on the use of emotion-related information to help guide an optimal blend of short-term and long-term considerations. They may be overly swayed by the promise of immediate reward or a simple solution to a complicated problem (approaches that are commonly used in fraudulent and misleading marketing practices), and fail to detect the longer-range adverse consequences of their actions. Moreover, they may fail to recognize the implausibility of any long-term benefit at all (as is the case for many telemarketing schemes). This was postulated as a direct consequence of neurological dysfunction in systems that are critical for bringing emotion-related signals to bear on decision making. Interestingly, these same brain regions have been implicated in functional neuroimaging studies investigating purchase decisions (Knutson, Rick, Wimmer, Prelec, & Loewenstein, 2007), decision making under uncertainty (Bechara et al., 2000), and decision making under risk (Weller, Levin, Shiv, & Bechara, 2007), among healthy younger adults.

The Frontal Aging Hypothesis

Researchers have suggested that areas of the brain implicated in the SMH are more affected by aging than other areas of the brain. One theory, referred to as the frontal aging hypothesis (West, 1996), proposes that some older people have disproportionate age-related changes of frontal lobe brain structures and of associated cognitive abilities. This theory has gained support from several sources of evidence, including neuropsychological, electrophysiological, neuroanatomical, and functional neuroimaging studies.

Neuropsychological studies have demonstrated similarities in the behavioral presentation of older adults and patients with acquired lesions of the prefrontal cortex, such as deficits in cognitive flexibility (Salthouse, Atkinson, & Berish, 2003), planning (Allain et al., 2005; Sorel & Pennequin, 2008), attention and inhibition (Braver et al., 2001), perseverative behavior (Gunning-Dixon & Raz, 2003), self-monitoring (Ridderinkhof, Span, & Van Der Molen, 2002), and decision making (Denburg, Tranel, et al., 2005; Denburg, Cole, et al., 2007). Electrophysiological studies, utilizing event-related brain potentials, have also supported the notion of disproportionate frontal lobe decline with age (Fabiani, Friedman, & Cheng, 1998).

Further evidence for differential aging of the frontal lobe, and specifically the prefrontal cortex, has been demonstrated through various neuroanatomical studies (e.g., Cowell et al., 1994; DeCarli, Murphy, McIntosh, & Horwitz, 1994; Haug & Eggers, 1991; Murphy et al., 1996; Salat, Kaye, & Janowsky, 1999; Sullivan et al., 2001; Waldemar et al., 1991). To illustrate, Raz et al. (1997) conducted a volumetric magnetic resonance imaging (MRI) study of adults ranging in age from 18 to 77. General linear model analyses revealed that the greatest age effects occurred in prefrontal cortex gray matter (*r*age, prefrontal volume = −0.55), with an average rate of volumetric decline of 4.9% per decade. Consistent with the Raz et al. (1997) findings, Salat et al. (1999) also found that the prefrontal cortex exhibited greater sensitivity to aging than the rest of the cerebral cortex. Both of these studies state that the underlying mechanism driving such prefrontal degeneration with age is currently unknown, although altered neurotransmitter systems have been proposed as one potential explanation. Similarly, Jernigan et al. (2001) examined the age-related volume loss of each cerebral lobe in a large sample of adults aged 30–99, and found that the frontal lobes were disproportionately affected by cortical volume loss and increased white matter abnormality.

Few longitudinal studies have been conducted to assess brain volume changes associated with normal aging. Resnick, Pham, Kraut, Zonderman, and Davatzikos (2003) followed 92 healthy, non-demented individuals (mean age of 70) participating in the Baltimore Longitudinal Study of Aging over a 5-year period, procuring cerebral MRIs at baseline,

3-year, and 5-year intervals. Participants lost an average of 5.4 cm^3 in brain volume and gained an average of 1.4 cm^3 of ventricular volume per year. Reductions in frontal lobe volume were most salient, with particular decrement of the orbital and inferior frontal cortices. A reduction in parietal lobe volume was found next, further followed by reductions in the temporal and occipital lobes. These results suggest that there are significant reductions in brain volume with normal aging, and the frontal lobes may be more susceptible to such changes. Given the central role that the frontal lobes play in decision making (Kable & Glimcher, 2007; Rangel, Camerer, & Montague, 2008) and related theories such as the SMH (Damasio, 1994), this raises the concern that these reductions in brain volume may lead to impaired decision making and hints at the importance of designing tests to identify these impairments.

The Creation of the Iowa Gambling Task

The pervasive real-world decision-making deficits of patients with lesions to the VMPC, such as Phineas Gage (see Damasio, 1994; Tranel, 1994, for reviews), have been elusive to capture with standard neuropsychological testing. It was against this backdrop that Bechara, Damasio, Damasio, and Anderson (1994) developed the test now known as the IGT, which finally did correlate with such patients' deficits in their everyday lives.

The IGT (Bechara, 2007) provides a close analog to real-world decision making by factoring in reward, punishment, and unpredictability. The task is designed to create a conflict between the lure of immediate reward and delayed, probabilistic punishment. The IGT is a computer-administered test in which participants make 100 card selections from four decks of cards, taking about 10–15 min to administer. On each trial, choosing a card gives an immediate monetary reward. At unpredictable points, the selection of some cards results in losing a sum of money. Two decks are predetermined to provide relatively lower immediate gain and even lower long-term loss, yielding an overall net gain of money (i.e., decks C and D, dubbed "the good decks"); the other two decks are predetermined to provide relatively higher immediate gain but even higher long-term loss, yielding an overall net loss of money (i.e., decks A and B, dubbed "the bad decks"). Participants are not informed of the number of trials or the gain/loss schedule.

Participants are instructed that they should try to win as much money as possible and avoid losing as much as possible. They are told that they are free to switch from any deck to another at any time, as often as they wish, that they will not know when the game will end (after 100 trials), and that they should keep playing until the computer stops. They are given the following hint: Some decks are worse than the others. You may find all of them bad, but some are worse than the others. No matter how much you find yourself losing, you can still win if you stay away from the worst decks.

An overall score provides a single indicator of whether the participant's decision making was advantageous or disadvantageous. The total score is calculated subtracting the number of selections from the disadvantageous decks, from the number of selections from the advantageous deck, i.e., [(deck C′ +deck D′) – (deck A′ +deck B′)]. A positive total score indicates advantageous decision making, whereas a negative total score indicates disadvantageous decision making. Poor performance on the IGT would seem to be a promising test for age-related changes in decision making given its ability to detect abnormal decision making related to VMPC damage and prior research suggesting the VMPC is disproportionately affected by aging.

RESEARCH ON AGING

Iowa Gambling Task Studies

IGT Behavioral. Impaired decision making on the IGT among a subgroup of seemingly healthy older adults has been documented by Denburg and colleagues (Denburg, Recknor, et al., 2006; Denburg, Tranel, et al., 2005). In their first study (Denburg, Tranel, et al., 2005) comparing IGT performance of healthy (with no diagnosed neurological or psychiatric disease) older adults ($n=40$; aged 56–85 years) to healthy younger adults ($n=40$; aged 26–55 years), the authors reported that the performance of about one-third of seemingly healthy older adults (a replication study yielded a very similar rate of impairment; Denburg, Recknor, et al., 2006) on the task is akin to that of neurological patients with VMPC injury: both exhibit a preference for choices that lead to high immediate reward but greater long-term punishment. This seemingly healthy subgroup is referred to as the "impaired" decision makers[1]. They contrast with a subgroup of older adults—deemed "unimpaired"—who perform normally on the task and select responses that have small immediate, but higher long-term reward. Of note, none of the younger participants qualified as impaired. IGT performance for the groups of participants is depicted in Figure 1. The y-axis of this graph represents the net advantageous choices

[1] Denburg, Tranel, et al. (2005), Denburg, Recknor, et al. (2006), and Denburg, Cole, et al. (2007) have taken the aforementioned overall score a step further, by evaluating whether the total score differed significantly from zero (using the binomial test), and in which direction (Siegel, 1956, p. 37), ultimately classifying participants as impaired (significantly different than zero in the negative direction) or unimpaired (significantly different than zero in the positive direction).

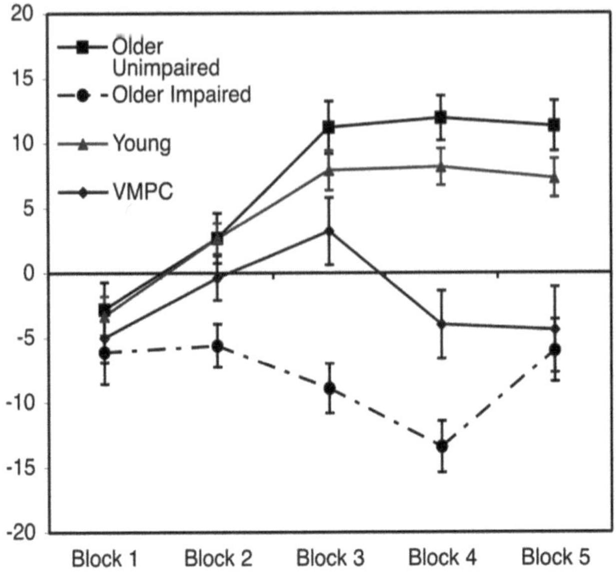

FIGURE 1 Decision-making performance on the Iowa Gambling Task in the older unimpaired and older impaired, young, and ventromedial prefrontal cortex (VMPC) participants, graphed as a function of trial block (±SEM).

of the subjects (that is, the number of choices from good decks minus the number of choices from bad decks), and the x-axis displays the 100 decks choices in five blocks of 20 selections each. For perspective, we have also plotted the performance of a group of patients with stable focal lesions of the VMPC. This demonstrates that the older unimpaired group is at least as good as normal, healthy younger adults, and the impaired group is at least as bad (if not worse) as the VMPC patient group.

The impaired older group was compared to the unimpaired older group on a variety of demographic variables (e.g., age, education, sex distribution) and neuropsychological test scores (e.g., attention, working memory, language, anterograde memory, psychomotor speed, and executive functions) with no significant differences emerging. These studies (Denburg, Tranel, et al., 2005; Denburg, Recknor, et al., 2006) clearly demonstrate that there is a substantial subset of older adults who are susceptible to decision-making deficits in spite of age-appropriate scores across all manner of neuropsychological tests. The remainder of this chapter will deal with our ongoing efforts to distinguish these two groups of seemingly healthy older adults (i.e., older-unimpaired vs older-impaired participants).

IGT Psychophysiological. The results of the previous IGT behavioral study were extended to include psychophysiological measurements (Denburg, Recknor, et al., 2006), building upon prior work that had shown that lesions of the VMPC interfered with participants' ability to generate discriminatory skin conductance responses (SCRs) prior to card selection in the IGT (Bechara, Damasio, Tranel, & Damasio, 1997). Denburg, Recknor, et al. (2006) sought to determine whether a disruption in the anticipatory SCR might explain the deficit in the subset of older adults who were impaired on the IGT. The results of this study revealed that older adults who were unimpaired on the IGT generated anticipatory SCRs that were capable of discriminating between good and bad decks. By contrast, the anticipatory SCRs of older adults who were impaired on the IGT did not discriminate between good and bad decks. This lack of discriminatory SCRs provides another link between the significant subset of older adults that are impaired on the IGT and patients with stable focal lesions of the VMPC. It is interesting to note, however, that the anticipatory SCRs generated by the unimpaired older adults (Denburg, Recknor, et al., 2006) were different than those generated by young adults (Bechara et al., 1997). While younger adults generate higher SCR values in anticipation of selections from the disadvantageous decks, the unimpaired older adults generate higher SCR values prior to selections from the advantageous deck.

From the point of view of the SMH, it seems plausible that the normal aging process may interfere with the ability to assign somatic markers. The third of older adults who fail the IGT may be failing for the same reason that VMPC patients fail: aging may reduce these individuals' ability to assign somatic markers to outcomes. Those older adults who are able to perform well on the IGT do so using apparently reversed somatic markers. Rather than marking the bad decks in a negative way, they are positively marking the good decks to facilitate approach. The use of positive rather than negative somatic markers in later life is in line with research demonstrating a positivity bias associated with older age (Carstensen & Charles, 1999; Mather & Carstensen, 2003). Perhaps there is a natural shift in decision-making behavior from avoiding negative stimuli to seeking out positive stimuli, and this process is disrupted somehow in the impaired older adults.

Hypersensitivity to Reward. Additional evidence for this shift toward positive stimuli among older adults comes from performance on an alternative version of the IGT, referred to as Variant E′F′G′H′. Like Original A′B′C′D′, Variant E′F′G′H′ contains four decks each with an equal number of cards, is administered on a computer, allows participants to pick from any deck they wish, and ends after 100 card selections (Bechara, 2007; Bechara et al., 2000). Unlike Original A′B′C′D′, this version always delivers an immediate punishment followed, intermittently, by a delayed reward. The game is rigged such that the decks with the larger immediate punishment (decks E and G) also yield a larger delayed reward, while the decks with the smaller immediate punishment (decks F and H) yield a smaller delayed reward. If more cards are chosen from decks E and G (the "good" decks), there will be a net gain in money; however, a greater number of picks from decks F and H (the "bad" decks) will result in a net loss of money.

To perform advantageously on E′F′G′H′ IGT, one must choose high initial punishment with higher delayed reward versus low initial punishment with lower delayed reward. Bauer et al. (2013) found that older adults performed better on the Variant IGT than on the Original IGT. That is, younger adults perform comparably and advantageously on both versions of the IGT, whereas older adults' performance on E′F′G′H′ significantly outpaces their performance on A′B′C′D′, with E′F′G′H′ being advantageous and not reliably different than their younger counterparts performance (Bauer et al., 2013). In summary, the findings point to an age-related increase in hypersensitivity to reward. This explanation would account for the apparent tendency for older adults to perform less well on the IGT when the contingencies call for opting against higher upfront reward (as in A′B′C′D′), and to perform better when the contingencies call for opting for higher long-term reward (as in E′F′G′H′).

Neuroimaging Studies

To complement neuropsychological studies, our team has used neuroimaging to explore the inner workings of the brains of older impaired decision makers. Comparing the brain MRI results of 20 impaired older adults with those of 20 unimpaired older adults, we found that the impaired group displayed a comparative thinning of left rostral anterior cingulate, an area within the broader region of the VMPC (Denburg, 2009). This region is critical for complex, emotion-related decision making (Gläscher et al., 2012). Of note, there were no group differences in temporal lobe regions.

We have also used fluorodeoxyglucose-positron emission tomography (FDG-PET) to examine the brain's metabolism and cell functioning. Our resting FDG-PET imaging study involved 48 older adults, 24 with impaired decision making and 24 with unimpaired decision making, as measured by the IGT. Results indicated that older impaired decision makers had lower metabolism in medial prefrontal regions (activity in this area covaries with emotional regulation, self-awareness, social conduct, and subjective value) as compared to older unimpaired decision makers. Such regions include the frontal inferior operculum, frontal superior medial gyri, and anterior cingulate. In addition, lower metabolism in the insula (activity in this area covaries with interoceptive awareness and body representation) among the impaired decision makers was observed (Denburg & Harshman, 2010). Notably, there were no group differences in medial temporal lobe brain regions that are associated with learning and memory (Scoville & Milner, 1957).

These FDG-PET results link intriguingly to our overall framework for explaining why some older adults seem to have impaired decision-making abilities: Several areas of their brains have lower metabolism compared with the brains of older adults who are unimpaired. These anterior brain regions, which include those that are critical for decision making and representing emotional states, belong to the brain circuitry involved in the SMH. Equally noteworthy, the impaired and unimpaired groups show no consistent metabolic or structural differences in their temporal lobe structures, including medial temporal lobe sectors that are important for memory. These findings, which support our neuropsychological and MRI results, suggest that abnormalities in areas involved in emotions and complex decision making—rather than areas involved in memory—may make some older adults especially susceptible to fraud. These findings are significant because they suggest that older adults who make poor decisions are not "demented," but rather display relatively localized abnormalities in regions of the prefrontal cortex known previously to be important for judgment and making complex decisions, including consumer decisions (Knutson et al., 2008).

A recent study by Halfmann, Hedgcock, Bechara, and Denburg (2014) further confirmed differing neurofunctional patterns between older impaired versus older unimpaired decision makers. Using functional magnetic resonance imaging (fMRI), two groups of older adults, previously categorized as impaired ($n=15$) or unimpaired ($n=16$) based on A′B′C′D′ IGT performance, were administered an alternative version of the IGT, developed to reduce practice effects, termed K′L′M′N′ (Xiao et al., 2013), in which the differences between the advantageous and disadvantageous decks are considerably more subtle than in A′B′C′D′. These two groups did not differ in their performance on standard neuropsychological instruments (e.g., attention, memory, processing speed).

Here, we highlight two of the findings of Halfmann et al. (2014): (1) The older impaired group showed relatively greater activation than the older unimpaired group in more anterior brain regions (e.g., the VMPC) during the early (prechoice) phase of the IGT; and (2) the older impaired group showed relatively greater activation than the older unimpaired group in more posterior brain regions (e.g., the precuneus activity in this area covaries with mental imagery, self-consciousness, and source memory) during the later (prefeedback and feedback) phases of the IGT. We believe the aforementioned differences in compensatory mechanisms (e.g., VMPC) during the early (prechoice) phase, and differences in reward processing (e.g., posterior cingulate cortex—functional data are more mixed, but activity covaries with mind-wandering and emotional memory—and precuneus) during the later (feedback) phase likely contribute to the observed behavioral disparities in decision making on the IGT. We additionally note that the neurofunctional differences we observed between older impaired and unimpaired decision makers largely occurred in the absence of differences in regions that subserve working memory or motor functions (e.g., dorsolateral prefrontal cortex and parahippocampal gyrus). This, along with the previously described findings, provides strong evidence linking IGT-associated decision-making impairments in seniors to emotional-processing deficits that are localized in the VMPC.

Consumer Decision-Making Studies

While the previously discussed laboratory tests and psychophysiological measures are useful at determining the correlates of age-related changes in decision making, experimenters ultimately want to confirm that these findings translate to real-world situations. To that end, we have created a novel consumer task, entitled Advertising Task (Denburg, Cole, et al., 2007). This task is based on a set of real advertisements that had been deemed deceptive by the Federal Trade Commission (FTC, 1991, 1998). These advertisements were deemed deceptive for a number of reasons, ranging from the withholding of crucial information about the product to the use of biased graphs. All advertisements were recreated in printed form, as would be found in a magazine or newspaper. A counterpart was created for each of the deceptive advertisements, which disclosed the important product information that had been withheld. The advertisements were then separated into two booklets composed of one-half deceptive, or limited-disclosure, ads, and the other half of nondeceptive, or full-disclosure, ads. Following an incidental presentation of the advertisement stimuli to participants, comprehension of the ad's claims and interest in purchasing the product are assessed in a questionnaire format.

Lesion Patient Performance. Asp and colleagues (2013) sought to identify a neuroanatomical correlate for vulnerability to consumer fraud among neurological patients with acquired, focal brain lesions. Eighteen patients with VMPC damage, 21 patients with lesions outside of the prefrontal cortex, and 10 healthy, age- and education-matched comparison participants were presented the Advertising Task. The behavioral results indicated that patients with damage to the VMPC demonstrated reliably poorer comprehension of the ad's claims and endorsed more intention to purchase the products, relative to the brain-damaged control and healthy comparison groups. A lesion overlap map of those who performed abnormally on a version of our advertising task revealed that the greatest overlap was in the lower medial prefrontal areas. This study serves as an anatomical cross-validation of the basic theme of this work, that is, that the prefrontal cortex is crucial to effective consumer decision making.

Older Adult Performance. Denburg, Cole, et al. (2007) tested the hypothesis that those older adults who were impaired on the IGT would also fail to make appropriate decisions in more complex and realistic circumstances.

Here, the Advertising Task was administered to a group of young (unimpaired) gamblers and two groups of older adult decision makers, one with impaired IGT performance and one unimpaired on the IGT, in such a way that each individual participant was only exposed to one version of each ad.

As can be seen in Figure 2(A) and (B), the younger, older impaired, and older unimpaired were indistinguishable in terms of comprehension of the ads claim and purchase intentions in the nondeceptive condition (i.e., when the stimuli are entirely forthcoming, with no deceptive content). By contrast, the older impaired decision makers demonstrated poorer comprehension of deceptive ads and were more likely to say that they would purchase the product featured in them, compared with unimpaired decision makers (both old and young).

This is exactly what criminals would like to happen: That their deception promotes a miscomprehension of what the product can and cannot do, coupled with an increased desire to purchase the product. More generally, this study provides direct evidence that the subset of older adults with "impaired" decision-making abilities is more vulnerable to real-word fraudulent advertising.

Taken together, the studies with the Advertising Task provide evidence that older adults with impaired IGT performance, as well as neurological patients with acquired damage to the VMPC, demonstrate real-world deficits in consumer decision making. Furthermore, the data demonstrate that the VMPC is critical for providing the skepticism needed to identify misleading information in advertisements. In fact, preliminary evidence from an fMRI study fMRI demonstrated that increased susceptibility to deception was correlated with less activity in the VMPC (Koestner, Hedgcock, Halfmann, & Denburg, 2013). Finally, while this

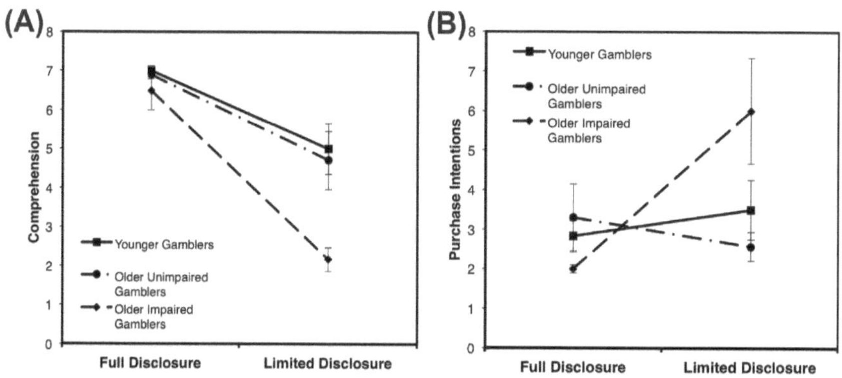

FIGURE 2 Mean comprehension of claims response (A) and purchase intentions response (B). Data are presented by group (older unimpaired vs older impaired vs younger) and by advertisement version (full disclosure vs limited disclosure).

particular study only shows that older impaired decision makers are more susceptible to deceptive advertisements, it leaves open room for future research to determine the full extent of these individuals' real-world disabilities.

Financial Decisions

Temporal Discounting. Many of the decisions faced by older adults (e.g., retirement savings) involve weighing future outcomes versus immediate desires. People often prefer smaller, immediate gains ($20 today) over larger, delayed gains ($25 a month from now), a preference behavior termed "temporal" or "time discounting." Temporal discounting also occurs in the domain of losses: Individuals tend to assign a larger subjective cost to sooner, smaller losses than later, but objectively larger losses. In other words, individuals tend to have difficulty delaying gratification and would rather delay negative consequences. This has largely been studied in younger adults, with greater rates of temporal discounting predicting an array of negative real-world outcomes such as credit card and debt behavior (Meier & Sprenger, 2010), credit scores (Meier & Sprenger, 2012), mortgage behaviors (Johnson, Atlas, & Payne, 2011), and job performance (Burks, Carpenter, Götte, & Rustichini, 2012). Temporal discounting need not be about money—it could be about food, exercise, or vaccinations. Optimal decision making is likely a function of knowing how to balance gratification and loss.

Halfmann, Hedgcock, and Denburg (2013) examined older individuals who performed either advantageously or disadvantageously on the IGT, and found that disadvantageous performance on the IGT was associated with steeper rates of discounting. As shown in Figure 3, older impaired adults tended to choose the later, larger option more frequently in the loss condition (Figure 3(A)) and the sooner, smaller option more frequently in the gain condition (Figure 3(B)), relative to their older unimpaired counterparts. Thus, these data demonstrate that previously characterized aging trajectories (i.e., strong vs weak decisional capacity on the IGT, with weaker performance suggestive of compromised emotional processing) are associated with distinct patterns of preferences in intertemporal choice.

Several groups have investigated the importance of emotion to the temporal discounting of immediate and delayed gains. There is a concept, referred to as future anhedonia, in which delayed gains are perceived as fundamentally less emotionally salient than immediate gains. Among younger adults, Kassam, Gilbert, Boston, and Wilson (2008) asked participants to rate their affective reactions to positive present events, as well as positive future events. From these ratings, a future anhedonia index was calculated. They found that future anhedonia predicted the within-subject

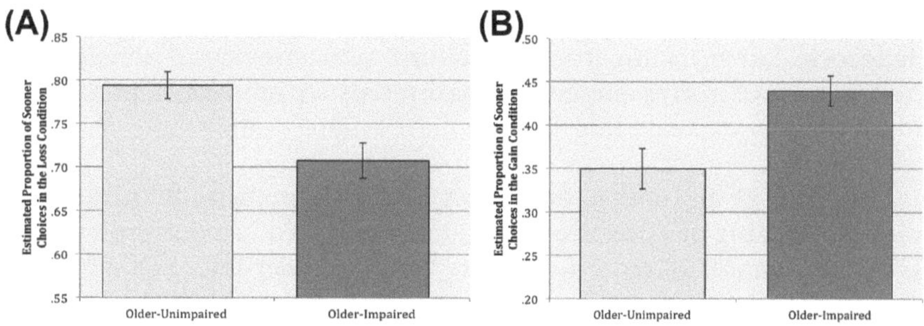

FIGURE 3 Estimated proportion of sooner choices (±SEM) in the loss condition (A) and gain condition (B). Data are presented by group (older unimpaired and older impaired adults).

rate of temporal discounting. Participants who expected to feel less pleasure in the future (i.e., future anhedonia) were less willing to wait for delayed gains.

This effect was replicated in a life-span sample of adults by Löckenhoff, O'Donoghue, and Dunning (2011). They showed that anticipation of future emotions modified the relationship between age and discounting, such that younger adults, compared to older adults, predicted future monetary gains would be less pleasing and less arousing the further in the future they occurred. Moreover, rather than cognitive factors influencing the relationship between age and discounting, dispositional affective factors such as self-reported emotional problems and social involvement were more likely to modify the relationship between age and discounting (Löckenhoff et al., 2011).

Taken together, the results of the aforementioned three studies suggest that intact emotional processing (as seen in older unimpaired and those adults with a lack of future anhedonia) is a crucial individual differences variable in intertemporal choice and is associated with reduced temporal discounting in older adults.

IGT Impairment Can Facilitate Certain Decisions

Many kinds of decisions are negatively impacted by age-related cognitive changes. But there are occasions when IGT impairment can actually signal improved decision making. Framing is an excellent example of how this can happen.

Framing Effects. Framing effects are decision biases that occur when objectively equivalent information is presented in either positive or negative terms. A classic example of the simplest type of framing—attribute framing—involves preference shifts for ground beef when the product is presented as percent lean versus percent fat (Levin, Schneider, & Gaeth, 1998). Prior research indicates that this decision bias is associated with emotional processing (De Martino, Kumaran, Seymour, & Dolan, 2006; Hedgcock, Levin, Halfmann, & Denburg, under review; Kahneman & Frederick, 2007). This suggests impairments in emotional processing might actually decrease this decision bias, making people more economically rational.

Hedgcock et al. (under review) tested this hypothesis by presenting attribute framing questions to older adults who were categorized by their IGT performance: 18 older unimpaired and 15 older impaired adults. It was predicted that the older impaired group would be *less* influenced by attribute framing (relative to the older unimpaired) as their previous failure on the IGT indicates impaired emotional processing. Results supported this prediction. Attribute valence (positive or negative) had a significant effect on preferences for older unimpaired participants but did not significantly affect older impaired participants.

In sum, this demonstrates that it is too simplistic to assume age-related cognitive changes will negatively affect all kinds of decisions. Rather, it is important to consider how specific cognitive changes will influence decision processing. For tasks such as the IGT, emotional processing improves task performance by biasing preferences away from disadvantageous decks. This means diminished emotional processing will lead to less preference shift toward good decks and lower payouts. But for tasks such as attribute framing, emotional processing hurts task performance by biasing preferences based on valence of terms. This means diminished emotional processing will lead to more consistent preferences that are less affected by framing.

Personality Traits

Investigations across the adult life span have identified personality as an important individual differences variable that is related to decision-making ability (e.g., Davis, Patte, Tweed, & Curtis, 2007). In our own work, we have shown that neuroticism (but not the remainder of the "big five" traits consisting of extraversion, openness, agreeableness, and conscientiousness) is relevant to complex decision making among older adults. Individuals high on trait neuroticism are prone to experience negative affective states, such as fear, sadness, embarrassment, guilt, and disgust. Neuroticism has also been shown to moderate brain activity to emotional stimuli (see Servaas et al., 2013, for an extensive meta-analysis on this topic). In our own work (Denburg et al., 2009), we found an interaction between IGT performance in older adults and trait neuroticism, whereby older adults with high trait neuroticism (as measured by the NEO-Five Factor Inventory or NEO-FFI) performed the most poorly on the IGT. By contrast, there was no significant relationship between trait neuroticism and IGT performance among younger adults.

We have also explored the contribution of personality factors to poor IGT performance in 58 healthy older adults ranging in age from 60 to 88 years. Rather than utilizing a self-report instrument of personality (e.g., NEO-FFI), Nguyen et al. (2013) sought out the perspective of an informant. The source of information is a relevant issue to older adults with age-related brain changes, as we know that brain-damaged individuals can be inaccurate secondary to reductions in insight (e.g., Leathem, Murphy, & Flett, 1988; Prigatano & Schacter, 1991). Moreover, Cummings et al. (1994) demonstrated that valid ratings can be achieved by knowledgeable informants utilizing rating scales with behavioral guidelines.

The *Iowa Scales of Personality Change* (ISPC; Barrash, Anderson, Hathaway-Nepple, Jones, & Tranel, 1997) is a behavior-rating scale that assesses personality changes associated with acquired neuropathological conditions (e.g., stroke, tumor, traumatic brain injury), as rated by an informant, typically a family member or close friend. Two ratings are made for each of the 30 personality characteristics: "before" (typical functioning over the adult years prior to the onset of a neuropathological condition) and "now" (typical functioning over the past several months, after the onset of a neuropathological condition). For the present study with healthy older adults, the ISPC was modified to reflect a developmental perspective (Denburg & Barrash, 2007). In this adaptation, all references to a "neurological condition" were removed, "before" ratings explicitly reflected typical personality functioning over the middle-aged years, and "now" ratings explicitly reflected typical personality functioning over the past several months.

The results indicated that it was not personality disturbances generally (even such characteristics as irascibility, disturbed social behavior, and distress), but rather disturbances in executive personality characteristics specifically, that were related to compromised decision making. More precisely, disturbances in executive personality characteristics—lack of planning, poor judgment, lack of persistence, perseveration, lack of initiative, impulsivity, and indecisiveness—were significantly associated with decision-making deficits on the IGT.

In sum, trait neuroticism and executive personality disturbances may reflect neurological "soft" signs indicative of decline in prefrontal brain regions, which in turn place older adults at risk for compromised real-world decision making. Support for this notion comes from the epidemiologic literature in which trait personality has been associated with dementia. A meta-analysis conducted by Low, Harrison, and Lackersteen (2013) revealed that neuroticism was associated with an increased risk of dementia, while conscientiousness was protective (openness was possibly protective, and agreeableness and conscientiousness were unrelated to dementia risk).

CONCLUSIONS AND IMPLICATIONS

Conclusions

In conclusion, deficits in emotional signaling caused by disproportionate age-related change in the ventromedial sector of the prefrontal cortices contribute to decision-making impairments that put some elderly people at risk for faulty real-world decision making (but see Hedgcock et al., under review, discussed previously, for an exception to this notion). The idea that emotional signals are crucial for advantageous decision making, which is a central tenet of the SMH, provides a testable account of this phenomenon at both behavioral and neural levels, as witnessed by the empirical work reviewed in this chapter.

Could an older adult who exhibits poor decision making be in an early stage of Alzheimer's disease or at greater risk for developing the disease? Although we cannot definitively answer the second part of this question, our studies indicate that isolated impaired decision making among older adults is a discrete phenomenon. It is distinct from Alzheimer's disease in terms of the brain regions affected, the course and progression of the syndrome, and the likely brain abnormalities involved. Furthermore, its clinical symptoms appear to be far more subtle than those of a dementia (see "Nomenclature," below, for further discussion). Of note, we have followed longitudinally many of the older adults in our studies for a decade or more, and there has been no emergence of other forms of dementia, such as frontotemporal dementia, at a rate higher than would be expected for the general population.

There are several gaps in our program of research that we hope to flesh out in the future. One future direction is to expand our examination of middle-aged adults. For example, harkening back to our psychophysiological finding—that unimpaired older adults demonstrate a somatic signaling that is opposite to that found among unimpaired younger adults—it would be important to know at what age this reversal in emotional signaling occurs. We are also very interested in the management of decision-making dysfunction, be it pharmacologically (e.g., with a serotonin agonist) or psychologically (e.g., with evidence-based brief psychotherapy).

Implications

Nomenclature. In the related fields of clinical neuropsychology, behavioral neurology, and neuropsychiatry, the notion that normal, healthy older adults have age-related changes in their memory abilities is so widely accepted that there are multiple terms to characterize this phenomenon, including "age-associated memory impairment" (AAMI) and "benign senescent forgetfulness." Conversely, as of yet, a formal term for age-associated changes in decision making (and other cognitive abilities referable to the integrity of the brain's frontal lobe) has not emerged, and in fact, has hardly been discussed. Having such a term would undoubtedly help to facilitate research and funding, identify at-risk individuals, and influence public policy. In this vein, we would like to propose the rubric of *age-associated executive dysfunction (AAED)* to designate normal, healthy older adults who demonstrate disproportionate decline in decision making and other executive functions.

Identification. Identification is crucial. Identifying older adults at risk for bad decisions because their prefrontal cortex is declining should be prioritized at a level comparable to the early detection of cancer or heart disease. Once detected, such at-risk elders could be provided explicit assistance or could, in extreme circumstances, have their prerogative to make weighty decisions circumscribed or abrogated (e.g., decisions shifted to a conservator or power of attorney).

Unfortunately, identification remains very challenging. We cannot always rely on the older adult to report his or her own problems, and executive dysfunction may be more difficult to detect by others in day-to-day interactions, as problems with decision making, judgment, planning, and the like may be less obvious than other cognitive problems, such as forgetfulness. People with frontal lobe dysfunction also suffer frequently from impaired awareness and insight (also known as anosognosia); they may be unaware of their own deficits and the ways in which their behavior affects other people. Neurological patients with impaired awareness may deny that they have anything wrong with them, even though their deficits are patently obvious to everyone around them. These patients are particularly liable to place themselves in harm's way, and a significant number of older adults who have fallen victim to financial scams may have such impairment. This makes it more important—and at the same time very difficult—to detect a person's potential impairment.

One of the studies reviewed does offer some promise in terms of identification. Nguyen et al. (2013) suggest that spouses and other close family members can indeed identify and quantify executive personality deficits (e.g., indecisiveness, perseveration) in their loved ones, and that these collateral observations are predictive of poorer older adult decision making, as measured by the IGT. Given how difficult it is to detect risk for future victimization among seemingly healthy, normal older adults, identifying older individuals with such personality traits and providing them closer monitoring by professionals, family, and the legal system, may be a worthwhile first step toward the protection of vulnerable elders.

Acknowledgment

Supported by NIA Career Development Award (K01 AG022033) and DANA Foundation Program in Brain and Immuno-Imaging grant, to N.L.D.

References

Allain, P., Nicoleau, S., Pinon, K., Etcharry-Bouyx, F., Barre, J., Berrut, G., et al. (2005). Executive functioning in normal aging: A study of action planning using the zoo map test. *Brain and Cognition, 57*, 4–7.

Barrash, J., Anderson, S. W., Hathaway-Nepple, J., Jones, R. D., & Tranel, D. (1997). *The Iowa scales of personality change*. Iowa City: University of Iowa, Department of Neurology.

Bauer, A., Timpe, J., Edmonds, E. C., Bechara, A., Tranel, D., & Denburg, N. L. (2013). Myopia for the future or hypersensivity to reward? Performance of older adults on two versions of the Iowa Gambling Task. *Emotion, 13*, 19–24.

Bechara, A. (2007). *Iowa Gambling Task (IGT) professional manual*. Lutz: Psychological Assessment Resources.

Bechara, A., Damasio, A. R., Damasio, H., & Anderson, S. W. (1994). Insensitivity to future consequences following damage to human prefrontal cortex. *Cognition, 50*, 7–15.

Bechara, A., Damasio, H., Tranel, D., & Damasio, A. R. (1997). Deciding advantageously before knowing the advantageous strategy. *Science, 275*, 1293–1295.

Bechara, A., Tranel, D., & Damasio, H. (2000). Characterization of the decision-making deficit of patients with ventromedial prefrontal cortex lesions. *Brain, 123*, 2189–2202.

Braver, T. S., Barch, D. M., Keys, B. A., Carter, C. S., Cohen, J. D., Kaye, J. A., et al. (2001). Context processing in older adults: Evidence for a theory relating cognitive control to neurobiology in healthy aging. *Journal of Experimental Psychology, 130*, 746–764.

Bruine de Bruin, W., Parker, A. M., & Fischhoff, B. (2012). Explaining adult age differences in decision-making competence. *Journal of Behavioral Decision Making, 25*, 352–360.

Burks, S., Carpenter, J., Götte, L., & Rustichini, A. (2012). Which measures of time preference best predict outcomes: Evidence from a large-scale field experiment. *Journal of Economic Behavior & Organization, 84*, 308–320.

Carstensen, L. L., & Charles, S. T. (1999). Emotion in the second half of life. *Current Directions in Psychological Science, 7*, 144–149.

Cowell, P. E., Turetsky, B. I., Gur, R. C., Grossman, R. I., Shtasel, D. L., & Gur, R. E. (1994). Sex differences in aging of the human frontal and temporal lobes. *Journal of Neuroscience, 14*, 4748–4755.

Cummings, J. L., Mega, M., Gray, K., Rosenberg-Thompson, S., Carusi, D. A., & Gombein, J. (1994). The neuropsychiatric inventory: Comprehension assessment of psychopathology in dementia. *Neurology, 44*, 2308–2314.

Damasio, A. R. (1994). *Descartes' error: Emotion, reason, and the human brain*. New York: Putnam.

Davis, C., Patte, K., Tweed, S., & Curtis, C. (2007). Personality traits associated with decision-making deficits. *Personality and Individual Differences, 42*, 279–290.

Death Planning Made Difficult. (2000). *The danger of living trust scams, hearing before the Special Committee on aging, United States Senate, 106th Cong., 2nd sess*. Washington, DC: U.S. Government Printing Office.

DeCarli, C., Murphy, D. G. M., McIntosh, A. R., & Horwitz, B. (1994). Discriminant analysis of Alzheimer's disease. *Archives of Neurology, 51*, 1088–1090.

Denburg, N. L. (May 2009). Neural basis of decision-making in aging. In *Invited talk presented at the NIA workshop on Advancing Integrative Psychological Research on Adaptive and Health Aging Preconference (APS)*, Berkeley, California.

Denburg, N. L., & Barrash, J. (2007). *Iowa scales of personality change: Adaptation for healthy adults*. Iowa City, Iowa: University of Iowa College of Medicine, Department of Neurology.

Denburg, N. L., Cole, C. A., Herandez, M., Yamada, T. H., Tranel, Bechara, A., et al. (2007). The orbitofrontal cortex, real-world decision making, and normal aging. *Annals of the New York Academy of Sciences, 1121*, 480–498.

Denburg, N. L., & Harshman, L. (2010). Why so many seniors get swindled: brain anomalies and poor decision-making in older adults. In *The Dana Foundation's cerebrum: Emerging ideas in brain science* (pp. 123–131). New York: Dana Press.

Denburg, N. L., Recknor, E. C., Bechara, A., & Tranel, D. (2006). Psychophysiological anticipation of positive outcomes promotes advantageous decision-making in normal older persons. *International Journal of Psychophysiology, 61*, 19–25.

Denburg, N. L., Tranel, D., & Bechara, A. (2005). The ability to decide advantageously declines prematurely in some normal older persons. *Neuropsychologia, 43*, 1099–1106.

Denburg, N. L., Weller, J. A., Kaup, A. R., LaLoggia, A., Yamada, T., Cole, C. A., et al. (2009). Poor decision-making among older adults is related to elevated levels of neuroticism. *Annals of Behavioral Medicine, 37*, 164–172.

Fabiani, M., Friedman, D., & Cheng, J. C. (1998). Individual differences in P3 scalp distribution in older adults, and their relationship to frontal lobe function. *Psychophysiology, 35*, 698–708.

Federal Trade Commission. (1991). *Federal trade commission decisions* (Vol. 114). Lewis Galoob Toys Inc. pp.187–217.

Federal Trade Commission Bureau of Consumer Protection. (1998). *Complying with the Made in USA Standard* (Federal Trade Commission Report).

Finucane, M. L., Slovic, P., Hibbard, J. H., Peters, E., Mertz, C. K., & MacGregor, D. G. (2002). Aging and decision-making competence: An analysis of comprehension and consistency skills in older versus younger adults considering health-plan options. *Journal of Behavioral Decision Making, 15*, 141–164.

Gläscher, J., Adolphs, R., Damasio, H., Bechara, A., Rudrauf, D., Calamia, M., et al. (2012). Lesion mapping of cognitive control and value-based decision making in the prefrontal cortex. *Proceedings of the National Academy of Sciences, 109*, 14681–14686.

Gunning-Dixon, F. M., & Raz, N. (2003). Neuroanatomical correlates of selected executive functions in middle-aged and older adults: A prospective MRI study. *Neuropsychologia, 41*, 1929–1941.

Halfmann, K., Hedgcock, W., Bechara, A., & Denburg, N. L. (2014). Functional neuroimaging of the Iowa Gambling Task in older adults. *Neuropsychology, 28*, 870–880.

Halfmann, K., Hedgcock, W., & Denburg, N. L. (2013). Age-related differences in discounting future gains and losses. *Journal of Neuroscience, Psychology, and Economics, 6*, 42–54.

Harlow, J. M. (1868). Recovery from the passage of an iron bar through the head. *Publications of the Massachusetts Medical Society, 2*, 327–347.

Haug, H., & Eggers, R. (1991). Morphometry of the human cortex cerebri and corpus striatum during aging. *Neurobiology of Aging, 12*, 336–338.

Hedgcock, W., Levin, I., Halfmann, K., & Denburg, N. The role of emotional processing in risk and attribute framing. under review.

Infogroup/ORC. (2010, June). Elder investment fraud and financial exploitation: A survey conducted for investor protection trust. Available from http://www.investorprotection.org/downloads/EIFFE_Survey_Report.pdf.

Jernigan, T. L., Archibald, S. L., Fennema-Notestine, C., Gamst, A. C., Stout, J. C., Bonner, J., et al. (2001). Effects of age on tissues and regions of the cerebrum and cerebellum. *Neurobiology of Aging, 22*, 581–594.

Johnson, E., Atlas, S., & Payne, J. (2011). *Time preferences, mortgage choice, and Strategic Default*. New York, NY: Columbia University, Columbia Business School. Unpublished manuscript.

Kable, J. W., & Glimcher, P. W. (2007). The neural correlates of subjective value during intertemporal choice. *Nature Neuroscience, 10*, 1625–1633.

Kahneman, D., & Frederick, S. (2007). Frames and brains: elicitation and control of response tendencies. *Trends in Cognitive Sciences, 11*, 45–46.

Kassam, K. S., Gilbert, D. T., Boston, A., & Wilson, T. D. (2008). Future anhedonia and time discounting. *Journal of Experimental Social Psychology, 44*, 1533–1537.

Kemp, B., & Liao, S. (2006). Elder financial abuse: Tips for the Medical Director. *Journal of the American Medical Directors Association, 7*, 591–593.

Knutson, B., Rick, S., Wimmer, G. E., Prelec, D., & Loewenstein, G. (2007). Neural predictors of purchases. *Neuron, 53*, 147–156.

Knutson, B., Wimmer, G. E., Rick, S., Hollon, N. G., Prelec, D., & Loewenstein, G. (2008). Neural antecedents of the endowment effect. *Neuron, 58*, 814–822.

Koestner, B., Hedgcock, W., Halfmann, K., & Denburg, N. L. (2013). Scamming depression era elders: Neuroanatomical basis for poor decision making among older adults. In *Paper presented at the annual meeting of the Association for Consumer Research,* Chicago, IL.

Leathem, J. M., Murphy, L. J., & Flett, R. A. (1998). Self- and informant-ratings on the patient compensation rating scale in patients with traumatic brain injury. *Journal of Clinical and Experimental Neuropsychology, 20*, 694–705.

Levin, I. P., Schneider, S. L., & Gaeth, G. J. (1998). All frames are not created equal: A typology and critical analysis of framing effects. *Organizational Behavior and Human Decision Processes, 76*, 149–188.

Löckenhoff, C. E., O'Donoghue, T., & Dunning, D. (2011). Age differences in temporal discounting: The role of dispositional affect and anticipated emotions. *Psychology and Aging, 26*, 274–284.

Low, L. F., Harrison, F., & Lackersteen, S. M. (2013). Does personality affect risk for dementia? A systematic review and meta-analysis. *American Journal of Geriatric Psychiatry, 21*, 713–728.

Martino, B., Kumaran, D., Seymour, B., & Dolan, R. J. (2006). Frames, biases, and rational decision-making in the human brain. *Science, 313*, 684–687.

Mather, M., & Carstensen, L. L. (2003). Aging and attentional biases for emotional faces. *Psychological Science, 14*, 409–415.

Meier, S., & Sprenger, C. (2010). Present-biased preferences and credit card borrowing. *American Economic Journal, 2*, 193–210.

Meier, S., & Sprenger, C. D. (2012). Time discounting predicts creditworthiness. *Psychological Science, 23*, 56–58.

MetLife mature market institute. (2011, June). The MetLife study of elder financial abuse: Crimes of occasion, desperation, and predation against america's elders. Available from https://www.metlife.com/assets/cao/mmi/publications/studies/2011/mmi-elder-financial-abuse.pdf.

Moye, J., & Marson, D. C. (2007). Assessment of decision-making capacity in older adults: An emerging area of practice and research. *Journals of Gerontology Series B: Psychological Sciences and Social Sciences, 62*, 3–11.

Murphy, D. G., DeCarli, C., McIntosh, A. R., Daly, E., Mentis, M. J., Pietrini, P., et al. (1996). Sex differences in human brain morphometry and metabolism: An in vivo quantitative magnetic resonance imaging and positron emission tomography study on the effect of aging. *Archives of General Psychiatry, 53*, 585–594.

National center on elder abuse. (2005). Elder abuse prevalence and incidence fact sheet. Available from http://www.ncea.aoa.gov/resources/publication/finalstatistics050331.pdf.

Nguyen, C. M., Barrash, J., Koenigs, A. L., Bechara, A., Tranel, D., & Denburg, N. L. (2013). Decision-making deficits in normal elderly persons associated with executive personality disturbances. *International Psychogeriatrics, 25*, 1811–1819.

Prigatano, G. P., & Schacter, D. L. (1991). *Awareness of deficit after brain injury: Clinical and theoretical issues*. New York: Oxford University Press.

Rangel, A., Camerer, C., & Montague, P. R. (2008). A framework for studying the neurobiology of value-based decision making. *Nature Reviews Neuroscience, 9*, 545–556.

Raz, N., Gunning, F. M., Head, D., Dupuis, J. H., McQuain, J., Briggs, S. D., et al. (1997). Selective aging of the human cerebral cortex observed in vivo: Differential vulnerability of the prefrontal gray matter. *Cerebral Cortex, 7*, 268–282.

Resnick, S. M., Pham, D. L., Kraut, M. A., Zonderman, A. B., & Davatzikos, C. (2003). Longitudinal magnetic resonance imaging studies of older adults: A shrinking brain. *The Journal of Neuroscience, 23*, 3295–3301.

Ridderinkhof, K. R., Span, M. M., & Van Der Molen, M. W. (2002). Perseverative behavior and adaptive control in older adults: Performance monitoring, rule induction, and set shifting. *Brain and Cognition, 49*, 382–401.

Ross, M., Grossmann, I., & Schryer, E. (2014). Contrary to psychological and popular opinion, there is no compelling evidence that older adults are disproportionately victimized by consumer fraud. *Perspectives of Psychological Science, 9*, 427–442.

Salat, D. H., Kaye, J. A., & Janowsky, J. S. (1999). Prefrontal gray and white matter volumes in healthy aging and Alzheimer's disease. *Archives of Neurology, 56*, 338–344.

Salthouse, T. A., Atkinson, T. M., & Berish, D. E. (2003). Executive functioning as a potential mediator of age-related decline in normal adults. *Journal of Experimental Psychology, 132*, 566–594.

Samanez-Larkin, G. R., Wagner, A. D., & Knutson, B. (2011). Expected value information improves financial risk taking across the adult life span. *Social Cognitive and Affective Neuroscience, 6*, 207–217.

Scoville, W. B., & Milner, B. (1957). Loss of recent memory after bilateral hippocampal lesions. *Journal of Neurology, Neurosurgery and Psychiatry, 20*, 11–21.

Servaas, M. N., van der Velde, J., Costafreda, S. G., Horton, P., Ormel, J., Riese, H., et al. (2013). Neuroticism and the brain: A quantitative meta-analysis of neuroimaging studies investigating emotion processing. *Neuroscience and Biobehavioral Reviews, 37*, 1518–1529.

Siegel, S. (1956). *Nonparametric statistics for the behavioral sciences*. New York: McGraw Hill.

Sorel, O., & Pennequin, V. (2008). Aging of the planning process: The role of executive functioning. *Brain and Cognition, 66*, 196–201.

Sullivan, E. V., Adalsteinsson, E., Hedehus, M., Ju, C., Moseley, M., Lim, K. O., et al. (2001). Equivalent disruption of regional white matter microstructure in ageing healthy men and women. *NeuroReport, 12*, 99–104.

Teuber, H. L. (1964). The riddle of frontal lobe function in man. In J. M. Warren, & K. Akert (Eds.), *The frontal granular cortex and behavior*. New York: McGraw-Hill.

Tranel, D. (1994). Acquired sociopathy: The development of sociopathic behavior following focal brain damage. In D. C. Fowles, P. Sutker, & S. H. Goodman (Eds.), *Progress in experimental personality and psychopathology research* (Vol. 17, pp. 285–311). New York: Springer.

Waldemar, G., Hasselbach, S., Anderson, A. R., Delecluse, F., Petersen, P., Johnsen, A., et al. (1991). 99mTc-*d,l*-HMPAO and SPECT of the brain in normal aging. *Journal of Cerebral Blood Flow Metabolism, 11*, 508–521.

Weller, J. A., Levin, I. P., Shiv, B., & Bechara, A. (2007). Neural correlates of adaptive decision making for risky gains and losses. *Psychological Science, 18*, 958–964.

West, R. (1996). An application of prefrontal cortex function theory of cognitive aging. *Psychological Bulletin, 120*, 272–292.

Xiao, L., Wood, S. M., Denburg, N. L., Moreno, G. L., Hernandez, M., & Bechara, A. (2013). Is there a recovery of decision-making function after frontal lobe damage? A study using alternative versions of the Iowa Gambling Task. *Journal of Clinical and Experimental Neuropsychology, 35*, 518–529.

SECTION 2

BEHAVIORAL MECHANISMS

CHAPTER

6

Adaptive Decision Making and Aging

Rui Mata[1, 2], *Anika K. Josef*[2], *Patrick Lemaire*[3, 4]

[1]Department of Psychology, University of Basel, Basel, Switzerland; [2]Max Planck Institute for Human Development, Berlin, Germany; [3]Université de Provence, Marseille, France; [4]Centre National de la Recherche Scientifique, Paris, France

It is a truism that different problems require different solutions. In other words, to maximize performance, individuals must select actions as a function of their fit to the problem at hand. But how does aging alter the ability to adapt behavior as a function of the problem? In this chapter, we adopt an ecological perspective on decision making that links life-span changes in core cognitive abilities to strategy use, and ultimately, decision performance in different environments or tasks. This perspective suggests that life-span changes in decision making may arise from changes in the ability to adaptively select and accurately execute decision strategies. In what follows, we first discuss the concept of decision strategies as well as potential effects of aging on strategy use. Second, we review similar concepts and empirical results from the aging literature on memory and arithmetic computation to help us inform decision-making research. Finally, we present a review of aging and adaptive decision making with an outlook on future research in this area.

AN ECOLOGICAL PERSPECTIVE ON LIFE-SPAN CHANGES IN STRATEGY USE

In Cicero's *de Senectute*, Cato the Elder explains to two younger men that the key to successful aging lies not in struggling to regain the strength of youth but in using the available resources adaptively: "Nor, again, do I now miss the bodily strength of a young man... You should use what you have, and whatever you may chance to be doing, do it with all

Aging and Decision Making
http://dx.doi.org/10.1016/B978-0-12-417148-0.00006-6

your might." Past and current research on aging emphasizes the importance of adaptation to the environment in dealing with changes brought about by aging (Bronfenbrenner, 1979; Lindenberger & Mayr, 2014). We aim to bring this adaptivity aspect to bear on the research on aging and decision making by introducing the perspective of ecological rationality (Gigerenzer & Todd, 1999; Mata, Pachur, et al., 2012). From this perspective, there is no domain-general answer to the question of how changes in cognitive capabilities—commonly, gain in childhood and adolescence but decline in old age—affect decision making. Our thesis is that the impact of changes in cognitive capabilities depends strongly on the demands of specific task environments and ecologies. In other words, the quality of decisions made by people of all ages is the result of how task demands and affordances interact with particular cognitive strategies. To better understand this interaction, we suggest, one needs to describe the structure of decision environments, the processes of strategy use, and the cognitive capacities that strategies exploit, including their developmental trajectories (see Figure 1).

Strategies can be defined as sequences of operations or processes that are goal-directed—that is, are aimed at accomplishing a particular task and therefore, mediate task performance (Pressley, Borowski, & Schneider, 1987; Reese, 1962). The strategy concept has been used to describe cognitive processes and mechanisms of human cognition in many domains including memory (Bjorklund & Harnishfeger, 1990; Dunlosky & Hertzog, 1998), arithmetic (Ashcraft, 1992; Lemaire, 2010), and decision making (Payne, 1976; Payne, Bettman, & Johnson, 1993). For example, use of different strategies has been found when participants encode pairs of words in associative recall tasks (Dunlosky & Hertzog, 1998), estimate the correct solution to an arithmetic problem in a computational estimation task (Duverne & Lemaire, 2004), mentally rotate objects (Cohen & Faulkner, 1983), verify sentences (Reder, 1982), integrate (e.g., add) multiple pieces of information in order to evaluate a decision alternative (Dawes, 1979), or reason about arguments (Bucciarelli & Johnson-Laird, 1999; Girotto & Gonzalez, 2001; Hartley & Anderson, 1983).

To summarize, the notion of ecological rationality sees decision making as the result of the fit between the human mind and the environment. In turn, the concept of strategy provides the mediating mechanism between environments and individuals' core abilities, such as attention and memory (Marewski & Schooler, 2011; Stevens & Hauser, 2004). There are a number of useful distinctions arising from the strategy framework; that is, the idea that behavior of agents can be understood as the deployment of different strategies (cf. Gigerenzer & Todd, 1999; Lemaire & Siegler, 1995; Payne et al., 1993; Siegler & Lemaire, 1997). One important distinction that can be made within this context is that between strategy selection and strategy execution. From an ecological perspective, each strategy may

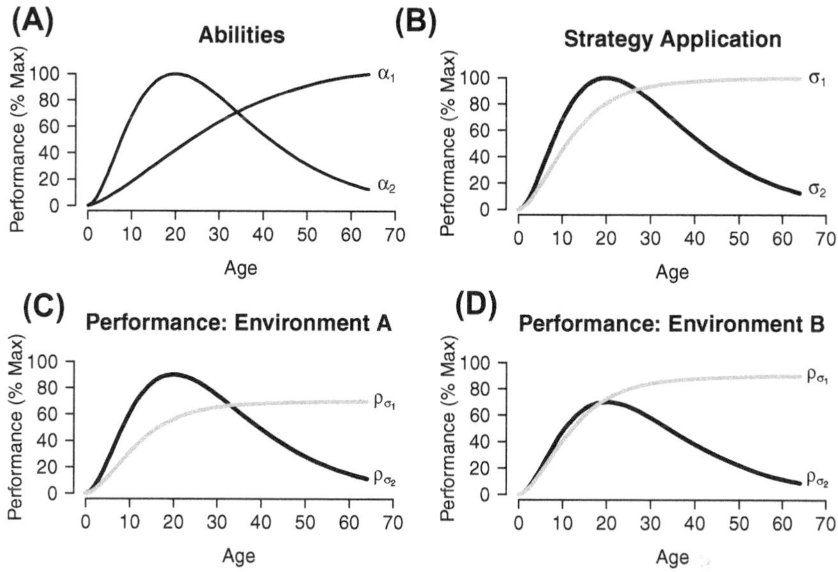

FIGURE 1 Decomposition of decision-making performance across the life span. (A) Distinct age-related patterns of change in basic cognitive abilities, skills, and knowledge, with some showing early peaks (e.g., fluid abilities; α_1) and, others, more protracted but sustained performance across the life span (e.g., crystallized abilities; α_2). (B) The pattern of performance for different decision strategies depends on which cognitive abilities, skills, or knowledge strategies rely on: Although some strategies may tap predominantly into early-peaking abilities (e.g., fluid abilities; σ_1), others may tap into both early- and late-peaking abilities (e.g., fluid and crystallized abilities; σ_2). (C, D) The final impact on performance depends on the strategy–environment fit, with some environments favoring one strategy over another and leading to different age-related patterns of decision performance, including cross-over (environment A) or dominance of particular strategies (environment B). Under the assumption that decision makers are adaptive, differential effectiveness of strategies should lead decision makers to select different strategies as a function of the environment and their own abilities.

be seen as occupying a particular niche that is the product of particular environmental characteristics as well as the core cognitive abilities that are available to exploit the former (Marewski & Schooler, 2011). Given a toolbox or repertoire of strategies, each fitting particular tasks or environments, it becomes crucial to adaptively select a strategy that suits the challenge at hand to do well in a particular situation—the issue of strategy selection. Another related but potentially orthogonal aspect of strategy use concerns the ability of agents to execute a strategy successfully—the issue of strategy execution; that is, the ability to carry out all subcomponents correctly, in the appropriate order, and at the right time. Note that, in principle, strategy selection and execution processes are dissociable: Agents may know which strategies to select and yet not be able to execute them correctly, or vice versa. More central to the issue of how aging impacts the use of decision strategies is the question of which cognitive mechanisms underlie these components of strategy use. In particular, do age-related changes in basic cognitive abilities impact strategy selection and execution and, if so, do they do so differentially?

In the remainder of this chapter, we first present two classes of abilities that plausibly underlie age differences in strategy selection and execution, cognitive control and reward processing, and then review work from the memory, arithmetic computation, and decision-making domains to evaluate the role of these cognitive processes in determining the link between aging and strategy use.

COGNITIVE AGING: THE ROLE OF COGNITIVE CONTROL AND REWARD PROCESSING

Aging is associated with a large range of structural and neuromodulatory brain changes, which in turn are associated with detectable decline in behavioral measures of fluid abilities, such as those measuring working-memory, episodic memory, or reasoning (Nyberg & Bäckman, 2010; Rodrigue & Kennedy, 2010; Verhaeghen & Salthouse, 1997). The links between these basic abilities and strategy use are not yet understood, but past work suggests that there are at least two general aspects of cognitive function that may lead to changes in strategy use: (1) cognitive control, including manipulation of information in working memory and the selective and strategic retrieval of information from long-term memory; and (2) reward processing, including the ability to compute prediction errors associated with learning from probabilistic feedback.

First, regarding cognitive control, there is some consensus that cognitive control involves fronto-parietal neural systems and that these may be significantly affected by aging. Cognitive control is an umbrella term for the system or class of processes that are involved in controlling or managing other cognitive processes such as maintaining and updating information in working memory, focusing attention in the face of interference, or the strategic retrieval of information from memory (e.g., Diamond, 2013; Gazzaley & Nobre, 2012). In this vein, cognitive control can be understood as the link between traditionally disparate cognitive domains or abilities, such as inhibitory function, memory, and potentially, decision making (Gazzaley & Nobre, 2012; Lenartowcz, Kalar, Congdon, & Poldrack, 2010; Ridderinkhof, Ullsperger, Crone, & Nieuwenhuis, 2004). Recent research shows that the ability to adapt behavior to specific task demands results from the flexible interaction of this fronto-parietal brain network with other brain regions (Cole et al., 2013). In turn, aging research has shown that cognitive control mechanisms may suffer from substantial age-related decline due to aging of frontal regions of the brain (West, 1996).

For example, researchers have suggested that age deficits in episodic and working memory may be explained, at least partly, by the impact of aging on the strategic manipulation and control of information guided by frontal structures (Sander, Werkle-Bergner, & Lindenberger, 2011; Shing, Werkle-Bergner, Li, & Lindenberger, 2008).

Second, regarding reward processing, results from behavioral experiments, computational modeling, and neuroimaging studies suggest that age-related deficits in reward processing are central to age differences in adapting decision behavior to specific task structures (Eppinger, Hämmerer, & Li, 2011). Recent work has directly related these limitations to dopaminergic function in striatal regions of the brain (Chowdhury et al., 2013; Samanez-Larkin, Kuhnen, Yoo, & Knutson, 2010). For example, Samanez-Larkin et al. (2010) examined age differences in dynamic financial decisions with functional neuroimaging: Older adults made more suboptimal choices than younger adults when choosing risky assets, and this age-related effect was mediated by a neural measure of temporal variability in nucleus accumbens activity, a neural structure related to reward processing. More generally, prior research on age differences in neural reward processing has revealed that the representation of reward magnitude in the striatum and medial prefrontal cortex remains intact in old age (Cox, Aizenstein, & Fiez, 2008; Samanez-Larkin et al., 2007; Samanez-Larkin et al., 2010), but that the computation of expected value during tasks that require probabilistic learning are disrupted in these same regions; however, it can be restored with dopaminergic supplementation in older adults (Chowdhury et al., 2013). All in all, age-related deficits in reward processing seem likely to affect adaptive behavior when representations must be built from feedback.

In sum, research on age-related cognitive change suggests that there are significant alterations of structural and neuromodulatory efficiency that may underlie age differences in cognitive control and learning. But what are the implications of such cognitive changes to adaptive strategy use? In what follows, we provide a first attempt at answering this question by considering the aging literature on strategy use in different domains. Our goal is to obtain a broad picture of the link between aging and strategy use, and to evaluate the extent to which deficits in cognitive control and reward processing may underlie age differences in strategy selection or execution.

AGING AND STRATEGY USE

Our main focus below is on reviewing the literature on aging and strategy use in the decision-making domain. However, we first review related work on memory and arithmetic computation. Indeed, there is considerable research in the latter areas using the strategy framework and thus concerned with identifying age differences in different aspects of strategy use, such as selection and execution. Unfortunately, there is little cross-talk between research areas, and so it is unclear to what extent the behavioral patterns and prevailing explanations generalize across domains. Yet the cognitive processes underlying strategy use in memory, arithmetic, and decision making likely overlap. Therefore, the review below offers an opportunity to assess the degree of overlap in findings and mechanisms of age differences in strategy use across domains.

Aging and Strategy Use in Memory

There is a long tradition of considering the role of strategies in the development of memory performance, as well as distinguishing different components of strategy use, such as selection and execution (Flavell, 1976; see Schneider, 2011, for an overview). Before we proceed, however, let us make a terminological clarification. The term *production deficiency* has been often used in memory research to refer to difficulties in generating (producing) a strategy for a given problem (cf. Schneider, 2011). This concept is analogous to the concept of strategy selection, albeit the former has the connotation that strategies are formed online rather than selected from a preexisting repertoire or toolbox (Gigerenzer & Todd, 1999). In turn, the concept of *utilization deficiency* has been used to refer to difficulties in the ability of individuals to produce adequate performance given that a particular strategy was used; we call this *strategy execution*. Note, however, that *mediation deficiency* has also been used in the memory literature to refer to the lack of strategic behavior in memory tasks (cf. Schneider, 2011). In what follows, we adopt the common usage in decision research of distinguishing between strategy selection and execution.

The concept of strategy in memory research is typically associated with mnemonic procedures devised to enhance memory performance during either encoding or retrieval. For example, different strategies may be used to encode pairs of words in an episodic memory task, such as when memorizing paired associates, including rote repetition, the use of imagery, or sentence generation. Research in this domain suggests that older adults engage in memory-relevant strategy processes less often and less efficiently than do younger adults, but there is still debate concerning the extent to which strategic processes can fully account for age differences in several aspects of memory functioning (see Hertzog & Dunlosky, 2004, for an overview). For example, Dunlosky and Hertzog (1998) (see also Touron & Hertzog, 2004; Touron, Hertzog, & Frank, 2011) showed that age differences in episodic memory are not fully described by a deficiency in older adults to select (produce) effective strategies and that other issues, namely, strategy execution (utilization) deficits, may be needed to account for age differences in memory performance. Indeed, most current views on memory performance assign "blame" to at least two components of memory. Specifically, aging is thought to impact both the strategic manipulation and control of information (strategic component) and the basic encoding and storage of information as a bound memory representation (associative component; Bouazzaoui et al., 2010; Sander et al., 2011; Shing et al., 2008). Whereas the strategic component is thought to be more localized in frontal brain areas, the associative memory components are thought to be posterior (parietal, temporal), and it is commonly assumed that the posterior activations during memory retrieval are controlled by the prefrontal cortex (e.g., Badre & Wagner, 2014; Buckner & Wheeler, 2001). These views dovetail nicely with the cognitive control hypothesis, which suggests that age differences in frontal brain areas are responsible for age differences in strategy use, such as those strategies involved in memory encoding and retrieval.

In sum, the literature on age differences in strategy use in memory suggests that age differences in decision performance may be partly attributed to differences in the selection and execution of different strategies. Importantly, the deficits in strategy selection and execution are partly attributable to age-related deficits in cognitive control abilities and thus go beyond aging decline in associative memory.

Aging and Strategy Use in Arithmetic

Strategic variations and age-related differences have been the object of numerous investigations in arithmetic. Studies have shown that both young and older participants use a wide variety of strategies to accomplish arithmetic tasks, whether they have to find the exact (e.g., $8 \times 7 = 56$) or approximate (e.g., $23 \times 47 = 1000$) answers to problems. Previous research also found that young and older adults differ in some but not in other arithmetic tasks in terms of which strategy they use, how often they use each available strategy, and how they execute and select strategies.

Regarding the repertoire of strategies, Lemaire and Lecacheur (2007) identified the same set of nine strategies to solve two-digit addition problems (e.g., $23 + 58$) in groups of young and older adults. These nine strategies included strategies such as rounding both operands down (i.e., doing $20 + 50 = 70 + 3 + 8 = 70 + 11 = 81$), sometimes both operands up (i.e., $30 + 60 = 90 - 9 = 81$), sometimes one operand up (i.e., $23 + 60 = 83 - 2 = 81$), sometimes one operand down (i.e., $20 + 58 = 78 + 3 = 81$). Lemaire and Arnoud (2008), however, found that individual older adults tended to use only a subset of these nine strategies and overall fewer relative to young adults. Similarly, Duverne and Lemaire (2004) found that young adults used two types of verification strategies for arithmetic problems, namely the plausibility strategy for problems such as $8 + 4 < 59$ (true/false?) and the exhaustive verification strategy for problems such as $8 + 4 < 13$, whereas older adults used only one (exhaustive verification) strategy. Thus, age-related differences in the repertoire of strategies used are often found in the arithmetic domain.

More often reported in the literature are age-related differences in strategy distributions. Even when young and older adults use the same set of strategies, they may use each available strategy in different proportions and show different strategy preferences, above and beyond older adults tending to more often use the easier strategy. For example, in a series of experiments on numerosity estimation tasks (i.e., in which participants are shown collections of dots on a computer screen and have to quickly estimate the number of dots, without counting the dots exactly), Gandini and colleagues investigated strategy distributions while controlling strategy repertoire by allowing participants to use only one of two available strategies on each problem (Gandini, Lemaire, Anton, & Nazarian, 2008; Gandini, Lemaire, & Dufau, 2008; Gandini, Lemaire, & Michel, 2009). The authors found that young adults used the perceptual strategy (i.e., scanning the whole pattern or a subset of dots, searching a corresponding numerosity in memory, and adding or subtracting a small amounts to this retrieved numerosity before stating a response) and the anchoring strategy (i.e., counting groups of dots and adding the number of groups before estimating the remaining dots) equally often whereas older adults used the perceptual strategy more often than the anchoring strategy. Such age differences in strategy distributions have been found in a number of other arithmetic studies (e.g., Geary & Lin, 1998; Lemaire, Arnaud, & Lecacheur, 2004).

In almost all studies assessing age differences in strategy execution, older adults were less efficient (either slower or less accurate, or both) than young adults. These differences were found even when strategy selection biases (i.e., differences over participants and/or over items in strategy use) were controlled via the choice/no-choice method proposed by Siegler and Lemaire (1997). In this method, participants are tested under a choice condition (in which they can choose whichever strategy they want among available strategies on each problem) and under no-choice conditions (in which they are asked to use a given strategy on all problems). For example, in their studies on numerosity estimation, Gandini et al. (Gandini, Lemaire, Anton, et al., 2008; Gandini, Lemaire, & Dufau, 2008; Gandini et al., 2009) found that older adults were slower than young adults while executing the anchoring strategy but both age groups were equally fast when executing the perceptual strategy. These age differences in strategy execution have also been found when participants are asked to calculate the exact or approximate answer to simple (e.g., 3×6) or more complex (e.g., 43×28) problems (e.g., Ardiale & Lemaire, 2013; Geary & Lin, 1998; Lemaire & Hinault, 2014; Uittenhove & Lemaire, 2013).

Finally, age differences have been found in strategy selection. For example, when asked to select the best strategy for each problem during a computational estimation task, older adults were less able to select the best strategy than young adults, and tended to repeatedly use the same strategy, even when it would have been better to switch (e.g., Ardiale & Lemaire, 2013; Lemaire & Leclère, 2014). To illustrate, Lemaire et al. (2004) asked young and older adults to find approximate products for arithmetic problems (e.g., 46 × 52). For each problem, participants were asked to choose the best between two strategies, the rounding-up and rounding-down strategies. As the names suggest, the rounding-up strategy involves rounding both operands up (e.g., 50 × 60), whereas the rounding-down strategy involves rounding both operands down (e.g., 40 × 50). The two strategies have, however, distinct ecologies or niches: The rounding-down strategy yields the best product for problems involving smaller unit-digits (<5, small-unit problems), such as 51 × 62, whereas the rounding-up strategy is best for problems involving larger unit digits (>5, large-unit problems), such as 57 × 69. Lemaire and colleagues found that young adults selected the best strategy for each problem type significantly more often than did older adults (65% vs 57%). These results match other findings in memory research suggesting that older adults show reduced meta-awareness of when particular strategies should be deployed (e.g., Brigham & Pressley, 1988).

The mechanisms of age differences in strategies are still under investigation, but some findings suggest that cognitive control deficits may be one source of age differences in arithmetic problem-solving. For example, Duverne and Lemaire (2004) found that 70% of age-related variance in strategy use in arithmetic problem-solving tasks is mediated by processing speed, a fluid ability measure. Similarly, Hodzik and Lemaire (2011) found that 91% of age-related variance in strategy repertoire (i.e., mean number of strategies used by individuals) and 44% of age-related variance in strategy selection (i.e., mean number of best strategy use on each problem) were accounted for by general executive control processes (e.g., inhibition, switching). One open issue is the exact mechanism whereby cognitive control limits available strategies, and whether it does so by affecting strategy selection, strategy execution, or both.

In sum, the literature on age differences in strategy use in arithmetic suggests that age differences may be attributed to differences in strategy use, including the adaptive selection and efficient execution of specific strategies. Importantly, the strong association between individual differences in strategy use and fluid cognitive abilities supports the idea that cognitive control abilities may underlie age differences in strategy selection and execution.

AGING AND STRATEGY USE IN DECISION MAKING

The strategy approach has a long tradition in decision research, with various strategies having been proposed, each with its particular cognitive demands and domain of execution (see Shah & Oppenheimer, 2008, for an overview). But what are the mechanisms underlying the adaptive selection of decision strategies? Decision research has proposed cost–benefit approaches to explain how people select from a repertoire of strategies (e.g., Beach & Mitchell, 1978). According to this view, decision makers weigh the different costs (e.g., the cognitive effort and time involved in executing a strategy) against the benefits (e.g., its accuracy in making decisions) to make a decision about which strategy to select. In line with this idea, research has shown that, for example, in conditions under which the selection of complex decision strategies is cognitively costly (e.g., under time pressure or when search in memory is necessary), people rely on simpler strategies that reduce cognitive load (e.g., Bröder & Schiffer, 2003; Ford, Schmitt, Schechtmann, Hults, & Doherty, 1989; Payne, Bettmann, & Johnson, 1988, 1993). In some cases, this cost–benefit calculus may be learned on a trial-by-trial basis, when decision makers learn about the relative value of particular strategies over time. In this case, strategy selection may be considered a reinforcement learning process at the level of strategies, and formal theories have been proposed to account for this process (Rieskamp & Otto, 2006).

What about age differences in strategy use? One intuition is that aging may lead to increased reliance on simpler strategies. Anecdotal evidence supports this view: Franz Müntefering, a leading political figure in Germany, when asked, at age 67, how he coped with his job, answered that "although one is no longer so fast, or innovative, one knows the shortcuts" (Haselberger & Solms-Laubach, 2012). Earlier work identified age differences in either information search or final choices, which are possible indicators of strategy selection (e.g., Johnson, 1990; see Mather, 2006, for an overview). However, only more recently has there been resurgent interest in this line of work. More recent studies have systematically varied task demands, used specially designed stimuli, and employed more specific strategy assessments (e.g., via verbal protocols or computational modeling) to discriminate between strategies and thus more reliably capture age differences in strategy selection (e.g., Mata, Schooler, & Rieskamp, 2007; Queen, Hess, Ennis, Dowd, & Grühn, 2012; Worthy & Maddox, 2012). As an overview, Table 1 provides a list of decision strategies and their niches of execution, as well as some of our own studies that have investigated age differences as a function of task characteristics. We also provide references for studies investigating the neural bases of these strategies because, as we will argue later, this is a promising avenue for future work aimed at understanding age differences in strategy use.

TABLE 1 Overview of Prototypical Decision Strategies, Their Ecological Niches, and Example Studies Investigating Age Differences and Neural Correlates of Strategy Use

Strategy Description (*Seminal Study*)	Ecological Niche	Differences Between Young and Older Adults	Neural Correlates
RECOGNITION If one of two alternatives is recognized, infer that it has the higher value on the criterion (Goldstein & Gigerenzer, 2002).	Little knowledge available, validity of recognition is larger than chance	Older adults show a tendency to rely on recognition (Pachur, Mata, & Schooler, 2009).	Volz et al. (2006)
TAKE-THE-BEST To infer which of two alternatives has the higher value, (1) search through cues in order of validity, (2) stop search as soon as a cue discriminates, and (3) choose the alternative this cue favors (Gigerenzer & Goldstein, 1996).	High cue redundancy	Older adults rely more on take-the-best (Mata et al., 2007).	Khader et al. (2011); Gluth et al. (2014)
TALLYING To infer which of two alternatives has the higher value, count the number of positive cues of each alternative and choose the one with the higher sum (Dawes, 1979).	Low cue redundancy, uncertainty about the cue weights	Older adults rely more on tallying (Mata, von Helversen, & Rieskamp, 2010).	Gluth et al. (2014)
WEIGHTED ADDITIVE To infer which of two alternatives has the higher value, multiply each cue value by the respective cue weight, sum the results for each alternative, and choose the one with the higher sum (Payne et al., 1993).	Low cue redundancy, good knowledge of cue importance	Older adults rely less on the weighted additive strategy (Mata et al., 2007; 2010).	—

Pachur et al. (2009) investigated age differences in the adaptive use of recognition in decision making. Specifically, Pachur and colleagues examined this issue by asking younger and older adults to make inferences regarding pairs of cities ("Which city has more inhabitants?") and infectious diseases ("Which disease is more prevalent?"). A prominent model of a simple inference strategy, the recognition heuristic (Goldstein & Gigerenzer, 2002), assumes that in those cases for which individuals recognize only one of the objects they may base their judgments on whether or not the options are recognized (see Table 1). This heuristic or strategy often leads to accurate inference because it exploits the phenomenon that known objects differ from unknown ones in statistically systematic ways in many real-world environments (e.g., larger cities, more successful athletes, and higher mountains tend to be recognized more often; Pachur, Todd, Gigerenzer, Schooler, & Goldstein, 2011). However, this is not true for all environments, and indeed recognition validity is low (about 0.6) in the case of disease prevalence (compared to above 0.9 in the cities environment). The main question of interest was whether young and older adults showed similar levels of *environment* or *task adaptivity*, in particular, whether participants chose the recognized object more often in the cities relative to the diseases environment. Pachur et al. found that both young and older participants chose recognized objects more frequently over unrecognized ones in a domain with high recognition validity (cities) than in a domain with low recognition validity (diseases), and thus that both younger and older adults were adaptive decision makers. However, older adults also showed a (weak) tendency to use the recognition cue more than younger adults.

Similar age differences have been reported regarding more complex strategies. Mata et al. (2007) asked older adults to make inferences about which of two diamonds is more expensive based on a number of cues (see Figure 2). Mata and colleagues asked participants to make inferences in an environment in which either all cues were equally predictive of the criterion (equal validities), or alternatively, some cues were significantly more informative than others (dispersed validities). Using a simple strategy, such as take-the-best, would yield the higher payoff in the dispersed validities condition. A weighted-additive strategy, which weights the attribute values based on how well they predict price, would yield the higher payoff in the equal-validities environment. Participants were classified according to which strategy described their decisions best. The results suggest that both young and older adults were able to adjust their strategy selection as a function of task structure. However, older adults showed a tendency to rely on simpler strategies regardless of environment (see Figure 3). In fact, such a pattern of age differences may extend to other inference problems, such as estimation and categorization tasks, with older adults defaulting to less cognitively demanding strategies,

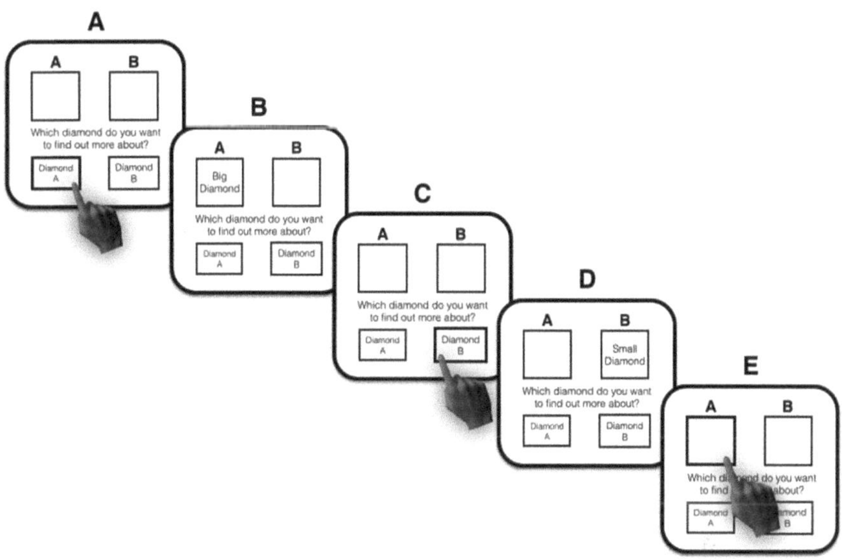

FIGURE 2 Experimental display and example of executing the take-the-best strategy in Mata et al. (2007). Mata et al. conducted an experiment in which the participants had to infer which of two diamonds was more expensive. When making their inferences, participants were able to look up information about each diamond using a computerized display (eight dichotomous attributes, such as size, cut, clarity). (A) The participant presses a button to see information concerning Diamond A. (B) The participant observes the cue value for 2 s. (C) The participant presses a button to see information concerning Diamond B. (D) The participant observes the cue value for 2 s. (E) The participant chooses Diamond A by pressing the appropriate button.

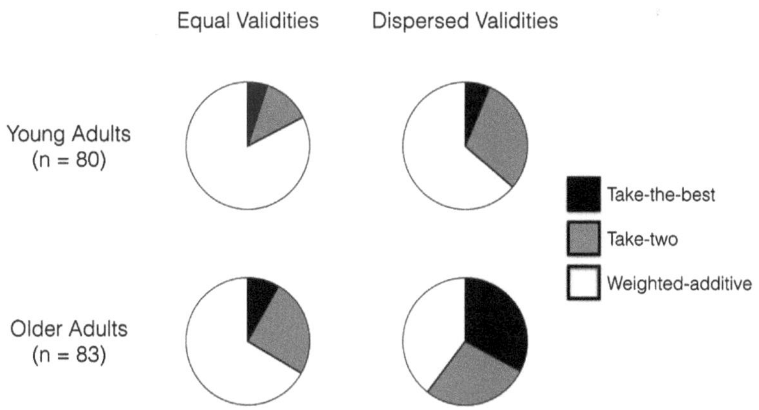

FIGURE 3 Proportion of young and older adults classified as users of different strategies in Mata et al. (2007). The results show that older adults are adaptive decision makers but rely more on simpler strategies relative to young adults.

for example, those that do not rely heavily on memory retrieval (Mata, von Helversen, Karlsson, & Cüpper, 2012).

It is plausible to assume that cognitive control deficits brought about by aging may underlie the increased tendency to rely on simpler strategies. After all, reliance on simple strategies has been related to individual differences in fluid abilities, such as working memory (Mata et al., 2007). However, several mechanisms may underlie such deficits, including failure to identify environment–strategy fit, difficulty integrating costs and benefits of particular strategies, and an inability to execute particular strategies. Unfortunately, to our knowledge, there are no studies that have explicitly addressed each of these mechanisms. Future studies employing the choice/no-choice method (Siegler & Lemaire, 1997)—that is, in which participants are tested under a choice condition (in which they can select which strategy to execute) and under a no-choice condition (in which they are asked to execute a specific strategy)—could be particularly useful in distinguishing the impact of strategy execution on selection, and vice versa.

Age-related changes in reward processing may also affect strategy selection. Mata et al. (2010) investigated the ability of younger and older adults to adapt their decision strategies as a function of environment structure when provided with massive performance feedback. Participants made inferences about which of three stocks would be more profitable given a number of cues. After an initial block of choices without feedback, participants received trial-by-trial feedback in 170 inferences. Other work with a similar task suggests that reinforcement learning at the level of strategies provides a good description of how participants adjust behavior through reward-based processes (Rieskamp & Otto, 2006). Also, as expected, learning in the task seems to have a distinct neural signature associated with prediction errors in striatal structures (Gluth, Rieskamp, & Buechel, 2014). Mata et al. (2010) showed that, although both younger and older adults were adaptive in choosing a strategy that matched the task environment, older adults showed poorer learning relative to younger adults, particularly in an environment favoring the use of a more cognitively demanding strategy, the weighted-additive rule, which requires extensive information integration (see Figure 4). The results from Mata et al. (2010) match other work using simpler probabilistic learning tasks focusing on model-free learning that show that age-related changes in reward processing can lead to failures in adapting behavior to the statistical structure of the environment, possibly due to deficits in dopaminergic neuromodulation (e.g., Chowdury et al., 2013).

Decision researchers have investigated the cognitive demands of executing particular decision strategies (e.g., Bettman, Johnson, & Payne, 1990). However, only a few studies have investigated age differences in strategy execution. Those studies that have explicitly instructed young and older adults to apply specific decision strategies suggest that aging

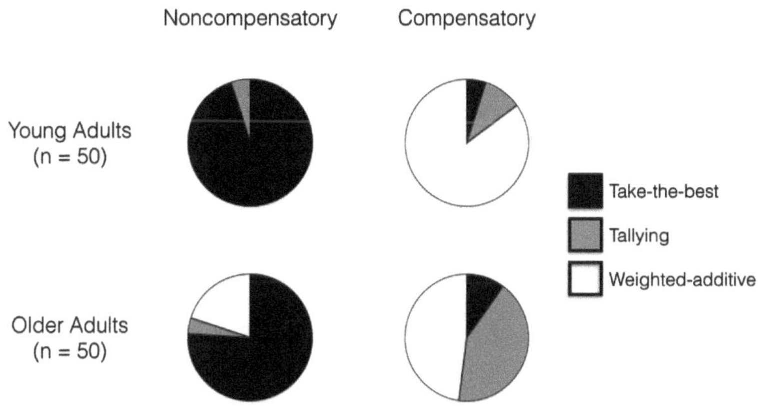

FIGURE 4 Proportion of young and older adults classified as users of different strategies after extensive training through performance feedback in Mata et al. (2010). The results show that older subjects learn to use strategies adaptively but have difficulties executing cognitively demanding strategies, such as a weighted-additive strategy.

is associated with error rates (Bruine de Bruin, Parker, & Fischhoff, 2007). However, these studies have not typically considered the role of strategy or interactions with task complexity. The study by Mata et al. (2010) described above relied on computational modeling to decompose the decision process of younger and older adults, which included a strategy execution component. The results suggest that age differences do differ by strategy: Older adults showed increased strategy execution errors relative to younger adults, particularly in an environment favoring complex strategies that require extensive integration and weighing of information.

Executing decision strategies may be particularly effortful and error prone when this involves manipulating and retrieving information from memory (Bröder & Schiffer, 2003). Khader et al. (2011) monitored the activation of specific representations of attribute knowledge with functional magnetic resonance imaging (fMRI) while participants made decisions using take-the-best. The amount of information required for a decision was reflected in activation of the dorsolateral prefrontal cortex and this activation modulated posterior areas responsible for memory storage. Given older adults' difficulties in strategic retrieval and manipulation of information (Park & Reuter-Lorenz, 2009; Shing et al., 2008), it is natural to assume that age-related deficits in cognitive control have a direct impact on strategy execution in decisions from memory.

One open issue in the literature is to what extent age differences in information search and strategy selection change as a function of the number of options in the decision task. In general, empirical results concerning the role of number of options is equivocal. The too-much-choice hypothesis (Iyengar & Lepper, 2000) predicts that people forego choice or choose simpler options as set sizes increase. However, recent analyses suggest that choice overload is not to be taken for granted but could depend on particular details of the task and perhaps on individuals' abilities (Hills, Noguchi, & Gibbert, 2013; Scheibehenne, Greifeneder, & Todd, 2010). Results of a meta-analysis with a small number of studies suggest that older adults search less information relative to younger adults before making a decision, and that this difference may increase when informational demands are high (Mata & Nunes, 2010). Likewise, studies have consistently found that older adults often prefer having less choice relative to younger adults (Mikels, Reed, & Simon, 2009). However, such effects are not always found (e.g., Queen et al., 2012) and the mechanisms underlying age differences are not well understood (cf., Reed, Mikels, & Lockenhoff, 2013). Some have suggested that age differences arise only in situations that are of low-motivational investment for older adults (Hess, Queen, & Ennis, 2013). Other work found that incidental positive affect may also account for age differences in information search (von Helversen & Mata, 2012). Overall, the heterogeneous findings suggest that considerable work still needs to be done to uncover the causes underlying age differences in choice-rich environments.

In sum, the literature on age differences in strategy use in decision making suggests that there are significant age differences in the adaptive selection and efficient execution of decision strategies. The results from this literature further emphasize the potential moderating role of both environment and strategy characteristics; specifically, age differences seem to be particularly evident in those tasks or for those strategies that have high memory demands or require learning from probabilistic feedback. These results favor theories that emphasize the role of age differences in cognitive control and reward processing on age differences in the use of decision strategies.

IMPLICATIONS OF AGE DIFFERENCES IN STRATEGY SELECTION AND EXECUTION

Judging from the average age of people in the *Forbes* 2013 *World's Most Powerful People*—61 years—political and economic power is concentrated in the hands of people who are, on average, considerably older than the general population (Howard, 2013). Older adults' overrepresentation in influential roles may be intensified in the future by demographic aging across the globe (Christensen, Doblhammer, Rau, & Vaupel, 2009). The extent to which older adults rely on simpler strategies that ignore information could have important implications for a number of domains, including consumer (e.g., Johnson, 1990), financial (Agarwal, Driscoll, Gabaix, & Laibson, 2009), and health domains (e.g., Szrek & Bundorf, 2011).

Against this backdrop, the following question is more pertinent than ever: Given that, as we have seen above, aging is associated with decline in many cognitive abilities and these may lead to changes in strategy selection and execution, how do these changes impact decision quality?

The ecological rationality framework proposes that reliance on simpler strategies does not necessarily lead to diminished decision performance (Gigerenzer & Todd, 1999; see Figure 1). Indeed, the ecological perspective gives room to the idea that simple cognitive mechanisms can exploit the structure of the environment in which they operate to achieve successful outcomes (see Table 1 for an overview of ecologies in which the strategies discussed here perform well). The question that one must ask, however, is to what extent the natural environments that young and older adults encounter in their daily lives are amenable to the successful use of simple strategies.

Mata and Nunes (2010) used simulation methods to investigate the possible consequences of relying on simpler strategies in the consumer domain. They used data from a range of products (e.g., home appliances, credit cards) under the assumption that decision makers use different strategies varying in whether they make use of little or all information available. The results of their simulations suggest that less may be enough—older adults may lose less than 10% of value on average by selecting simpler strategies, a significant yet relatively small decrease in choice quality. Unfortunately, we still know little about the statistical structure of many other real-world environments faced by young and older adults. Future work is needed to conduct systematic environment analysis and assess the performance of the strategies that are likely available to older adults. One particularly important step in this regard is to evaluate to what extent strategy-execution deficits may lead to interesting trade-offs such that decision makers are better off using simple, less error-prone strategies, relative to complex strategies that could, in principle, be more accurate but also lead to higher error rates.

SUMMARY AND CONCLUSION

Research on aging and strategy use in the memory, arithmetic, and decision-making domains suggests that there are significant age differences in strategy use. Overall, both young and older adults seem to adapt their behavior to task characteristics. However, older adults seem to rely more on simpler strategies and make more execution errors relative to young adults. The extent to which strategy selection of simple strategies is an adaptive decision based on a cost–benefit computation or an inability to use more complex strategies is, however, an open question. Also, the neural mechanisms underlying age differences in such aspects are not completely understood, and considerable work is needed to understand the boundary conditions of adaptive strategy selection. More importantly, the implications for real-world decision making are yet to be determined. Although simple strategies may do well in some environments, it remains an open question to what extent particular simple strategies allow older adults to achieve satisfactory decisions in real-world environments.

References

Agarwal, S., Driscoll, J. C., Gabaix, X., & Laibson, D. I. (2009). The age of reason: Financial decisions over the life cycle with implications for regulation. *Brookings Papers on Economic Activity*, *2*, 51–117.

Ardiale, E., & Lemaire, P. (2013). Effects of execution duration on within-item strategy switching in young and older adults. *Journal of Cognitive Psychology*, *25*, 464–472.

Ashcraft, M. H. (1992). Cognitive arithmetic: A review of data and theory. *Cognition*, *44*, 75–106.

Badre, D., & Wagner, A. D. (2014). Left ventrolateral prefrontal cortex and the cognitive control of memory. *Neuropsychologia*, *45*, 2883–2901.

Beach, L. R., & Mitchell, T. R. (1978). A contingency model for the selection of decision strategies. *Academy of Management Review*, *3*, 439–449.

Bettman, J. R., Johnson, E. J., & Payne, J. W. (1990). A componential analysis of cognitive effort in choice. *Organizational Behavior and Human Decision Processes*, *45*, 111–139.

Bjorklund, D. F., & Harnishfeger, K. K. (1990). The resources construct in cognitive development: Diverse sources of evidence and theory of inefficient inhibition. *Developmental Review*, *10*, 48–71.

Bouazzaoui, B., Isingrini, M., Fay, S., Angel, L., Vanneste, S., Clarys, D., et al. (2010). Aging and self-reported internal and external memory strategy uses: The role of executive functioning. *Acta Psychologica*, *135*(1), 59–66.

Brigham, M. C., & Pressley, M. (1988). Cognitive monitoring and strategy choice in younger and older adults. *Psychology and Aging*, *3*, 249–257.

Bröder, A., & Schiffer, S. (2003). Take the best versus simultaneous feature matching: Probabilistic inferences from memory and effects of representation format. *Journal of Experimental Psychology: General*, *132*, 277–293.

Bronfenbrenner, U. (1979). *The ecology of human development: Experiments by nature and design.* Cambridge, MA: Harvard University Press.

Bruine de Bruin, W., Parker, A. M., & Fischhoff, B. (2007). Individual differences in adult decision-making competence. *Journal of Personality and Social Psychology*, *92*, 938–956.

Bucciarelli, M., & Johnson-Laird, P. N. (1999). Strategies in syllogistic reasoning. *Cognitive Science*, *23*, 247–303.

Buckner, R. L., & Wheeler, M. E. (2001). The cognitive neuroscience of remembering. *Nature Reviews Neuroscience*, *2*, 624–634.

Chowdhury, R., Guitart-Masip, M., Lambert, C., Dayan, P., Huys, Q., Düzel, E., et al. (2013). Dopamine restores reward prediction errors in old age. *Nature Neuroscience*, *16*, 648–653.

Christensen, K., Doblhammer, G., Rau, R., & Vaupel, J. W. (2009). Ageing populations: The challenge ahead. *The Lancet*, *374*, 1196–1208.

Cohen, G., & Faulkner, D. (1983). Age differences in performance on two information-processing tasks: Strategy selection and processing efficiency. *Journal of Gerontology*, *38*, 447–454.

Cole, M. W., Reynolds, J. R., Power, J. D., Repovs, G., Anticevic, A., & Braver, T. S. (2013). Multi-task connectivity reveals flexible hubs for adaptive task control. *Nature Neuroscience*, *16*, 1348–1355.

Cox, K. M., Aizenstein, H. J., & Fiez, J. A. (2008). Striatal outcome processing in healthy aging. *Cognitive, Affective, and Behavioral Neuroscience, 8*, 304–317.

Dawes, R. M. (1979). The robust beauty of improper linear models. *American Psychologist, 34*, 571–582.

Diamond, A. (2013). Executive functions. *Annual Review of Psychology, 64*, 135–168.

Dunlosky, J., & Hertzog, C. (1998). Aging and deficits in associative memory: What is the role of strategy production? *Psychology and Aging, 13*, 597–607.

Duverne, S., & Lemaire, P. (2004). Age-related differences in arithmetic problem-verification strategies. *Journal of Gerontology: Psychological Sciences, 59B*, 135–142.

Eppinger, B., Hämmerer, D., & Li, S.-C. (2011). Neuromodulation of reward-based learning and decision making in human aging. *Annals of the New York Academy of Sciences, 1235*, 1–17.

Flavell, H. P. (1976). Metacognitive aspects of problem solving. In L. Resnick (Ed.), *The nature of intelligence* (pp. 231–236). Hillsdale, NJ: Lawrence Erlbaum.

Ford, J. K., Schmitt, N., Schechtman, S. L., Hults, B. M., & Doherty, M. L. (1989). Process tracing methods: Contributions, problems, and neglected research questions. *Organizational Behavior and Human Decision Processes, 43*, 75–117.

Gandini, D., Lemaire, P., Anton, J.-L., & Nazarian, B. (2008). Neural correlates of approximate quantification strategies in young and older adults: An fMRI study. *Brain Research, 1246*, 144–157.

Gandini, D., Lemaire, P., & Dufau, S. (2008). Older and younger adults' strategies in approximate quantification. *Acta Psychologica, 129*, 175–189.

Gandini, D., Lemaire, P., & Michel, B. F. (2009). Approximate quantification in young, healthy older adults', and Alzheimer patients. *Brain and Cognition, 70*, 53–61.

Gazzaley, A., & Nobre, A. C. (2012). Top-down modulation: Bridging selective attention and working memory. *Trends in Cognitive Sciences, 16*, 129–135.

Geary, D. C., & Lin, J. (1998). Numerical cognition: Age-related differences in the speed of executing biologically primary and biologically secondary processes. *Experimental Aging Research, 24*, 101–137.

Gigerenzer, G., & Goldstein, D. G. (1996). Reasoning the fast and frugal way: Models of bounded rationality. *Psychological Review, 103*, 650–669.

Gigerenzer, G., Todd, P. M. (1999). Fast and frugal heuristics: The adaptive toolbox. In G. Gigerenzer, P. M. Todd, & the ABC Research Group, *Simple heuristics that make us smart* (pp. 3–34). New York: Oxford University Press.

Girotto, V., & Gonzalez, M. (2001). Solving probabilistic and statistical problems: A matter of information structure and question form. *Cognition, 78*, 247–276.

Gluth, S., Rieskamp, J., & Büchel, C. (2014). Neural evidence for adaptive strategy selection in value-based decision making. *Cerebral Cortex, 24*, 2009–2021.

Goldstein, D. G., & Gigerenzer, G. (2002). Models of ecological rationality: The recognition heuristic. *Psychological Review, 109*, 75–90.

Hartley, A. A., & Anderson, J. W. (1983). Task complexity and problem-solving performance in younger and older adults. *Journal of Gerontology, 38*, 72–77.

Haselberger, S., & Solms-Laubach, F. (July 17, 2012). *Franz Müntefering über seine Ehe, das Alter und den Tod.* [Franz Müntefering on his marriage, aging and death] Bild Zeitung. Retrieved from http://www.bild.de/politik/inland/franz-muentefering/spd-urgestein-im-bild-interview-was-ich-von-meiner-frau-lernen-kann-1-25185568.bild.html.

Helversen, B. von, & Mata, R. (2012). Losing a dime with a satisfied mind: Positive affect predicts less search in sequential decision making. *Psychology and Aging, 27*, 825–839.

Hertzog, C., & Dunlosky, J. (2004). Aging, metacognition, and cognitive control. In B. H. Ross (Ed.), *The psychology of learning and motivation: Advances in research and theory* (vol. 45, pp. 215–251). San Diego, CA: Academic Press.

Hess, T. M., Queen, T. L., & Ennis, G. E. (2013). Age and self-relevance effects on information search during decision making. *Journal of Gerontology: Psychological Sciences, 68B*, 703–711.

Hills, T. T., Noguchi, T., & Gibbert, M. (2013). Information overload or search-amplified risk? Set size and order effects on decisions from experience. *Psychonomic Bulletin and Review, 20*, 1023–1031.

Hodzik, S., & Lemaire, P. (2011). Inhibition and shifting capacities mediate adults' age-related differences in strategy selection and repertoire. *Acta Psychologica, 137*, 335–344.

Howard, C. (Ed.). (November 1, 2013). *The world's most powerful people 2013*. Forbes. Retrieved from http://www.forbes.com/powerful-people/.

Iyengar, S. S., & Lepper, M. R. (2000). When choice is demotivating: Can one desire too much of a good thing? *Journal of Personality and Social Psychology, 79*, 995–1006.

Johnson, M. M. S. (1990). Age differences in decision making: A process methodology for examining strategic information processing. *Journal of Gerontology, 45*, 75–78.

Khader, P. H., Pachur, T., Meier, S., Bien, S., Jost, K., & Rösler, F. (2011). Memory-based decision-making: Evidence for a controlled activation of memory representation. *Journal of Cognitive Neuroscience, 23*, 3540–3554.

Lemaire, P. (2010). Cognitive strategy variations during aging. *Current Directions in Psychological Science, 19*, 363–369.

Lemaire, P., & Arnaud, L. (2008). Young and older adults' strategies in complex arithmetic. *American Journal of Psychology, 121*, 1–16.

Lemaire, P., Arnaud, L., & Lecacheur, M. (2004). Adults' age-related differences in adaptivity of strategy choices: Evidence from computational estimation. *Psychology and Aging, 19*, 467–481.

Lemaire, P., & Hinault, T. (2014). Age-related differences in sequential modulations of poorer-strategy effects. *Experimental Psychology, 61*, 252–262.

Lemaire, P., & Lecacheur, M. (2007). Aging and numerosity estimation. *Journal of Gerontology: Psychological Sciences, 62B*, 305–312.

Lemaire, P., & Leclère, M. (2014). Strategy repetition in young and older adults: A study in arithmetic. *Developmental Psychology, 50*, 460–468.

Lemaire, P., & Siegler, R. S. (1995). Four aspects of strategic change: Contributions to children's learning of multiplication. *Journal of Experimental Psychology: General, 124*, 83–97.

Lenartowcz, A., Kalar, D. J., Congdon, E., & Poldrack, R. A. (2010). Towards an ontology of cognitive control. *Topics in Cognitive Science, 2*, 678–692.

Lindenberger, U., & Mayr, U. (2014). Cognitive aging: Is there a dark side to environmental support? *Trends in Cognitive Sciences, 18*, 7–15.

Marewski, J. N., & Schooler, L. J. (2011). Cognitive niches: An ecological model of strategy selection. *Psychological Review, 118*, 393–437.

Mata, R., von Helversen, B., Karlsson, L., & Cüpper, L. (2012). Adult age differences in categorization and multiple-cue judgment. *Developmental Psychology, 48*, 1188–1201.

Mata, R., von Helversen, B., & Rieskamp, J. (2010). Learning to choose: Cognitive aging and strategy selection learning in decision making. *Psychology and Aging, 25*, 299–309.

Mata, R., & Nunes, L. (2010). When less is enough: Cognitive aging, information search, and decision quality in consumer choice. *Psychology and Aging, 25*, 289–298.

Mata, R., Pachur, T., von Helversen, B., Hertwig, R., Rieskamp, J., & Schooler, L. J. (2012). Ecological rationality: A framework for understanding and aiding the aging decision maker. *Frontiers in Neuroscience, 6*, 19.

Mata, R., Schooler, L. J., & Rieskamp, J. (2007). The aging decision maker: Cognitive aging and the adaptive selection of decision strategies. *Psychology and Aging, 22*, 796–810.

Mather, M. (2006). A review of decision-making processes: Weighing the risks and benefits of aging. In L. L. Carstensen & C. R. Hartel (Eds.), *When I'm 64* (pp. 145–173). Washington, DC: The National Academies Press.

Mikels, J. A., Reed, A. E., & Simon, K. I. (2009). Older adults place lower value on choice relative to young adults. *Journal of Gerontology: Psychological Sciences, 64B*, 443–446.

Nyberg, L., & Bäckman, L. (2010). Memory changes and the aging brain: A multimodal imaging approach. In K. W. Schaie & S. L. Willis (Eds.), *Handbook of the psychology of aging* (7th ed., pp. 121–132). San Diego, CA: Elsevier Press.

Pachur, T., Mata, R., & Schooler, L. J. (2009). Cognitive aging and the adaptive use of recognition in decision making. *Psychology and Aging, 24*, 901–915.

Pachur, T., Todd, P. M., Gigerenzer, G., Schooler, L. J., & Goldstein, D. G. (2011). The recognition heuristic: A review of theory and tests. *Frontiers in Psychology, 2*, 147.

Park, D. C., & Reuter-Lorenz, P. (2009). The adaptive brain: Aging and neurocognitive scaffolding. *Annual Review of Psychology, 60*, 173–196.

Payne, J. W. (1976). Task complexity and contingent processing in decision making: An information search and protocol analysis. *Organizational Behavior and Human Performance, 16*, 366–387.

Payne, J. W., Bettman, J. R., & Johnson, E. J. (1988). Adaptive strategy selection in decision making. *Journal of Experimental Psychology: Learning, Memory, and Cognition, 14*, 534–552.

Payne, J. W., Bettman, J. R., & Johnson, E. J. (1993). *The adaptive decision maker*. New York: Cambridge University Press.

Pressley, M., Borkowski, J. G., & Schneider, W. (1987). Cognitive strategies: Good strategy users coordinate metacognition and knowledge. *Annals of Child Development, 4*, 89–129.

Queen, T. L., Hess, T. M., Ennis, G. E., Dowd, K., & Grühn, D. (2012). Information search and decision making: Effects of age and complexity on strategy use. *Psychology and Aging, 27*, 817–824.

Reder, L. M. (1982). Plausibility judgments versus fact retrieval: Alternative strategies for sentence verification. *Psychological Review, 89*, 250–280.

Reed, A. E., Mikels, J. A., & Löckenhoff, C. E. (2013). Preferences for choice across adulthood: Age trajectories and potential mechanisms. *Psychology and Aging, 28*, 625–632.

Reese, H. W. (1962). Verbal mediation as a function of age level. *Psychological Bulletin, 59*, 502–509.

Ridderinkhof, K. R., Ullsperger, M., Crone, E. A., & Nieuwenhuis, S. (2004). The role of the medial frontal cortex in cognitive control. *Science, 306*, 443–447.

Rieskamp, J., & Otto, P. E. (2006). SSL: A theory of how people learn to select strategies. *Journal of Experimental Psychology: General, 135*, 207–236.

Rodrigue, K. M., & Kennedy, K. M. (2010). The cognitive consequences of structural changes to the aging brain. In K. W. Schaie & S. L. Willis (Eds.), *Handbook of the psychology of aging* (7th ed., pp. 73–92). San Diego, CA: Elsevier Press.

Samanez-Larkin, G. R., Gibbs, S. E. B., Khanna, K., Nielsen, L., Carstensen, L. L., & Knutson, B. (2007). Anticipation of monetary gain but not loss in healthy older adults. *Nature Neuroscience, 10*, 787–791.

Samanez-Larkin, G. R., Kuhnen, C. M., Yoo, D. J., & Knutson, B. (2010). Variability in nucleus accumbens activity mediates age-related suboptimal financial risk taking. *Journal of Neuroscience, 30*, 1426–1434.

Sander, M. C., Werkle-Bergner, M., & Lindenberger, U. (2011). Binding and strategic selection in working memory: A lifespan dissociation. *Psychology and Aging, 26*, 612–624.

Scheibehenne, B., Greifeneder, R., & Todd, P. M. (2010). Can there ever be too much choice? Meta-analytic review of choice overload. *Journal of Consumer Research, 37*, 409–425.

Schneider, W. (2011). Memory development in childhood. In U. Goswami (Ed.), *The Wiley-Blackwell handbook of childhood cognitive development* (2nd ed., pp. 347–376). London: Wiley.

Shah, A. K., & Oppenheimer, M. (2008). Heuristics made easy: An effort-reduction framework. *Psychological Bulletin, 134*, 207–222.

Shing, Y. L., Werkle-Bergner, M., Li, S.-C., & Lindenberger, U. (2008). Associative and strategic components of episodic memory: A lifespan dissociation. *Journal of Experimental Psychology: General, 137*, 496–513.

Siegler, R. S., & Lemaire, P. (1997). Older and younger adults' strategy choices in multiplication: Testing predictions of ASCM using the choice/no-choice method. *Journal of Experimental Psychology: General, 126*, 71–92.

Stevens, J. R., & Hauser, M. D. (2004). Why be nice? Psychological constraints on the evolution of cooperation. *Trends in Cognitive Sciences, 8*, 60–65.

Szrek, H., & Bundorf, M. K. (2011). Age and the purchase of prescription drug insurance by older adults. *Psychology and Aging, 26*, 308–320.

Touron, D. R., & Hertzog, C. (2004). Distinguishing age differences in knowledge, strategy use, and confidence during strategic skill acquisition. *Psychology and Aging, 19*, 452–466.

Touron, D. R., Hertzog, C., & Frank, D. (2011). Eye movements and strategy shift in skill acquisition: Adult age differences. *Journal of Gerontology: Psychological Sciences, 66B*, 151–159.

Uittenhove, K., & Lemaire, P. (2013). Strategy sequential difficulty effects vary with working-memory and response-stimulus-intervals: A study in arithmetic. *Acta Psychologica, 143*, 113–118.

Verhaeghen, P., & Salthouse, T. A. (1997). Meta-analyses of age-cognition relations in adulthood: Estimates of linear and nonlinear age effects and structural models. *Psychological Bulletin, 122*, 231–249.

Volz, K. G., Schooler, L. J., Schubotz, R. I., Raab, M., Gigerenzer, G., & von Cramon, D. Y. (2006). Why you think Milan is larger than Modena: Neural correlates of the recognition heuristic. *Journal of Cognitive Neuroscience, 18*, 1924–1936.

West, R. L. (1996). An application of prefrontal cortex function theory to cognitive aging. *Psychological Bulletin, 120*, 272–292.

Worthy, D. A., & Maddox, W. T. (2012). Age-based differences in strategy use in choice tasks. *Frontiers in Neurosciences, 5*, 145.

CHAPTER

7

Aging, Memory, and Decision Making

Fabio Del Missier[1, 2], *Timo Mäntylä*[2], *Lars-Göran Nilsson*[2, 3, 4]

[1]Department of Life Sciences, Psychology Unit, University of Trieste, Trieste, Italy; [2]Department of Psychology, Stockholm University, Stockholm, Sweden; [3]ARC, Karolinska Institutet Stockholm, Stockholm, Sweden; [4]UFBI, Umeå University, Umeå, Sweden

INTRODUCTION

Researchers in cognitive aging have devoted much effort in trying to understand how and why memory processes change across the adult life span (e.g., Park et al., 2002, 1996; Rönnlund, Nyberg, Bäckman, & Nilsson, 2005). The investigation of the relationship between aging and judgment and decision making, however, has attracted relatively less interest, even if this research is quickly growing and a number of studies have provided an initial body of valuable evidence (for reviews see Mather, 2006; Peters & Bruine de Bruin, 2012; Peters, Hess, Västfjäll, & Auman, 2007; Strough, Karns, & Schlosnagle, 2011).

Within this latter research stream, limited effort has been devoted to understanding how aging affects judgment and decision making through changes in memory processes. This is not surprising, considering the limited attention generally paid to the role of memory processes in judgment and decision-making literature, especially in the early years of this research. More recently, interest in the role of specific memory and attentional processes in judgment and decision making has grown, promoting the accumulation of empirical evidence and fostering the proposal of memory-based theories (for reviews of older and more recent work, see, e.g., Alba, Hutchinson, & Lynch, 1991; Del Missier et al., 2013; Dougherty, Gronlund, & Gettys, 2003; Weber, Goldstein, & Barlas, 1995).

Aging and Decision Making
http://dx.doi.org/10.1016/B978-0-12-417148-0.00007-8

Thus, the recent developments in research on aging and decision making and on the memory bases of decision making have set the stage for integrative studies aimed at shedding light on how age-related changes in judgment and decision making are linked to age-related changes in memory processes. In this chapter, we provide our contribution to this endeavor by scrutinizing the complex relationships between aging, memory, and judgment and decision making. In particular, we identify empirical generalizations through an integrative review of research findings and discuss their theoretical and applied implications.

Our analysis follows a classification of memory topics functional to the exploration of age–memory relationships on the one hand, and memory–decision-making relationships on the other (Table 1).[1] We adopt this classification for the sake of organization and without endorsing a particular hypothesis on the architecture of human memory. The chapter reviews the main age-related changes in different aspects of memory functioning and shows how these changes affect judgment and decision making. In the final section of the chapter, we highlight promising avenues for future investigation.

AGE-RELATED CHANGES IN MEMORY FUNCTIONING AND THEIR INFLUENCE ON JUDGMENT AND DECISION MAKING

Working Memory

Getting older is associated with many changes in memory functioning (see Table 1). However, the clearest age-related differences are apparent in working memory and episodic memory tasks, which often show worse performance in older adults (e.g., Nilsson et al., 2004; Park et al., 2002; Salthouse, 2004; Verhaeghen & Salthouse, 1997). Age differences have been observed in various memory span measures for verbal materials, ranging from tasks requiring mere maintenance (short-term memory span) to tasks

[1] There are different definitions of basic memory constructs (see Baddeley, Eysenck, & Anderson, 2009). However, short-term memory is usually referred to as maintenance of a limited amount of information for short time-frames (seconds), with working memory usually implying also active processing. Episodic memory refers to contextualized memories associated with a specific form of awareness (autonoetic). Mental simulation is related to the processes that allow simulating future events and situations. Semantic memory is usually associated with conceptual knowledge and related language knowledge. Nondeclarative and implicit memories refer to experiences or learning outcomes that cannot be verbally reported but affect behavior, and include procedural memory, classical conditioning, and processes supporting repetition priming.

TABLE 1 Summary of the Main Age-Related Differences in Memory

Memory Topic	Main Age-Related Differences
Working memory and short-term memory	Worse performance in older adults, with stronger effects for working memory measures.
Episodic memory and mental simulation	Worse performance in older adults, with stronger effects in free recall (vs recognition) and in recollection (vs familiarity). Greater proneness to false memory and misinformation effects in older adults. Fewer episodic details in retrospective memory and mental simulation, but more semantic and external elements.
Emotional aspects of memory	Positivity biases in older adults' episodic and autobiographic memory.
Semantic memory	Performance increase over adulthood for vocabulary and general knowledge. Decline at very old age. Some problems in accessing words and slower access to semantic memory.
Implicit and nondeclarative memory	Small differences in measures of implicit memory (e.g., repetition priming) and learning, stable mere exposure effect, age-related differences in classical conditioning (reduced priming effects and less effective learning/conditioning when age differences are present).

requiring both maintenance and processing (working memory). However, meta-analytic works indicate that age-related effects are stronger in working memory tasks than in simple maintenance tasks, with reordering tasks (backward digit span) falling in between (Bopp & Verhaeghen, 2005; see also Verhaeghen, Marcoen, & Goosens, 1993; Verhaeghen & Salthouse, 1997). Research has also shown age-related differences in working memory tasks for visuospatial information (e.g., Jenkins, Myerson, Joerding, & Hale, 2000; Kemps & Newson, 2006; Park et al., 2002; Salthouse, 1995).

Working Memory and Decision Making. A number of dual-task and individual-differences studies carried out in young adults suggest that working memory and related executive control processes support judgment and decision making in tasks requiring extensive processing and thoughtful evaluation of information about options, while the same processes seem to be less relevant to tasks that can be successfully completed by using less demanding strategies. Dual-task experiments show that under high cognitive load posed by a concurrent task, participants tend to rely on simpler but less effective judgment and evaluation strategies or emotion-based choice processes (e.g., De Neys & Verschueren, 2006; De Neys, 2006; Hinson, Jameson, & Whitney, 2003; Shiv & Fedorikhin, 1999). These findings suggest that working-memory resources are necessary to articulate a preference or judgment when these need to be based on a more thoughtful consideration of information. Individual-differences studies show that participants with greater working memory capacity provide probability judgments more consistent with probability theory (i.e., less subadditive; Dougherty & Hunter, 2003) and that better executive functioning is associated with better results on cognitively demanding judgment and decision-making tasks (Del Missier, Mäntylä, & Bruine de Bruin, 2010, 2012; Parker & Fischhoff, 2005).

Starting from these investigations, it can be hypothesized that an age-related decline will be observed in cognitively taxing judgment and decision-making tasks, and that this decline will be at least partially mediated by an age-related decline in working memory. Preliminary, indirect support for this hypothesis was provided by an individual-differences study (Bruine de Bruin, Parker, & Fischhoff, 2012), which showed that age-related decline in two cognitively demanding tasks of the Adult Decision-Making Competence battery (A-DMC; Bruine de Bruin, Parker, & Fischhoff, 2007) is mediated by fluid intelligence.[2] These tasks were Resistance to Framing (measuring, within subjects, resistance to the improper influence of variations in the decision problem description; see also Stanovich & West, 2008) and Applying Decision Rules (assessing the ability to apply decision procedures to multiattribute choice problems). However, this study did not include specific measures of working memory.

A relevant investigation was carried out on a population-based sample of Swedish adults between 25 and 80 years of age (Del Missier et al., 2013). In this study, multiple measures of individual differences in working memory, semantic memory, and episodic memory were collected, together with the whole set of A-DMC tasks. A main hypothesis of the study was that working memory supports performance in three of the more cognitively demanding A-DMC tasks (Resistance to Framing, Applying Decision Rules, and Under/Overconfidence—measuring calibration of confidence in knowledge), but it is not so strongly involved in the other tasks of the battery. Moreover, an age-related decline was expected in these three demanding A-DMC tasks, which was supposed to be at least partially mediated by an age-related decline in working memory.

[2] For a detailed description of the whole A-DMC battery, which aims to measure main aspects of decision-making competence, see Strough, Parker, and Bruine de Bruin (this volume). It is worth mentioning that validation studies showed that A-DMC performance is able to predict real-word decision outcomes (e.g., Bruine de Bruin et al., 2007).

Structural equation modeling showed that the best measurement model of memory variables was composed of three latent variables (working memory, semantic memory, and episodic memory), which were positively correlated (see also Nyberg, 1994; Nyberg et al., 2003; Rönnlund et al., 2005). As expected, only working memory and episodic memory were negatively related with age. Structural models linking specific memory latent variables with A-DMC measures showed that individual differences in working memory were positively related with performance in the three more cognitively demanding A-DMC tasks, but not with the other A-DMC tasks. Mediation models tested the hypothesis that the negative relations between age and performance in these tasks are (at least partly) explained by an age-related decline in working memory. They showed that the negative effect of age on Resistance to Framing and Under/Overconfidence was completely mediated by the negative effect of age on working memory and by the positive relationship between working memory and decision-making performance, while a trend toward partial mediation was apparent in the case of Applying Decision Rules (but see Bruine de Bruin et al., 2012. for different findings on the Under/Overconfidence task).

However, there is the possibility that the negative relation between age and decision making observed in some A-DMC tasks is not explained by the working memory decline but by the negative effects of aging on alternative determinants of cognitive processing. Cognitive aging researchers proposed that age-related differences in complex cognitive tasks can be traced back to age-related declines in diverse general factors, which include sensory functioning (Lindenberger & Baltes, 1997), processing speed (Salthouse, 1996), working memory (Mayr & Kliegl, 1993), and inhibition (Hasher & Zacks, 1988). Processing speed explains a large fraction of variance in complex tasks (e.g., Park et al., 2002; Salthouse, 1996), but it seems that performance on more complex tasks can be better explained by processing speed *and* working memory predictors, and the contribution of working memory increases with task complexity (Kliegl, Mayr, & Krampe, 1994; Mayr & Kliegl, 1993; Nettelbeck & Rabbitt, 1992; Park et al., 1996).

Following this work, Del Missier et al. (2014) carried out a study to disentangle the relative contributions of sensory functioning, processing speed, and working memory on the age-related decline in the three A-DMC tasks previously identified as more cognitively demanding (Del Missier et al., 2010, 2012, 2013; see also Bruine de Bruine et al., 2007, 2012). The critical hypothesis was that, even after controlling for the influence of the age-related decline in sensory functioning and processing speed, working memory still plays a significant role in explaining the age-related decline in decision-making performance. This hypothesis was rooted in the consideration that the A-DMC tasks investigated require cognitive operations of information integration and memory updating, together with task-related attention focusing, goal management, and inhibition (Del Missier et al., 2010, 2012), and that these operations are central to working memory functioning.

The data collection included two working memory measures, three measures of processing speed, and a series of different measures of sensory functioning for audition, vision, and olfaction. Resistance to Framing, Applying Decision Rules, and Under/Overconfidence scores were the criterion decision-making variables. As expected, all predictors were positively related with decision-making measures, with slightly stronger correlations for working memory. Age was negatively related both with decision-making performance and with measures of the three general age-related factors, with stronger correlations for processing speed.

Mediation testing using structural equation modeling produced consistent results for the A-DMC tasks. In particular, after considering all the effects of sensory functioning, processing speed, and working memory, no significant direct effects of sensory functioning and processing speed on decision-making performance were detected. Additionally, in each A-DMC task, the two indirect paths connecting age and decision making (but not involving sensory functioning) conveyed stronger indirect effects than the ones including the sensory paths, with the age→working memory→decision making path contributing more than any other. The results were robust even after the inclusion of education in the models as a control variable for cohort effects (see Rönnlund et al., 2005). Moreover, removing the working memory latent variable or removing the specific age→working memory link from the models led to significant decreases in fit and predictive capacity. To summarize the findings of this study, working memory seems to act both as a *direct* mediator of age effects on decision making and as a *target* of lower-level effects of sensory functioning and processing speed. Age-related declines in sensory functioning and processing speed seem to have a less important and indirect role in the complex judgment and decision-making tasks considered in this research.

Episodic Memory

Age-related differences have been observed in episodic memory (e.g., Nilsson et al., 1997; Park et al., 2002; Salthouse, 2005; Salthouse et al., 2003; Verhaeghen & Salthouse, 1997), with worse performance in older adults. Some findings suggest stronger age-related effects in recall tasks (e.g., Craik, Byrd, & Swanson, 1987; Craik & McDowd, 1987; Kemps & Newson, 2006; Nyberg et al., 2003), possibly because of age-related deficits in self-initiated processing and recoding operations (e.g., Craik &

McDowd, 1987; Craik, 1983).[3] Studies on recognition show that aging negatively affects recollection (conscious retrieval of an episode and its details), while familiarity (not based on retrieval of specific information but on a sense of knowing) seems to be less affected, even if the evidence supporting this latter conclusion is not univocal (e.g., Light, Prull, La Voie, & Healy, 2000; Yonelinas, 2002). Older adults' problems in recollection partially reflect poor encoding (less frequent adoption of elaborative encoding strategies), although retrieval problems are also probably involved. In their meta-analysis, Spencer and Raz (1995) also observed that memory for context of a message (e.g., perceptual, spatial, and temporal aspects) is more vulnerable to aging than memory for its content, with stronger effects for contextual features that were more likely to have been encoded independently from content.

The observation that older adults encounter more problems than younger adults in recollecting an event with its episodic context (e.g., where and when the event took place) and in accessing the source of information (e.g., who said something) suggests that older adults may rely more on general familiarity (Grady & Craik, 2000). This may contribute to explaining why older adults are more prone to source memory failures, false memories, and familiarity-related errors after repeated presentations of information (Jacoby, 1999a; Schacter, Koutstaal, & Norman, 1997).

Interestingly, age-related differences have been observed not only in autobiographic memory but also in imagination. In particular, older adults produce fewer episodic details than younger adults both when remembering the past and imagining the future, with an increased number of external and semantic elements (e.g., Addis, Wong, & Schacter, 2008; Levine, Svoboda, Hay, Winocur, & Moscovitch, 2002).

Episodic Memory and Decision Making. Although age-related changes in episodic memory have the potential to affect decision making in different

[3] Cross-sectional and longitudinal studies offer different pictures of age-related changes in episodic memory (Rönnlund et al., 2005), with cross-sectional data showing an earlier onset and smoother decline, and longitudinal data highlighting a steeper decline with a much later onset. Cross-sectional studies on cognitive functioning (e.g., Salthouse, 1998, 2005; Schaie, 2005) generally show monotonic declines in performance starting in early adulthood (20s–30s), with longitudinal investigations showing a much later (>55–60) and sometimes less pronounced decline (Rönnlund et al., 2005; Schaie, 2005). These differences can be due to peculiar factors affecting cross-sectional designs (e.g., cohort effects associated with changes in the social and cultural environment) and longitudinal designs (e.g., retest and attrition effects). These methodological issues suggest caution in the generalization of the findings, which are mainly based on cross-sectional designs. They also suggest adopting research designs that include longitudinal and cross-sectional data and allow for the main confounding factors to be taken into account (see e.g., Rönnlund et al., 2005; Salthouse, 2009).

ways, research on this topic is particularly scarce. We will now consider: (1) the multiple effects of declining recollection versus relatively better preserved familiarity on judgments and decisions, (2) the influence of learning and memory effects in risky choice tasks, and (3) the consequences of age-related differences in future simulation for planning.

Less effective recollection contributes to strengthening older adults' hindsight bias in some circumstances (Bayen, Erdfelder, Bearden, & Lozito, 2006; Bayen, Pohl, Erdfelder, & Auer, 2007; Bernstein, Erdfelder, Meltzoff, Peria, & Loftus, 2011).[4] Similarly, less effective encoding and recollection processes, together with emotion-related factors, might contribute to older adults' stronger positivity biases for past choices (Mather & Johnson, 2000), with the decline of executive control processes also playing a role (Mather & Johnson, 2003).[5] The age-related strengthening of these biases may improperly boost older adults' confidence in their judgment and decision-making skills and reduce their capacity to learn from the past.

A decreased ability in recalling specific features of options, together with reduced working memory and executive control, may also lead to changes in older adults' decision-making strategies. Older decision-makers may rely more on global or gist-based judgments or impressions (Mather & Johnson, 2003; Reyna & Brainerd, 2011) or adopt simpler decision strategies that focus on fewer criteria or pieces of information. Although these strategies may reduce cognitive effort and be effective in some environments, they may also lead to poorer outcomes when more complex trade-offs or precise discriminations are required (e.g., Mata, Schooler, & Rieskamp, 2007; Mata, von Helversen, & Rieskamp, 2010).

Encoding and recollection problems may also harm estimation and judgment based on episodic memory. This may happen, in particular, when encoding requires attention and/or when estimation is based on cognitively demanding retrieval strategies (Brown, 2002). The Recognizing Social Norms task of the A-DMC battery asks respondents to estimate the social norms of their group of pairs in relation to some more or less undesirable behaviors (e.g., stealing under certain circumstances; not holding the door open for people). Performance in this task is assumed to rely on episodic memory, as a repository of information derived from observed behaviors or instances related to the social norms (for the role

[4] The hindsight bias (Fischhoff, 1975) is the tendency to overestimate the quality of past estimates of an outcome after receiving actual outcome information (for instance, an estimate of 31% of votes to a given party, before the election, may be recalled as 34% after hearing that the party had 35% of the votes; Blank, Fischer, & Erdfelder, 2003).

[5] The positivity bias for past choices is a memory distortion that favors chosen options over rejected options (see also the section on emotional aspects of memory).

of perceived experience on social norms, e.g., Cialdini, Kallgren, & Reno, 1991). Del Missier et al. (2013) found that performance in the Recognizing Social Norms task depends on two contrasting age-related influences: a negative indirect effect stemming from age-declining episodic memory and a direct positive influence of age, which was interpreted as an effect of older adults' increased social competence and skills (e.g., Hess, Osowski, & Leclerc, 2005).

Declining recollection and relatively preserved familiarity may boost the use of familiarity-based strategies and enhance familiarity-related effects in older adults. For instance, familiarity may boost the illusion of truth (repeated statements are perceived as more valid than novel ones, even for statements that are explicitly identified as false on initial presentation (e.g., Begg, Anas, & Farinacci, 1992) with stronger effects observed in older adults (Skurnik, Yoon, Park, & Schwarz, 2005; but cf. Parks & Toth, 2006). These effects may be moderated by the number of repetitions (massive repetition may backfire: Briñol & Petty, 2009) and by the extent of processing (Moons, Mackie, & Garcia-Marques, 2009). Ironically, repeatedly identifying a claim as false helped older adults remember it as false in the short term, but made them more likely to remember it as true after a 3-day delay (Skurnik et al., 2005). This effect reflected increased familiarity with the claim but decreased recollection of the claim's context.

If older individuals are less able to recollect the source and the context of a message as well as content-related detailed information, which are fundamental to judge its credibility, it can be hypothesized that misleading advertising or political communication may have stronger effects on older adults' decision making. If this were to be the case, given that repeatedly identifying a claim as false may even backfire, it may be worth exploring the possibility of providing older adults with effective retrieval cues or with easy-to-use fact-checking tools.

Additionally, given that older adults seem to be more prone to false memory effects and have greater susceptibility to misinformation, they may be victims of fraudulent schemes that capitalize on these memory weaknesses (Jacoby & Rhodes, 2006). For instance, older adults may be led to falsely believe that they have expressed interest in a product on a previous occasion in order to persuade them to buy the product (for other examples, see Jacoby, 1999b; Jacoby & Rhodes, 2006). However, there is still no clear evidence supporting the claim that older adults are more prone to fraud (Ross, Grossmann, & Schryer, 2014), and older adults' vulnerability may not depend only on memory factors (see e.g., Castle et al., 2012). In any case, specific programs may reduce the probability of adults becoming fraud victims via warning, getting individuals to generate advice for others about how to avoid scams, and demonstrating how easy it is to fall prey to a fraud (Mather, 2006).

Older adults' learning and memory difficulties also may explain their lower performance in decision making tasks involving learning. A meta-analysis carried out by Mata, Josef, Samanez-Larkin, and Hertwig (2011) comprised a number of aging studies on risky decision making. Older adults were found to be more risk-seeking than young adults in the Iowa Gambling task (IGT) and more risk-averse in the Balloon Analog Risk Task, which are behaviors associated with lower performance in these tasks, while no age-related differences were detected in description-based (i.e., noninteractive) risky tasks not involving demanding probability/reward trade-offs between the options. This pattern of findings was interpreted as indicative of less effective learning and memory processes in older adults in tasks where probabilities and potential outcomes are not explicitly provided (see also Henninger, Madden, & Huettel, 2010).[6] However, these studies have not made clear the specific role of age-related episodic memory changes in risky choices involving learning, and understanding the specific memory processes involved in these tasks may represent a future research goal.

Age-related differences in the simulation of future scenarios may have implications for decision making. Taylor, Pham, Rivkin, and Armor (1998) showed that students who simulated important steps for success on an exam (process simulation) were more successful and less prone to the planning fallacy[7] than students who simulated how good they would feel if they received a high grade (outcome simulation). Sheldon, McAndrews, and Moscovitch (2011) showed that older adults generate fewer task-relevant episodic steps when simulating solutions to ill-defined problems. Converging evidence comes from the studies on implementation intentions in older adults (e.g., Liu & Park, 2004), which suggests that forming a detailed plan, specifying how, where, and when a desired behavior will be completed in the future, can enhance goal achievement (see also Schacter, 2012). Thus, it might be worth testing whether older adults' less specific and less episodic-based simulation of the steps needed to carry out a task may enhance the planning fallacy. On the other hand, older

[6] Although existing findings on the role of cognitive processes in the IGT and in similar tasks are not fully consistent and different stances on the processes involved in these tasks remain, a reasonable interim conclusion is that diverse kinds of processes can be at work in complex, experience-based, emotionally laden tasks, and that specific age-related changes in these processes may bring both negative (e.g., less effective memory and learning processes) and positive (e.g., more accurate evaluation) consequences for performance (see e.g., Wood, Busemeyer, Koling, Cox, & Davis, 2005).

[7] The planning fallacy (Kahneman & Tversky, 1979) consists in underestimating the time needed to complete a future task (e.g., writing a paper, completing an origami, filling out a tax form).

adults may capitalize on their experience of life situations and better emotion regulation skills, and thus be more capable at predicting their future emotional responses (Lachman, Röcke, Rosnick, & Ryff, 2008; Nielsen, Knutson, & Carstensen, 2008; Scheibe, Mata, & Carstensen, 2011), although it is unclear if this holds only for positive events (for a short review, see also Löckenhoff, 2011).

Emotional Aspects of Memory

Clear evidence exists for age-related differences in remembering valenced stimuli and information. While young adults have the tendency to remember more negative than positive information, older adults do not show this bias toward negative information, and they sometimes remember more positive than negative information (Charles, Mather, & Carstensen, 2003). This shift in the ratio of positive to negative material processed in memory (and attention) is called the positivity effect (Mather & Carstensen, 2005). Positively biased memory in older adults has been observed both in autobiographical reports and in laboratory studies, even if the effect has not been observed in some decision contexts (Depping & Freund, 2013). Some studies employing divided attention manipulations and individual differences suggest that preserved cognitive control is needed to ensure emotion-regulation success in older adults (Mather & Carstensen, 2005; Mather & Knight, 2005). This implies that older adults need to have cognitive control resources and the freedom to selectively process information in order to expose positivity biases (see Kryla-Lighthall & Mather, 2009).[8] Socioemotional selectivity theory has explained these findings by referring to the individual's adaptations to his or her life course, with the reduction in time horizons strengthening the motivation to preserve emotional balance (vs knowledge-related goals), and leading to a greater focus on emotion regulation and positive aspects of life (e.g., Carstensen, 2006). These changes are thought to affect attention and memory processes in a way that is functional to the maintenance of a positive emotional state.

Emotional Aspects of Memory and Decision Making. Older adults' focus on emotion regulation has implications for older adults' judgment and decision making. Probably the best-known example is the positivity bias for past choices. In a series of studies (e.g., Mather & Johnson, 2000), participants were asked to choose between two options that have positive and negative features. After a delay, participants were asked to indicate which

[8] However, these findings do not agree with the observation that positivity biases for past choices are negatively related with the efficiency of executive control processes (Mather & Johnson, 2000, 2003), pointing to the need for clarification of the role of cognitive control in different kinds of positivity biases.

option features had been associated with. In these studies, older adults had a stronger tendency to associate positive features with the chosen option and negative features with the rejected option, with this difference not simply due to poorer memory. However, when younger adults were asked to focus on their feelings after making the choices, they showed the same degree of positivity bias. According to Mather (2006), a potential implication of choice-supportive memory is that older adults are more likely to repeat the same choices. Although repeating a good choice may be a good strategy in many situations, this tendency may hinder adaptive behavior when priorities or criteria change.

Implicit and Nondeclarative Memory

Other aspects of memory functioning, such as implicit memory, seem to be less harmed by aging (Fleischman & Gabrieli, 1998; LaVoie & Light, 1994; Light et al., 2000). Age-related differences in implicit memory tasks are small compared to performance changes in recall and recognition (e.g., LaVoie & Light, 1994). Additionally, the mere exposure effect (mere repeated exposure to a stimulus enhances its evaluation) seems to be preserved in older adults (Wiggs, 1993). These findings may be interpreted in terms of relatively less impaired activation, familiarity, or perceptual fluency mechanisms versus more impaired context-dependent operations.

Implicit learning is thought to be relatively preserved in older adults (e.g., Prull, Gabrieli, & Bunge, 2000; Zacks, Hasher, & Li, 2000), even if age differences emerge when sequences with more complex statistical structures had to be learned implicitly (e.g., Curran, 1997; Howard & Howard, 1997) or after prolonged practice with an associative probabilistic learning task (Simon, Howard, & Howard, 2011). Moreover, the type of implicit learning task may moderate age-related differences (e.g., Howard & Howard, 2012). Interestingly, other processes usually grouped under the broad umbrella of nondeclarative memory, like classical conditioning, show age-related differences (e.g., Gabrieli, 1998).

Implicit Processes and Decision Making. Implicit learning and memory have been linked to intuitive judgment and decision-making heuristics and social heuristics. In particular, according to Lieberman (2000), the "similarity between intuition and implicit learning suggests that it may be fruitful to consider intuition as the subjective experience associated with the use of knowledge gained through implicit learning" (p. 109). Other scholars in the judgment and decision-making field suggest instead that intuitive heuristics may be supported by a variety of processes, including implicit learning, associative learning, conditioning, emotion-related processes, proceduralization of knowledge, perceptual judgment, pattern-matching, and accumulation mechanisms (for a review, see Glöckner & Witteman, 2010). If intuition depends on less cognitively demanding processes that are relatively less harmed by aging, older adults' performance should be spared when a judgment or decision-making task can be successfully completed by relying on these processes (Peters et al., 2007). Queen and Hess (2010) presented evidence supporting this view, but more research is needed to strengthen it and to qualify the specific intuitive processes involved in different tasks. On the other hand, more reliance on simple and intuitive judgment and decision-making heuristics may sometimes backfire, exposing older adults to biases associated with an improper use of these heuristics (e.g., Finucane & Gullion, 2010).

Various studies showed that implicit learning and implicit memory components contribute to performance in dynamic control environments, in which cue–criterion (or stimulus–response) relationships are very difficult to grasp (e.g., a simulated sugar factory whose production level needs to be controlled; Berry & Broadbent, 1984, 1987). According to Dienes and Fahey (1995, 1998), control tasks governed by highly salient rules are handled by learning the rules, while control tasks in which the rules are very difficult to understand are controlled via instance-based learning. This means that when the "rules of the game" are very hard to grasp, situational cues will trigger associatively stored situation–response pairs, and these will be used to guide behavior, including control decisions to be taken.

Interestingly, a distinction between rule-based and instance-based representation emerged also in the field of multiple cue judgment. Juslin, Karlsson, and Olsson (2008) showed that in environments requiring an additive integration of cues in order to reach an accurate judgment, individuals are able to abstract explicitly the linear combination of cues. However, individuals are also able to express their judgment in environments with nonadditive cue combination, nonlinear relations, and intercue correlation by resorting to implicit exemplar memory. Following some findings that showed that categorization tasks are usually handled by exemplar memory while linear multiple-cue judgment is primarily driven by rule-based processing (Juslin, Olsson, & Olsson, 2003), Mata, von Helversen, Karlsson, and Cüpper (2012) examined adult age differences in these two tasks. They found that both older and young adults relied on rule-based processes in the multiple-cue judgment task. However, in the categorization task, young adults resorted to exemplar-based and similarity-based processing while the majority of older adults relied on rule-based processes. Moreover, older adults relying on rule-based processing showed a lower level of performance. These findings suggest that we cannot take for granted the possibility that older adults may effectively switch to (allegedly) better-preserved instance-based processing. Furthermore, controlled processing may be involved in exemplar-based multiple-cue judgment tasks (e.g., Juslin et al., 2008). Thus, further research on rule/instance shifts in older adults and on the cognitive load of instance-based processing is needed to clarify these issues.

Semantic Memory

Performance in knowledge-based measures of semantic memory (as vocabulary tests or test of general knowledge) seems to improve with age or at least it is well preserved up to old age (e.g., Rönnlund et al., 2005; Salthouse et al., 2003; Verhaeghen, 2003). Performance in other tasks, like semantic priming and comprehension (but only after controlling for memory for the presented information), seems to be age invariant (for a review, see Burke, MacKay, & James, 1999). However, age-related differences favoring young adults are usually found in comprehension tasks in which remembering is required, and this may have consequences for real-world situations in which older adults have to draw inferences from remembered information. Interestingly, multiple-choice vocabulary tests seem to yield a larger advantage for older adults (vs younger adults) than production tests (i.e., choose a synonym vs define a word), suggesting that although older adults may have a richer pool of words and concepts available in semantic memory, they may need stronger cues to access it (Verhaeghen, 2003). This is compatible with studies showing older adults' word-finding difficulties (e.g., Burke et al., 1999; MacKay & Abrams, 1996). Moreover, older adults show a slower access to semantic memory in some tasks (e.g., sentence verification: Baddeley, Emslie, & Nimmo-Smith, 1992). However, despite these difficulties, adults regularly working on crossword puzzles show the highest level of performance in their 60s and 70s (Salthouse, 2004), suggesting that older adults may successfully overcome their difficulties in tasks in which they have accrued relevant knowledge and experience.

Semantic Memory and Decision Making. Some empirical evidence suggests that knowledge and experience can be beneficial for older adults' judgment and decision making in some contexts. Older adults show preserved decision-making capacity in familiar environments and problems that allow exploiting acquired experience and knowledge (e.g., Fisk & Rogers, 2000). Two studies (Kim & Hasher, 2005; Tentori, Osherson, Hasher, & May, 2001) showed that older adults are less prone to the biasing influence of an asymmetric-dominated option in a grocery-store context. A potential explanation is that older participants had greater experience in this domain, although alternative explanations are possible (e.g., Kim & Hasher, 2005). Meyer, Russo, and Talbot (1995) and Meyer and Pollard (2004) showed that older women's decisions in the health domain (e.g., breast cancer) were as good as younger women's, but older women sought less information and were faster, due to better knowledge of the disease. Two recent individual-differences studies (Del Missier et al., 2013; Li, Baldassi, Johnson, & Weber, 2013) used semantic memory and crystallized intelligence measures as proxies for more specific measures of decision-related knowledge (e.g., economic rules, probability-related knowledge, etc.), and found that individuals with better scores in the semantic/crystallized measures showed better performance in decision-making tasks requiring the ability to resist sunk costs, to express consistent judgments of risk perception, and to exhibit less temporal discounting. Li et al. (2013) also showed that age-related knowledge increases compensated for age-related decreases in fluid ability in some of the tasks they investigated (see also Samanez-Larkin, 2013).

However, when presented with new and complex decision problems, older adults show lower comprehension and are less able to apply decision strategies (Bruine de Bruin et al., 2012; Del Missier et al., 2013; Finucane & Gullion, 2010; Finucane, Mertz, Slovic, & Schmidt, 2005), even when the problems refer to domains that they should find familiar (e.g., health, nutrition, economy). Thus, it seems that older adults need to be able to transfer their knowledge and experience into the specific problems that have to be solved in order to show better performance. This may allow them to reduce the complexity of the task or to avoid decision-related biases.

Another implication for decision making stems from preserved sematic priming in older adults. These preserved effects suggest that priming manipulations targeted at increasing the accessibility of specific options (Nedungadi, 1990) or attributes (Mandel & Johnson, 2002) in choice are likely to affect also older adults. Moreover, considering that older adults tend to generate fewer options (Del Missier & Terpini, 2009) and to seek less information in decision making, they might even show a stronger tendency to stick to the information made more accessible by priming manipulations.

AGING, MEMORY, AND DECISION MAKING: WHERE DO WE GO FROM HERE?

In this chapter, we provided a nonexhaustive review of the research linking aging, memory, and decision making. The overall picture shows that aging is associated with many changes in memory processes, which can influence judgment and decision making in complex ways, with different aspects of memory functioning contributing selectively to different tasks, and multiple aspects potentially contributing to the same task. Moreover, other cognitive and noncognitive factors related to age can play a role (e.g., processing speed, social competence, emotion regulation). Therefore, performance on a specific judgment and decision-making task will depend on a complex interplay of the factors that are needed to perform that task with a given strategy. The good news is that now we are sufficiently aware of the role of these factors, including memory-based ones, to start unraveling the complex skein of the multiple influences underlying older adults' decision making.

The review also highlighted various issues that are still underinvestigated, poorly understood, or almost completely neglected. First, the role of visuo-spatial memory processes in judgment and decision making has been almost neglected. Several aspects of episodic memory are under-investigated or poorly understood in the context of decision making, including the consequences of older adults' greater reliance on familiarity (vs recollection) for judgments and decisions, the episodic substrate of memory-based estimation and future planning, and the specific nature of age-related differences in learning processes supporting experience-based decisions. Underinvestigated topics in semantic memory comprise the specific effects (and nature) of knowledge and experience in judgment and decision making and the influence of accessibility-related manipulations on older adults' decisions. Finally, more research is definitely needed on the role of nondeclarative memory processes in intuitive decisions and in complex experience-based decision tasks. However, considering the progress recently made, we are confident that research on aging, memory, and decision making will shed light on these and other issues in the near future.

Acknowledgment

This work is supported by grants for the projects *Aging and Decision-Making Competence* (Riksbankens Jubileumsfond, Sveriges Riksbanken), *Decision-Making Abilities Across the Adult Life Span* (Wenner Gren Foundation), and by an *FRA* grant (University of Trieste, 2011–2013). The Betula project is supported by the Swedish Research Council. Corresponding author: Fabio Del Missier, Department of Life Sciences, University of Trieste, Via Weiss 21, I-34128 Trieste (TS), Italy. E-mail: delmisfa@units.it.

References

Addis, D. R., Wong, A. T., & Schacter, D. L. (2008). Age-related changes in the episodic simulation of future events. *Psychological Science, 19*, 33–41.

Alba, J. W., Hutchinson, J. W., & Lynch, J. G., Jr. (1991). Memory and decision making. In H. H. Kassarjian, & T. S. Robertson (Eds.), *Handbook of consumer theory and research* (pp. 1–49). New York, NY: Prentice Hall.

Baddeley, A., Emslie, H., & Smith, I. N. (1992). *The speed and capacity of language-processing test*. Bury St. Edmunds, England: Thames Valley Test Company.

Baddeley, A., Eysenck, M. W., & Anderson, M. C. (2009). *Memory*. New York, NY: Psychology Press.

Bayen, U. J., Erdfelder, E., Bearden, J. N., & Lozito, J. P. (2006). The interplay of memory and judgment processes in effects of aging on hindsight bias. *Journal of Experimental Psychology: Learning, Memory, and Cognition, 32*, 1003–1018.

Bayen, U. J., Pohl, R. F., Erdfelder, E., & Auer, T. S. (2007). Hindsight bias across the life span. *Social Cognition, 25*, 83–97.

Begg, I. M., Anas, A., & Farinacci, S. (1992). Dissociation of processes in belief: Source recollection, statement familiarity, and the illusion of truth. *Journal of Experimental Psychology: General, 121*, 446–458.

Bernstein, D. M., Erdfelder, E., Meltzoff, A. N., Peria, W., & Loftus, G. R. (2011). Hindsight bias from 3 to 95 years of age. *Journal of Experimental Psychology: Learning, Memory, and Cognition, 37*, 378.

Berry, D. C., & Broadbent, D. E. (1984). On the relationship between task performance and associated task knowledge. *The Quarterly Journal of Experimental Psychology: Human Experimental Psychology, 36*(A), 209–231.

Berry, D. C., & Broadbent, D. E. (1987). The combination of explicit and implicit learning processes in task control. *Psychological Research, 49*, 7–15.
Blank, H., Fischer, V., & Erdfelder, E. (2003). Hindsight bias in political elections. *Memory, 11*, 491–504.
Bopp, K. L., & Verhaeghen, P. (2005). Aging and verbal memory span: A meta-analysis. *Journal of Gerontology: B Series, 60*, 223–233.
Briñol, P., & Petty, R. E. (2009). Persuasion: Insights from the self-validation hypothesis. In M. P. Zanna (Ed.), *Advances in experimental social psychology* (Vol. 41) (pp. 69–118). New York: Academic Press.
Brown, N. R. (2002). Encoding, representing, and estimating event frequencies: A multiple strategy perspective. In P. Sedlmeier, & T. Betsch (Eds.), *Frequency processing and cognition* (pp. 37–53). New York: Oxford University Press.
Bruine de Bruin, W., Parker, A. M., & Fischhoff, B. (2007). Individual differences in adult decision-making competence. *Journal of Personality and Social Psychology, 92*, 938–956.
Bruine de Bruin, W., Parker, A. M., & Fischhoff, B. (2012). Explaining adult age differences in decision-making competence. *Journal of Behavioral Decision Making, 25*, 352–360.
Burke, D. M., MacKay, D. G., & James, L. E. (1999). Theoretical approaches to language and aging. In T. J. Perfect, & E. A. Maylor (Eds.), *Models of cognitive aging* (pp. 204–237). Oxford, England: Oxford University Press.
Carstensen, L. L. (2006). The influence of a sense of time on human development. *Science, 312*, 1913–1915.
Castle, E., Eisenberger, N. I., Seeman, T. E., Moons, W. G., Boggero, I. A., Grinblatt, M. S., et al. (2012). Neural and behavioral bases of age differences in perceptions of trust. *Proceedings of the National Academy of Sciences, 109*, 20848–20852.
Charles, S. T., Mather, M., & Carstensen, L. L. (2003). Aging and emotional memory: The forgettable nature of negative images for older adults. *Journal of Experimental Psychology: General, 132*, 310–324.
Cialdini, R. B., Kallgren, C. A., & Reno, R. R. (1991). A focus theory of normative conduct: A theoretical refinement and reevaluation of the role of norms in human behavior. In L. Berkowitz (Ed.), *Advances in experimental social psychology* (Vol. 24) (pp. 201–234). San Diego, CA: Academic Press.
Craik, F. I. M. (1983). On the transfer of information from temporary to permanent memory. *Philosophical Transactions of the Royal Society of London, B302*, 341–359.
Craik, F. I., Byrd, M., & Swanson, J. M. (1987). Patterns of memory loss in three elderly samples. *Psychology and Aging, 2*, 79–86.
Craik, F. I. M., & McDowd, J. M. (1987). Age differences in recall and recognition. *Psychology and Aging, 13*, 474–479.
Curran, T. (1997). Effects of aging on implicit sequence learning: Accounting for sequence structure and explicit knowledge. *Psychological Research, 60*, 24–41.
De Neys, W. (2006). Automatic–heuristic and executive–analytic processing during reasoning: Chronometric and dual-task considerations. *Quarterly Journal of Experimental Psychology, 59*, 1070–1100.
De Neys, W., & Verschueren, N. (2006). Working memory capacity and a notorious brain teaser. *Experimental Psychology, 53*, 123–131.
Del Missier, F., Mäntylä, T., & Bruine de Bruin, W. (2010). Executive functions in decision making: An individual differences approach. *Thinking & Reasoning, 16*, 69–97.
Del Missier, F., Mäntylä, T., & Bruine de Bruin, W. (2012). Decision-making competence, executive functioning, and general cognitive abilities. *Journal of Behavioral Decision Making, 25*, 331–351.
Del Missier, F., Mäntylä, T., Bruine de Bruin, W., Hansson, P., Parker, A., & Nilsson, L.-G. (2014). *Unraveling the aging skein: Disentangling multiple age-related influences on decision making*. Manuscript in preparation.
Del Missier, F., Mäntylä, T., Hansson, P., Bruine de Bruin, W., Parker, A., & Nilsson, L.-G. (2013). The multifold relationship between memory and decision making: An individual-differences study. *Journal of Experimental Psychology: Learning, Memory, and Cognition, 39*, 1344–1364.

Del Missier, F., & Terpini, C. (2009). Part-set cuing in option generation. *Memory & Cognition, 37*, 265–276.

Depping, M. K., & Freund, A. M. (2013). When choice matters: Task-dependent memory effects in older adulthood. *Psychology and Aging, 28*, 923–936.

Dienes, Z., & Fahey, R. (1995). Role of specific instances in controlling a dynamic system. *Journal of Experimental Psychology: Learning, Memory, and Cognition, 21*, 848–862.

Dienes, Z., & Fahey, R. (1998). The role of implicit memory in controlling a dynamic system. *Quarterly Journal of Experimental Psychology, 51A*, 593–614.

Dougherty, M. R. P., Gronlund, S. D., & Gettys, C. F. (2003). Memory as a fundamental heuristic for decision making. In S. L. Schneider, & J. Shanteau (Eds.), *Emerging perspectives on judgment and decision research* (pp. 125–164). New York: Cambridge University Press.

Dougherty, M. R. P., & Hunter, J. E. (2003). Hypothesis generation, probability judgment, and individual differences in working memory capacity. *Acta Psychologica, 113*, 263–282.

Finucane, M. L., & Gullion, C. M. (2010). Developing a tool for measuring the decision-making competence of older adults. *Psychology and Aging, 25*, 271–288.

Finucane, M. L., Mertz, C. K., Slovic, P., & Schmidt, E. S. (2005). Task complexity and older adults' decision-making competence. *Psychology and Aging, 20*, 71–84.

Fischhoff, B. (1975). Hindsight is not equal to foresight: The effect of outcome knowledge on judgment under uncertainty. *Journal of Experimental Psychology: Human Perception and Performance, 1*, 288–299.

Fisk, A. D., & Rogers, W. A. (2000). Influence of training and experience on skill acquisition and maintenance in older adults. *Journal of Aging and Physical Activity, 8*, 373–378.

Fleischman, D. A., & Gabrieli, J. D. E. (1998). Repetition priming in normal aging and Alzheimer's disease: A review of findings and theories. *Psychology and Aging, 13*, 88–119.

Gabrieli, J. D. (1998). Cognitive neuroscience of human memory. *Annual Review of Psychology, 49*, 87–115.

Glöckner, A., & Witteman, C. (2010). Beyond dual-process models: A categorisation of processes underlying intuitive judgement and decision making. *Thinking & Reasoning, 16*, 1–25.

Grady, C. L., & Craik, F. I. (2000). Changes in memory processing with age. *Current Opinion in Neurobiology, 10*, 224–231.

Hasher, L., & Zacks, R. T. (1988). Working memory, comprehension, and aging: A review and a new view. In G. H. Bower (Ed.), *The psychology of learning and motivation* (Vol. 22) (pp. 193–225). San Diego, CA: Academic Press.

Henninger, D. E., Madden, D. J., & Huettel, S. A. (2010). Processing speed and memory mediate age-related differences in decision making. *Psychology and Aging, 25*, 262–270.

Hess, T. M., Osowski, N. L., & Leclerc, C. M. (2005). Age and experience influences on the complexity of social inferences. *Psychology and Aging, 20*, 447–459.

Hinson, J. M., Jameson, T. L., & Whitney, P. (2003). Impulsive decision making and working memory. *Journal of Experimental Psychology. Learning, Memory, and Cognition, 29*, 298–306.

Howard, J. H., & Howard, D. V. (1997). Age differences in implicit learning of higher order dependencies in serial patterns. *Psychology and Aging, 12*, 634–656.

Howard, D. V., & Howard, J. H., Jr. (2012). Dissociable forms of implicit learning in aging. In M. Naveh-Benjamin, & N. Ohta (Eds.), *Memory and aging: Current issues and future directions* (pp. 125–151). Psychology Press.

Jacoby, L. L. (1999a). Ironic effects of repetition: Measuring age-related differences in memory. *Journal of Experimental Psychology. Learning, Memory, and Cognition, 25*, 3–22.

Jacoby, L. L. (1999b). Deceiving the elderly: Effects of accessibility bias in cued-recall performance. *Cognitive Neuropsychology, 16*, 417–436.

Jacoby, L. L., & Rhodes, M. G. (2006). False remembering in the aged. *Current Directions in Psychological Science, 15*, 49–53.

Jenkins, L., Myerson, J., Joerding, J. A., & Hale, S. (2000). Converging evidence that visuospatial cognition is more age-sensitive than verbal cognition. *Psychology and Aging, 15*, 157–175.

Juslin, P., Karlsson, L., & Olsson, H. (2008). Information integration in multiple cue judgment: A division of labor hypothesis. *Cognition, 106*, 259–298.

Juslin, P., Olsson, H., & Olsson, A.-C. (2003). Exemplar effects in categorization and multiple-cue judgment. *Journal of Experimental Psychology: General, 132*, 133–156.

Kahneman, D., & Tversky, A. (1979). Intuitive prediction: Biases and corrective procedures. *TIMS Studies in Management Science, 12*, 313–327.

Kemps, E., & Newson, R. (2006). Comparison of adult age differences in verbal and visuospatial memory: The importance of "pure" parallel and validated measures. *Journal of Clinical and Experimental Neuropsychology, 28*, 341–356.

Kim, S., & Hasher, L. (2005). The attraction effect in decision making: Superior performance by older adults. *Quarterly Journal of Experimental Psychology, 58A*, 120–133.

Kliegl, R., Mayr, U., & Krampe, R. (1994). Time-accuracy functions for determining process and person differences: An application to cognitive aging. *Cognitive Psychology, 26*, 134–164.

Kryla-Lighthall, N., & Mather, M. (2009). The role of cognitive control in older adults' emotional well-being. In V. Berngtson, D. Gans, N. Putney, & M. Silverstein (Eds.), *Handbook of theories of aging* (2nd ed.) (pp. 323–344). Springer Publishing.

Lachman, M. E., Röcke, C., Rosnick, C., & Ryff, C. D. (2008). Realism and illusion in Americans' temporal views of their life satisfaction: Age differences in reconstructing the past and anticipating the future. *Psychological Science, 19*, 889–897.

LaVoie, D., & Light, L. L. (1994). Adult age differences in repetition priming: A meta-analysis. *Psychology & Aging, 9*, 539–553.

Levine, B., Svoboda, E., Hay, J. F., Winocur, G., & Moscovitch, M. (2002). Aging and autobiographical memory: Dissociating episodic from semantic retrieval. *Psychology & Aging, 17*, 677–689.

Li, Y., Baldassi, M., Johnson, E. J., & Weber, E. U. (2013). Complementary cognitive capabilities, economic decision making, and aging. *Psychology and Aging, 28*, 595–613.

Lieberman, M. D. (2000). Intuition: A social cognitive neuroscience approach. *Psychological Bulletin, 126*, 109–137.

Light, L. L., Prull, M. W., La Voie, D. J., & Healy, M. R. (2000). Dual-process theories of memory in old age. In T. J. Perfect, & E. A. Maylor (Eds.), *Models of cognitive aging* (pp. 238–300). New York: Oxford University Press.

Lindenberger, U., & Baltes, P. B. (1997). Intellectual functioning in old and very old age: Cross-sectional results from the Berlin aging study. *Psychology and Aging, 12*, 410–432.

Liu, L. L., & Park, D. C. (2004). Aging and medical adherence: The use of automatic processes to achieve effortful things. *Psychology and Aging, 19*, 318–325.

Löckenhoff, C. E. (2011). Age, time, and decision making: From processing speed to global time horizons. *Annals of the New York Academy of Sciences, 1235*, 44–56.

MacKay, D. G., & Abrams, L. (1996). Language, memory, and aging: Distributed deficits and the structure of new-versus-old connections. In J. E. Birren, & K. W. Schaie (Eds.), *Handbook of the psychology of aging* (4th ed.) (pp. 251–265). San Diego, CA: Academic Press.

Mandel, N., & Johnson, E. J. (2002). When web pages influence choice: Effects of visual primes on experts and novices. *Journal of Consumer Research, 29*, 235–245.

Mata, R., Josef, A. K., Samanez–Larkin, G. R., & Hertwig, R. (2011). Age differences in risky choice: A meta–analysis. *Annals of the New York Academy of Sciences, 1235*, 18–29.

Mata, R., Schooler, L. J., & Rieskamp, J. (2007). The aging decision maker: Cognitive aging and the adaptive selection of decision strategies. *Psychology and Aging, 22*, 796.

Mata, R., von Helversen, B., Karlsson, L., & Cüpper, L. (2012). Adult age differences in categorization and multiple-cue judgment. *Developmental Psychology, 48*, 1188–1201.

Mata, R., von Helversen, B., & Rieskamp, J. (2010). Learning to choose: Cognitive aging and strategy selection learning in decision making. *Psychology and Aging*, *25*, 299–309.

Mather, M. (2006). A review of decision making processes: Weighing the risks and benefits of aging. In L. L. Carstensen, & C. R. Hartel (Eds.), *When I'm 64* (pp. 145–173). Washington, DC: The National Academies Press.

Mather, M., & Carstensen, L. L. (2005). Aging and motivated cognition: The positivity effect in attention and memory. *Trends in Cognitive Science*, *9*, 496–502.

Mather, M., & Johnson, M. K. (2000). Choice-supportive source monitoring: Do our decisions seem better to us as we age? *Psychology and Aging*, *15*, 596–606.

Mather, M., & Johnson, M. K. (2003). Affective review and schema reliance in memory in older and younger adults. *American Journal of Psychology*, *116*, 169–189.

Mather, M., & Knight, M. (2005). Goal-directed memory: The role of cognitive control in older adults' emotional memory. *Psychology and Aging*, *20*, 554–570.

Mayr, U., & Kliegl, R. (1993). Sequential and coordinative complexity: Age-based processing limitations in figural transformations. *Journal of Experimental Psychology: Learning, Memory, & Cognition*, *19*, 1297–1320.

Meyer, B. J. F., & Pollard, C. A. (2004). Why do older adults make faster decisions about treatments for breast cancer? In *Paper presented at the cognitive aging conference, Atlanta, GA*.

Meyer, B. J. F., Russo, C., & Talbot, A. (1995). Discourse comprehension and problem solving: Decisions about the treatment of breast cancer by women across the life span. *Psychology and Aging*, *10*, 84–103.

Moons, W. G., Mackie, D. M., & Garcia-Marques, T. (2009). The impact of repetition-induced familiarity on agreement with weak and strong arguments. *Journal of Personality and Social Psychology*, *96*, 32–44.

Nedungadi, P. (1990). Recall and consumer consideration sets: Influencing choice without altering brand evaluations. *Journal of Consumer Research*, *17*, 263–276.

Nettelbeck, X., & Rabbitt, P. M. A. (1992). Aging, cognitive performance, and mental speed. *Intelligence*, *16*, 189–205.

Nielsen, L., Knutson, B., & Carstensen, L. L. (2008). Affect dynamics, affective forecasting, and aging. *Emotion*, *8*, 318–330.

Nilsson, L.-G., Adolfsson, R., Bäckman, L., de Frias, C. M., Molander, B., et al. (2004). Betula: A prospective cohort study on memory, health and aging. *Aging, Neuropsychology, and Cognition*, *11*, 134–148.

Nilsson, L.-G., Bäckman, L., Erngrund, K., Nyberg, L., Adolfsson, R., Bucht, G., et al. (1997). The Betula prospective cohort study: Memory, health, and aging. *Aging, Neuropsychology, and Cognition*, *4*, 1–32.

Nyberg, L. (1994). A structural equation modeling approach to the multiple memory systems question. *Journal of Experimental Psychology: Learning, Memory, and Cognition*, *20*, 485–491.

Nyberg, L., Maitland, S. B., Rönnlund, M., Bäckman, L., Dixon, R. A., Wahlin, Å., et al. (2003). Selective adult age differences in an age-invariant multifactor model of declarative memory. *Psychology and Aging*, *18*, 149–160.

Park, D. C., Lautenschlager, G., Hedden, T., Davison, N., Smith, A. D., & Smith, P. K. (2002). Models of visuospatial and verbal memory across the adult life span. *Psychology and Aging*, *17*, 299–320.

Park, D. C., Smith, A. D., Lautenschlager, G., Earles, J. L., Frieske, D., Zwahr, M., et al. (1996). Mediators of long-term memory performance across the life span. *Psychology and Aging*, *11*, 621–637.

Parker, A. M., & Fischhoff, B. (2005). Decision–making competence: External validation through an individual-differences approach. *Journal of Behavioral Decision Making*, *18*, 1–27.

Parks, C. M., & Toth, J. P. (2006). Fluency, familiarity, aging, and the illusion of truth. *Aging, Neuropsychology, and Cognition*, *13*, 225–253.

Peters, E. M., & Bruine de Bruin, W. (2012). Aging and decision skills. In M. K. Dhami, A. Schlottmann, & M. Waldmann (Eds.), *Judgment and decision making as a skill: Learning, development, and evolution* (pp. 113–139). New York, NY: Cambridge University Press.

Peters, E., Hess, T. M., Västfjäll, D., & Auman, C. (2007). Adult age differences in dual information processes and their influence on judgments and decisions: A review. *Perspectives on Psychological Science, 2*, 1–23.

Prull, M. W., Gabrieli, J. D. E., & Bunge, S. A. (2000). Age-related changes in memory: A cognitive neuroscience perspective. In F. I. Craik, & T. A. Salthouse (Eds.), *Handbook of aging and cognition* (2nd ed.) (pp. 91–153). Mahwah, NJ: Erlbaum.

Queen, T. L., & Hess, T. M. (2010). Age differences in the effects of conscious and unconscious thought in decision making. *Psychology and Aging, 25*, 251–261.

Reyna, V. F., & Brainerd, C. J. (2011). Dual processes in decision making and developmental neuroscience: A fuzzy-trace model. *Developmental Review, 31*, 180–206.

Rönnlund, M., Nyberg, L., Bäckman, L., & Nilsson, L.-G. (2005). Stability, growth, and decline in adult life span development of declarative memory: Cross-sectional and longitudinal data from a population-based study. *Psychology and Aging, 20*, 3–18.

Ross, M., Grossmann, I., & Schryer, E. (2014). Contrary to psychological and popular opinion, there is no compelling evidence that older adults are disproportionately victimized by consumer fraud. *Perspectives on Psychological Science, 9*, 427–442.

Salthouse, T. A. (1995). Differential age-related influences on memory for verbal-symbolic information and visual-spatial information. *Journal of Gerontology: Psychological Sciences, 50B*, 193–201.

Salthouse, T. A. (1996). The processing-speed theory of adult age differences in cognition. *Psychological Review, 103*, 403–428.

Salthouse, T. A. (1998). Independence of age-related influences on cognitive abilities across the life span. *Developmental Psychology, 34*, 851–864.

Salthouse, T. A. (2004). What and when of cognitive aging. *Current Directions in Psychological Science, 13*, 140–144.

Salthouse, T. A. (2005). Relations between cognitive abilities and measures of executive functioning. *Neuropsychology, 19*, 532–545.

Salthouse, T. A. (2009). When does age-related cognitive decline begin? *Neurobiology of Aging, 30*, 507–514.

Salthouse, T. A., Atkinson, T. M., & Berish, D. E. (2003). Executive functioning as a potential mediator of age-related cognitive decline in normal adults. *Journal of Experimental Psychology: General, 132*, 566–594.

Samanez-Larkin, G. R. (2013). Financial decision making and the aging brain. *APS Observer, 26*, 30–33.

Schacter, D. L. (2012). Adaptive constructive processes and the future of memory. *American Psychologist, 67*, 603–613.

Schacter, D. L., Koutstaal, W., & Norman, K. A. (1997). False memories and aging. *Trends in Cognitive Sciences, 1*, 229–236.

Schaie, K. W. (2005). *Developmental influences on adult intelligence: The Seattle longitudinal study.* New York: Oxford University Press.

Scheibe, S., Mata, R., & Carstensen, L. L. (2011). Age differences in affective forecasting and experienced emotion surrounding the 2008 US presidential election. *Cognition & Emotion, 25*, 1029–1044.

Sheldon, S., McAndrews, M. P., & Moscovitch, M. (2011). Episodic memory processes mediated by the medial temporal lobes contribute to open ended problem solving. *Neuropsychologia, 49*, 2439–2447.

Shiv, B., & Fedorikhin, A. (1999). Heart and mind in conflict: The interplay of affect and cognition in consumer decision making. *Journal of Consumer Research, 26*, 278–292.

Simon, J. R., Howard, J. H., & Howard, D. V. (2011). Age differences in implicit learning of probabilistic, unstructured sequences. *Journals of Gerontology, Series B: Psychological Sciences and Social Sciences, 66*, 32–38.

Skurnik, I., Yoon, C., Park, D. C., & Schwarz, N. (2005). How warnings about false claims become recommendations. *Journal of Consumer Research, 31*, 713–724.

Spencer, W. D., & Raz, N. (1995). Differential effects of aging on memory for content and context: A meta-analysis. *Psychology and Aging, 10*, 527–539.

Stanovich, K. E., & West, R. F. (2008). On the relative independence of thinking biases and cognitive ability. *Journal of Personality and Social Psychology, 94*, 672–695.

Strough, J., Karns, T. E., & Schlosnagle, L. (2011). Decision-making heuristics and biases across the life span. *Annals of the New York Academy of Sciences, 1235*, 57–74.

Taylor, S. E., Pham, L. B., Rivkin, I. D., & Armor, D. A. (1998). Harnessing the imagination: Mental simulation, self-regulation, and coping. *American Psychologist, 53*, 429–439.

Tentori, K., Osherson, D., Hasher, L., & May, C. (2001). Wisdom and aging: Irrational preferences in college students but not older adults. *Cognition, 81*, 87–96.

Verhaeghen, P. (2003). Aging and vocabulary score: A meta-analysis. *Psychology and Aging, 18*, 332–339.

Verhaeghen, P., Marcoen, A., & Goosens, L. (1993). Facts and fiction about memory aging: A quantitative integration of research findings. *Journal of Gerontology: Psychological Sciences, 48*, 157–171.

Verhaeghen, P., & Salthouse, T. A. (1997). Meta-analyses of age-cognition relations in adulthood: Estimates of linear and non-linear age effects and structural models. *Psychological Bulletin, 122*, 231–249.

Weber, E. U., Goldstein, W. M., & Barlas, S. (1995). And let us not forget memory: The role of memory processes and techniques in the study of judgment and choice. *The Psychology of Learning and Motivation, 32*, 33–81.

Wiggs, C. L. (1993). Aging and memory for frequency of occurrence of novel, visual stimuli: Direct and indirect measures. *Psychology and Aging, 8*, 400–410.

Wood, S., Busemeyer, J., Koling, A., Cox, C. R., & Davis, H. (2005). Older adults as adaptive decision makers: Evidence from the Iowa gambling task. *Psychology and Aging, 20*, 220–225.

Yonelinas, A. P. (2002). The nature of recollection and familiarity: A review of 30 years of research. *Journal of Memory and Language, 46*, 441–517.

Zacks, R. T., Hasher, L., & Li, K. Z. H. (2000). Human memory. In F. I. Craik, & T. A. Salthouse (Eds.), *The handbook of aging and cognition* (2nd ed.) (pp. 93–357). Mahwah, NJ: Lawrence Erlbaum.

CHAPTER

8

Complementary Contributions of Fluid and Crystallized Intelligence to Decision Making Across the Life Span

Lisa Zaval[1,3], *Ye Li*[2], *Eric J. Johnson*[3], *Elke U. Weber*[3]

[1]Department of Psychology, Columbia University, New York, NY, USA; [2]School of Business Administration, University of California, Riverside, CA, USA; [3]Center for Decision Sciences, Columbia University, New York, NY, USA

BETTER OR WORSE OFF?

In November 2013, 61 percent of voters in New York rejected a proposed amendment to their state Constitution, which would have raised the mandatory retirement age to 80 for judges of the New York Supreme Court and Court of Appeals. Proponents of the amendment had argued that the existing age limit of 70, set after the Civil War, had become outdated in a modern era of antibiotics and cataract surgery, and had led to the unnecessary exclusion of experienced legal experts on the bench. Opponents, meanwhile, were concerned about age-related declines in mental acuity. Thus, behind this debate stood a deeper question: Could these veterans of the law make sound decisions, or would they be encumbered by slower cognitive functioning due to the aging process?

It is an unfortunate, but well documented, fact of life that some cognitive abilities diminish with age. Yet it is also true that as people get older, they gain more life experience. Whether in their personal or professional lives, people continuously accumulate new knowledge and experience,

Aging and Decision Making
http://dx.doi.org/10.1016/B978-0-12-417148-0.00008-X

and recent research indicates that this accumulated life experience may counteract age-related cognitive declines.

This chapter explores the interplay between the fluid cognitive declines in older adults and their higher levels of crystallized intelligence, and how these two factors impact decision-making ability in everyday life. We first review literature on cognitive capabilities across the adult life span, and propose the hypothesis that *experience and accumulated knowledge may help compensate for declining fluid cognitive function* in decision making across the life span. We then discuss the role of domain-specific experience in context-specific tasks and everyday problem solving. Finally, we close with implications for public policy, particularly for the design of effective decision-making environments for older adults.

COGNITIVE CAPABILITIES AND DECISION MAKING ACROSS THE ADULT LIFE SPAN

The concept of aging has long given rise to conflicts in public perception: Although people believe in the adage that age brings knowledge, we also observe that older adults suffer from a decline in many cognitive abilities. Yet researchers have found mixed evidence regarding older adults' decision-making abilities. While there are many domains in which older adults are worse than younger adults, there are also domains in which they perform as well or better, depending on the type of decision (for a meta-analysis, see Thornton & Dumke, 2005).

What makes a "good" decision? For many decisions, economics prescribes a normatively correct choice. For example, people should never value a 50/50 gamble between $50 and $100 less than they value $50 (yet they do; Gneezy, List, & Wu, 2006). Even for decisions where individual preferences may affect what is deemed "correct" for the individual—for example, intertemporal choices (e.g., a choice between $50 today or $100 in a year)—economics suggests that some choices (e.g., $50 today, since $100 in a year provides a 100% interest rate) are suboptimal because they are inconsistent with other available options (e.g., borrowing at a lower interest rate; Frederick, Loewenstein, & O'Donoghue, 2002). On the other hand, it is important to note that decisions may not always be intended to maximize expected or net present utility, but rather to satisfy other criteria, such as minimizing expected loss or producing a quick resolution.

Some examples of decision making that seems to worsen with age include the suboptimal choices made when the number of alternative options increases (Besedes et al., 2012), and excessive risk aversion across certain domains (Mata, Josef, Samanez-Larkin, & Hertwig, 2011; Qian & Weber, 2008; Rolison, Hanoch, Wood, & Liu, 2013). Other research finds that decision-making skills improve with age: For example, older adults make more accurate evaluations of their own knowledge (Kovalchik, Camerer, Grether, Plott, & Allman, 2005), are better at avoiding the influence of irrelevant options on choices (Kim & Hasher, 2005), and are better at discontinuing unprofitable investments (Bruine de Bruin, Parker, & Fischhoff, 2012; Strough, Karns, & Schlosnagle, 2011; Strough, Mehta, McFall, & Schuller, 2008). Some of these age-related changes in decision capacity are functional and adaptive, whereas others may lead to decision-making patterns that leave older adults open to suboptimal or even dangerous outcomes. This discrepancy in the literature is puzzling: What might account for the conflicting pattern of the effect of age on decision-making quality?

The concepts of *fluid intelligence* and *crystallized intelligence* are useful in an attempt to reconcile these conflicting views of the effect of aging on decision making. Fluid and crystallized intelligence are two components of general intelligence that were originally identified by Cattell (1971, 1987).

Fluid intelligence (G_f) is defined as reasoning ability, and the ability to generate, transform, and manipulate different types of novel information in real time. Cross-sectional and longitudinal comparisons of adults at different ages have shown that a wide range of cognitive capabilities related to fluid intelligence decline steadily across the adult life span, including performance on tasks involving memory, reasoning, and processing speed (e.g., Salthouse, 2004, 2010; Schaie, 1993). In fact, cross-sectional studies of intelligence indicate that the average 60-year-old will have lost more than one standard deviation in fluid intelligence since the time they were 20 (e.g., Salthouse, 2004, 2010). These studies have found that all aspects of fluid intelligence decline nearly linearly with age starting from early adulthood, including processing speed and efficiency (Li et al., 2004; Salthouse, 1994, 1996), working memory (McArdle, Ferrer-Caja, Hamagami, & Woodcock, 2002; Salthouse, 1992), attention, and problem solving (Craik & Salthouse, 2000). These declines are especially noticeable when performing complex or novel tasks that require more active processing (Zacks, Hasher, & Li, 2000). This decline in fluid intelligence raises the question of if and how older adults can continue to make good decisions.

One way in which older adults may offset lower levels of fluid intelligence is by relying more heavily on their greater *crystallized intelligence*. Crystallized intelligence (G_c) is defined as an experienced-based knowledge component of intelligence that is acquired through interaction with one's environment. It reflects accumulated knowledge acquired through experience, culture, and prior learning. Crystallized intelligence is the result of accumulated life experiences, and the efficient processing and storage of accumulated information throughout a lifetime (Salthouse, 2004). This form of intelligence is often measured as knowledge, and appears to be linked to education, physical health, and general cognitive competence. It is dependent on a range of influences, including motivation, opportunity,

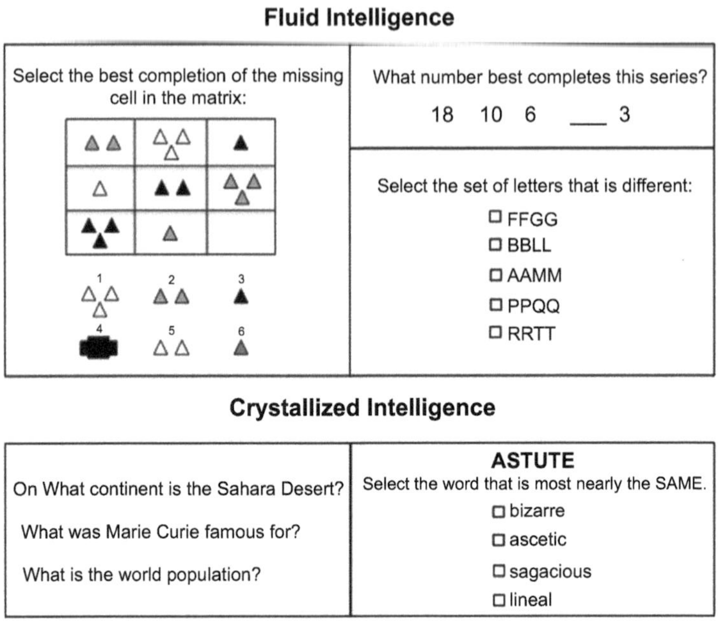

FIGURE 1 Sample items from five tasks used to measure fluid and crystallized intelligence: Raven's progressive matrices, Number series, Letter sets, WAIS III-information, and Shipley vocabulary.

and culture (Horn & Cattell, 1967). Crystallized intelligence thus signifies the acquisition and accumulation of practical experience and knowledge gained from a lifetime of practice dealing with varied tasks, situations, and challenges in everyday life (Glaser, 1984; Rowley & Slack, 2009). Indeed, those mental capabilities that depend most heavily on accumulated knowledge and experience, such as reading comprehension and vocabulary, improve across most of the life span (e.g., Salthouse, 2004). Researchers have also argued that crystallized intelligence is related to components of what may be referred to as *wisdom*, including the ability to view problems from multiple perspectives, accept compromise, and to recognize the limitations of one's own knowledge (Grossmann et al., 2010).

There are multiple ways of measuring cognitive capabilities. To obtain a global measure of crystallized intelligence, the standard practice in psychology is to assess vocabulary, analogies, and general knowledge. In contrast, fluid intelligence abilities are generally measured using cognitive functioning tasks that rely on working memory and abstract reasoning. Some of the differences in the types of standard cognitive tasks commonly used to measure fluid intelligence and crystallized intelligence are presented in Figure 1.

Decades of measurement using these tasks consistently support a widely documented cognitive aging pattern: whereas fluid intelligence

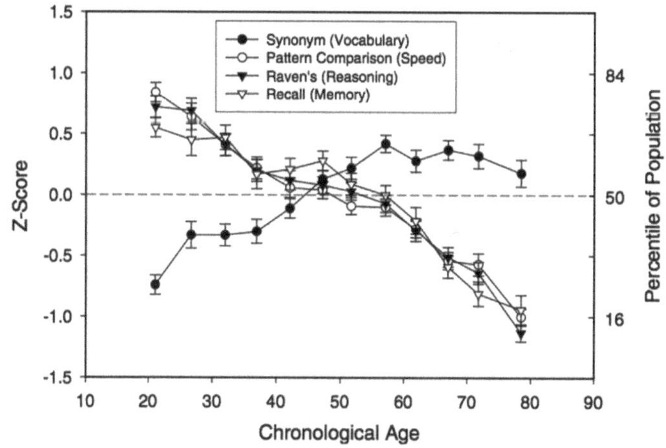

FIGURE 2 Age differences in fluid and crystallized intelligence. Means (and standard errors) of performance in four cognitive tests as a function of age. Each data point is based on between 52 and 156 adults. *From Salthouse (2010). Copyright © 2010 The International Neuropsychological Society. Reprinted with the permission of Cambridge University Press.* http://dx.doi.org/10.1017/S1355617710000706.

declines with age, crystallized intelligence increases across the adult life span into the 60s, after which it plateaus (see Figure 2). The combination of older adults' lower levels of fluid intelligence but higher levels of crystallized intelligence gives rise to the possibility that both forms of intelligence may contribute to the effect of age on decision performance, especially for decision tasks in which both the processing of new information and prior experience can contribute to forming a good decision. In the next section, we turn to the emerging research that has explored the effects of these two types of cognitive capabilities on decision quality.

COMPLEMENTARY COGNITIVE CAPABILITIES

The past several years have witnessed an expansion in research on the relationship between cognitive capabilities and aging, and in relating age differences in decision making to age differences in cognitive capabilities. An emerging theme in this area has been the emphasis on the theoretical importance of compensatory processes in understanding the effects of aging and decision making. That is, although fluid cognitive declines should generally lead to deterioration in decision quality, other capabilities may increase with age to compensate for those declines partially or completely, or even lead to age-related increases in decision quality. For example, some have suggested that older adults may rely more on affective or experiential processes to make decisions, rather than deliberative cognitive processes (e.g., Peters, Hess, Auman, & Västfjäll, 2007; Strough et al., 2011). For tasks where those affective or experiential processes can contribute to good decision making, declining cognitive abilities may therefore be offset by age differences in affective processing or experience with the task. Thus, research on aging and decision making cannot paint a full picture of age differences in decision making without understanding the underlying age-related changes in capability and reliance on these different processes.

One stream of research in this area has recently begun to empirically explore these potential interactions between cognitive and experiential processes, and their net influence on decision-making ability (e.g., Agarwal, Driscoll, Gabaix, & Laibson, 2009; Bruine de Bruin et al., 2012; Hansson, Rönnlund, Juslin, & Nilsson, 2008; Li, Baldassi, Johnson, & Weber, 2013; Peters & Bruine de Bruin, 2012). For example, Li et al. (2013) explored the possibility that higher levels of crystallized intelligence (i.e., experiential processes) provide an alternate pathway to good decisions, and that this may attenuate the effects of older adults' lower levels of fluid intelligence. Such compensation, which the authors termed the *complementary capabilities hypothesis*, was examined across a wide variety of important decisions from the judgment and decision-making literature: *temporal discounting* (how much less people value future consequences), *financial literacy* (understanding financial information and decisions), and *debt literacy* (understanding debt and interest rates). Li and colleagues related performance on these decision-making tasks to standard measures of fluid and crystallized intelligence. Interestingly, older adults performed as well as, or even better than, their younger counterparts in all four decision-making measures. The opposing age differences for fluid and crystallized intelligence with age, together with their positive relationships with decision performance, suggest how age differences in cognitive capabilities may underlay these age differences in decision performance (see Figure 3). For instance, for temporal discounting and financial literacy, the positive effect of age via crystallized intelligence perfectly offset the negative effect of age via fluid intelligence, leading to no net effect of age.

Findings from this research are consistent with the hypothesis that crystallized intelligence may represent a kind of *intellectual capital* that circumvents the diminished capabilities due to decreased fluid intelligence. The results lend empirical support to the notion that practical knowledge gleaned from a lifetime of decision-making experience may offset the declining ability to process and manipulate new information.

Importantly, the effect of age on decision quality depends on the *relative importance* of the two types of intelligence required for a particular decision. An increased level of crystallized intelligence may compensate for the negative effect of a deficit in fluid abilities on decision making—but only in situations in which the task can benefit from existing crystallized

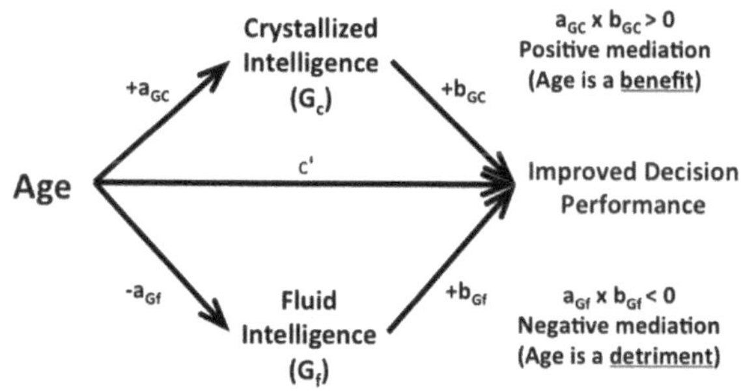

FIGURE 3 Complementary competencies hypothesis of age differences in decision performance as represented as a multiple pathway model from Li et al. (2013). As indicated by the positive paths on the right, both G_f and G_c should positively affect decision performance. However, because of opposing age trends (indicated by positive and negative paths on the left), the relationship between age and decision making requires understanding both pathways to good decisions. Using a notation similar to that of standard mediation analysis, the multiplicative product of age relationships with fluid and crystallized intelligence and their relationships with decision making shows the indirect effects of age on decision making ($a_i \times b_i$), and the remaining path as the direct effect (c') of age. *Copyright © 2013 by the American Psychological Association. Adapted with permission from Li, Y., Baldassi, M., Johnson, E. J., & Weber, E. U. (2013). Complementary cognitive capabilities, economic decision making, and aging.* Psychology and Aging, *28(3), 595.*

knowledge. If crystallized intelligence is a more important determinant of decision performance than fluid intelligence (e.g., filling out a tax return), we might expect older people to perform better than their younger counterparts. The opposite would be true for real-world tasks where fluid intelligence plays a more important role (such as learning how to operate a new smartphone). Finally, when a task depends about equally on fluid and crystallized abilities (such as driving a car, which depends on both driving experience and reaction time), the observed age trajectory might be relatively flat or even inverse-U-shaped.

Research has confirmed that the extent to which experience will attenuate age-related decline depends on the relationship between experience and decision performance on the task of interest. To illustrate, Bruine de Bruin et al. (2012) explored the relationships between age, cognitive capabilities, and a range of general decision-making capacities, including resistance to framing effects and under/over-confidence (i.e., the appropriateness of individuals' confidence in their knowledge). The authors determined that for decision tasks in which experience should impact performance (such as consistency in risk perception), task ability *did not decrease* with age. In contrast, for decision tasks in which prior experience should play no role (such as resistance to framing effects), performance *decreased* with age.

In addition to the literature assessing lab-based measures of decision making, there has been a recent emergence of studies testing the compensating capabilities framework within the context of real-world decision behaviors. Agarwal et al. (2009) studied the relationship between age and financial decision making using measures of 10 different types of credit behavior. The researchers predicted that the life-span pattern of financial performance should reflect a trade-off between rising financial experience and declining analytic ability. Consistent with these expectations, the researchers found a U-shaped age–price curve, with middle-aged adults borrowing at lower interest rates and paying fewer late fees compared to both younger and older adults. To better appreciate the magnitude of the effect of age, they found that for home-equity lines of credit, the average 75-year-old paid about $265 more each year compared to the average 50-year-old, whereas the average 25-year-old paid about $295 more. The authors argue that the middle-age peak in performance may be due to younger borrowers having high degrees of cognitive ability but relatively little financial experience, whereas older borrowers maintain a high degree of accumulated financial experience, but decline in their cognitive capacity.

The hypothesis that life-span changes in crystallized and fluid intelligence could explain age-related differences in real-world financial behaviors was corroborated in a study that combined web-based measures of cognitive ability with field observations of individuals' economic performance (Li et al., in press). Using a diverse sample of 478 adults between ages 18 and 86, the researchers combined multiple standard measures of crystallized and fluid intelligence with credit scores from a major credit reporting bureaus. Importantly, the researchers collected data on two different types of crystallized intelligence: (1) *domain-general* crystallized intelligence, measured using standard tests of vocabulary and general knowledge (as depicted in Figure 1); and (2) financial *domain-specific* crystallized intelligence, measured using a financial literacy test (Fernandes, Lynch, & Netemeyer, 2014; Lusardi & Mitchell, 2007). (A sample item from this test asks whether stocks, bonds, or savings accounts provides the highest fluctuations in returns over time.) Findings revealed that although the domain-specific measure of crystallized intelligence was positively related to higher credit scores and offset the negative influence of declining fluid intelligence, the measures of *general* crystallized intelligence were not similarly predictive. These results are consistent with the notion that crystallized intelligence may compensate for declines in fluid intelligence, but only for decisions relating to the specific domains in which the person has greater knowledge. Most importantly for public policy, the results suggest that, notwithstanding a general decline in the abilities associated with fluid intelligence, those older adults who possess high domain-specific crystallized intelligence, in the form of accumulated financial knowledge, may be finding an alternative cognitive pathway to making good financial decisions.

Practical Implications: Job Performance

Outside of the laboratory, perhaps the largest body of research examining real-world decision performance across age groups has been in studies of job performance. Because general cognitive capabilities are often a good predictor of performance in most job categories, an older adult who is able to compensate for fluid intelligence deficits should be able to maintain high work performance in life. Much of the research in this field finds no relationship between age and performance, supporting the perspective that crystallized abilities may help to offset cognitive decline across a range of domains in everyday life (McEvoy & Cascio, 1989). Because successful job performance depends both on the processing of new information as well as prior experience, the life-span pattern of job performance may reflect the tradeoff between rising prior experience and declining analytic function. What appears to be no relationship between chronological age and performance may actually depend on the relative contribution of fluid and crystallized intelligence on the specific task at hand. However, it is also important to mention that older adults may be able to compensate for cognitive deficits in everyday problem solving using techniques unrelated to expertise. In a recent review, Salthouse (2012) argues that relatively stable levels of functioning in job performance may also reflect the fact that everyday functioning may not require maximal levels of performance, as well as the contributions of noncognitive traits (e.g., personality) to success.

PRACTICAL DECISION MAKING AND THE ROLE OF DOMAIN-SPECIFIC EXPERIENCE

As we have seen, a growing body of research indicates that increased crystallized intelligence helps mitigate decreases in cognitive ability as measured by fluid intelligence. However, the precise ways in which crystallized intelligence makes this contribution have yet to be fully determined. We know little about which abilities are actually captured by standard measures of general crystallized intelligence (using tests of vocabulary and general knowledge), and how these abilities contribute to good decisions. As such, there is a need for more empirical research on the conceptualization and measurement of crystallized abilities.

Crystallized intelligence may encompass one or more of a number of abilities that contribute to improved decision making. These components may include (1) *domain-specific knowledge* (i.e., semantic knowledge about a domain); (2) *domain-specific expertise* (i.e., reduced information use and more efficient processing obtained from expert skill in a particular domain); and (3) *domain-general principles* (e.g., improved decision skills gained from years of practice, such as eliminating irrelevant or dominated alternatives in a choice task and identifying redundant information). To illustrate how each component may contribute to decision making, consider as an example how each contributes to a choice among different health insurance plans: *Domain-specific knowledge* about each type of cost (e.g., premium or deductible) seems essential to making an optimal choice. *Domain-specific expertise* derived from years of experience in choosing health care plans could allow one to develop efficient mental short-cuts in estimating annual costs for each plan. Finally, *domain-general principles* may include the ability to simplify decisions by finding redundancy between two dimensions, an ability gleaned from accumulated life experience in making multi-attribute decisions across many domains.

Given the varied components that comprise crystallized intelligence, how might each work to improve decision quality among older adults? Two possible interpretations have been suggested (e.g., Kim & Hasher, 2005). One is the more general domain experience view, which suggests that older adults are generally more skilled at making practical decisions compared with their younger, less experienced counterparts, and that this experience aids decision making globally across several contexts. In contrast, the domain-specific expertise/knowledge view argues that an older adult will be better in making decisions *only in those specific domains* in which they have greater knowledge or expertise. As we have seen, this latter view was supported by Li et al. in press, who found that domain-specific crystallized intelligence, in the form of financial literacy, offset cognitive declines for financial decision making. This perspective suggests that age-related cognitive declines may be attenuated by domain-specific experiences in decision tasks that are familiar and highly practiced.

A substantial amount of research has been conducted to find evidence for this type of attenuation across numerous domains. One way in which the domain-specific framework is commonly investigated is by choosing a task on which age-related decline has been documented, and then altering this task so that performance is supported by domain-specific experience (e.g., Soederberg-Miller, 2009). To illustrate, Meinz (2000) tested pianists across a range of experience and ages on measures of music memory and perceptual speed (visually identifying similarities of musical chord pairs), skills that generally decline with age. Results revealed that higher levels of musical experience in the older participants did partially attenuate the negative effects of age on the memory and recall tasks.

Other research suggests that the extent to which experience will offset age-related decline in decision making depends on the relationship between experience and performance on the task of interest. In a study of marketplace decision making, Tentori, Osherson, Hasher, and May (2001) observed the product choices made by college students and older adults faced with hypothetical discount cards for supermarket products.

Across a series of experiments, the decisions made by the younger group consistently violated the test of regularity, while older adults showed no such tendency. (A decision maker is considered "irregular" if he would choose B from [A, B, C] but not from [A, B]; i.e., preferring apple in a choice between apple and banana, but banana in a choice among apple, banana, and orange). The authors suggested that accumulated shopping experience in grocery stores may train an individual to be cautious of framing effects and other contextual effects in judging the value of products, perhaps even reducing impulsive marketplace purchases. Thus, it is possible that the greater accumulated shopping experience of older adults might act as a buffer against cognitive decline, manifesting in more "regular" choices. However, it should be noted that follow-up work by Kim and Hasher (2005) suggests that a lifetime of experience may result in skilled decision making across a range of topic domains, independent of interest or experience level.

Additional results exploring the role of marketplace expertise are provided by List (2003), who shows that increased market experience eliminates an important economic phenomenon known as the endowment effect, whereby people demand a higher price for a product that they own than they would be willing to pay for a product that they do not own. Further, Johnson, Gächter, and Herrmann (2006) demonstrate that consumers who are more knowledgeable about an attribute show lower levels of loss aversion for that attribute. Such findings support that notion that domain expertise may be an important boundary condition for understanding age effects on adults' decisions.

Mechanisms

To understand how older adults use their lifetime of expertise and knowledge to overcome potential problem-solving deficits, it is important to consider some of the proposed mechanisms responsible for this compensation.

First, in order to better understand the mechanisms by which domain-specific experience enhances decision quality, we must also understand how individual, task, and contextual characteristics impact the fit between an individual and the task. Yoon, Cole, and Lee (2009) argue that this "person-context" fit is expected to be highest when specific task and contextual demands do not exceed an individual's basic cognitive capabilities (i.e., fluid intelligence). In these high-fit circumstances where the opportunity for effective decision making is high, older adults should not feel compelled to adapt their decision processes. In contrast, when the requirements imposed by the task and contexts exceed the cognitive resources available, older adults may feel the need to modify their problem-solving strategies. As fit decreases, older adults may begin to rely more on their experience and accumulated knowledge, allowing them to compensate for deficits in cognitive resources resulting from advanced age.

Second, although it seems obvious that increased knowledge is beneficial to the decision-making process, there is a potential problem: Additional knowledge, if not well structured, can make information more difficult to retrieve (McCloskey & Bigler, 1980; Myers, O'Brien, Balota, & Toyofuku, 1984; Radvansky, Spieler, & Zacks, 1993). A good example of this principle is demonstrated in research on the fan effect (Anderson, 1976), in which learning a larger set of facts about a particular category typically *increases* the amount of time it takes to later verify whether any one fact in the category is true (Anderson & Reder, 1999; Lewis & Anderson, 1976). The fan effect is reduced, however, when the facts that one learns are organized into subcategories (McCloskey & Bigler, 1980)—a type of organization that is particularly likely when an individual has expert knowledge in a given domain (Chase & Ericsson, 1981).

Thus, the effect of additional knowledge will depend upon the degree to which knowledge is *well-structured*. Researchers have proposed that with accumulated experience, elements of knowledge become increasingly interconnected and structured, and are integrated with past representations of knowledge to make processing faster and more efficient (e.g., Doane, Sohn, & Jodlowski, 2004). When older adults have vast knowledge to draw upon, representing the long-term product of processing, they may be able to use their highly structured retrieval structures to support decision making, despite working memory declines and other deficits (Ericsson & Kintsch, 1995; Miller, Cohen, & Wingfield, 2006). In this way, older adults' greater experience in a number of decision-making domains may be related to well-structured memory representations that provide a buffer against their susceptibility to fluid declines.

To understand how this knowledge may lead to more consistent preferences, we have developed a theory that relates memory organization to preference. This model, termed *query theory*, suggests that these failures of memory retrieval may be due to output interference, and that differences in memory search and retrieval should affect decision performance for a number of decision-making phenomena (see query theory and the preferences-as-memory framework; Johnson, Häubl, & Keinan, 2007; Weber et al., 2007). The effects of interference appear to increase with age, such as in short-term memory and Stroop tasks (Hedden & Park, 2001; Spieler, Balota, & Faust, 1996), directed forgetting tasks (Zacks, Radvansky, & Hasher, 1996), and resolving interference from competing memories (Healey, Ngo, & Hasher, 2014). Thus, the role of organization may play an important moderating role in assessing the interplay between aging, increased knowledge, and interferences on determining preferences.

A second stream of research, and one that may be highly relevant to the study of context-specific decision making by older adults, has looked at mechanisms employed by "experts" when making decisions within their domain of expertise. This research suggests that the decision-making advantages that experts exhibit can be attributed, in part, to their well-organized knowledge base (e.g., Chi, Glaser, & Farr, 1988), to distinctive encoding processes (Van Overschelde, Rawson, Dunlosky, & Hunt, 2005), and to memory-retrieval structures that connect the contents of working memory and long-term memory (Ericsson & Kintsch, 1995). The benefit of having expertise increases as tasks become more challenging, perhaps because these tasks involve processes that are more likely to be automatized (Beilock, Wierenga, & Carr, 2002). The expertise literature also demonstrates that experts tend to rely on less elaborative search when it is advantageous (Ericsson, Prietula, & Cokely, 2007). An analogy between this work and age differences in decision making can be drawn: Older adults may employ a similarly selective approach to decision making by not generating strategies that were previously determined to be unproductive. Indeed, a body of work has found that older adults exhibit a tendency to use less information to solve problems, which might reflect their greater expertise (Berg, Meegan, & Klaczynski, 1999; Meyer, Talbot, & Ranalli, 2007; Queen, Hess, Ennis, Dowd, & Grühn, 2012). Related research has also revealed that experts make better decisions in part because of effective attention allocation strategies (Ericsson et al., 2007). Notable examples in this area are studies examining aviation expertise. For example, Morrow et al. (2008) showed that expert pilots spent more time than novice pilots reading cues that were diagnostic for problem solving, which was associated with enhanced decision-making outcomes. Related research found that expert pilots made better decisions than novices in terms of speed and accuracy, as exhibited by their attention strategies in a simulated aviation environment (Schriver, Morrow, Wickens, & Talleur, 2008). Further work is needed to investigate whether this mechanism, involving the use of more efficient attention allocation for tasks requiring expertise, is also being employed by older adults when concentrating their attention to familiar, domain-specific tasks. Research that investigates age-differences in eye-tracking performance as a measure of attention may be particularly helpful in investigating this hypothesis further.

IMPLICATIONS FOR PUBLIC POLICY AND EFFECTIVE DECISION ENVIRONMENTS

The oldest baby-boomers are now in their late 60s, representing the vanguard of an unprecedented, yet highly foreseeable, increase in the country's senior population. The finding that older adults show improved decision-making capacity with increased domain-specific knowledge should be an important consideration for policy-makers as they contemplate the future effects of this demographic shift. Further, the hypothesis that the accumulation of knowledge and experience can offset lower levels of fluid intelligence in older adults has important policy implications for the design of effective decision environments and tools for older adults. Accumulating research suggests that there may be multiple pathways that lead to better decision making, relying on fluid intelligence, crystallized intelligence, or both. To broadly foster optimal decision making, policy-makers and task-designers should focus on ways to minimize the role of declining fluid intelligence, and maximize the impact of crystallized intelligence among both young adults and older adults.

Maximize Impact of Crystallized Intelligence

As Li et al. (2013) note, one way for task designers to enhance the role of crystallized knowledge is by providing decision environments that are analogous to similar environments in which experience already exists, so as to provide a more familiar and meaningful context. The influence of familiar context on task performance has been demonstrated in classic experiments using the Wason selection task, a test of reasoning in which the subject is asked to determine whether a condition rule is being violated (Wason, 1966). The thematic content of some rules elicits a high percentage of logical responses, whereas the content of other rules does not, consistent with the perspective that reasoning may be tied to context-specific experiences for those midlife and beyond (see, for example, Johnson-Laird & Byrne, 1991).

Another means by which to enhance and maintain crystallized intelligence well into our senior years is through education. In addition to the benefits of general education, research also indicates that adults who remain active in a specific domain may show reduced age-related decline compared with those who discontinue engagement in a domain as they increase in age (Meinz, 2000). Older adults may therefore be able to maintain a high level of performance by continuing to accrue relevant experience in their domain of expertise. Research should continue investigating the potential role of the continual availability of new experiences focused on knowledge-based domains for older adults.

With respect to designing better decision-making methods for younger adults, it would be wise to emphasize early training and experience. For example, for those younger adults lacking direct financial experience, various hands-on initiatives for gaining practical financial knowledge, such as effective money management practices, may be an important early start for making sound financial decisions throughout their lives. Unfortunately, there is at best mixed empirical evidence supporting the notion that financial education programs actually improve decision making (Fernandes et al., 2014). For example, in a series of studies on middle-aged adults, a one-time educational survey was not effective in improving 401(k) savings rates relative to a control group (Choi, Laibson, & Madrian, 2011). Thus, it would seem that a targeted lesson is unlikely to have a long-term influence on planning and saving rate behaviors. The complementary capabilities framework suggests that acquired knowledge gained through accumulated experiences, but not necessarily passive learning, may be a key driver in improving financial decision making.

Minimize Impact of Fluid Decline

At the same time, task designers should consider ways to minimize the impact of declining fluid intelligence among older adults by developing decision-making aids that could compensate for cases where older individuals show deficits or undesirable choice-situation sensitivities in their decision making. This goal might be accomplished by designing interventions that capitalize on other criteria that influence competencies relevant to decision and choice. For example, task designers could supplement scarce internal working memory with external memory aids to alleviate processing loads for older decision makers. Other external aids could be provided to older adults to ease the burden on their decreased fluid processing ability, such as a retirement spending calculator for savings and retirement decisions (Brustkern, Denning, & Mayer, 2005).

For task environments in which experience and accumulated knowledge are not particularly helpful, the use of institutional "nudges" to protect older adults and encourage better decisions may be advisable (Agarwal et al., 2009). Nudges can alter decision behavior in a predictable way without forbidding any options (Thaler & Sunstein, 2008), and a growing body of research demonstrates that gentle institutional nudges can improve decision making without mandating any specific choice (Johnson et al., 2012). Prominent examples in this literature include automatic enrollment (with the option to opt-out) in 401(k) plans (Choi, Laibson, Madrian, & Metrick, 2002) and organ donation programs (Johnson & Goldstein, 2003). One example of a policy domain in which decision architecture could be used to promote better decisions among older adults is that of Social Security, since almost half of all recipients currently claim their monthly retirement benefits immediately upon eligibility, which significantly reduces their lifetime payments (Muldoon & Kopcke, 2008). Suboptimal decision making in this context may be due to the fact that the claiming choice is inherently complex, requires multiple constraints to be solved simultaneously, and has not been experienced previously. Promisingly, recent research has demonstrated that by encouraging middle-aged and older adults to shift the implicit default from early to later claiming (by altering the order in which participants consider claiming options), the preferred claiming age can be significantly delayed (Appelt, Johnson, Knoll, & Westfall, 2011).

Given the strong evidence for cognitive decline, it would seem that research showing the benefits of aging through increased crystalized intelligence for certain decision-making tasks is important to policy. Direction for the development of interventions that can aid and improve decisions is an increasingly important contribution in an aging society that tries to shift important decisions (e.g., on pension investments and health care choices) from government agencies to individuals. Policy-makers and task-designers should also be mindful of the relative importance that crystallized and fluid intelligence may have on a given task, as this will impact the observed relationship between age and decision-making ability.

SUMMARY

Older adults are faced with an increasing number of important choices that impact their welfare, such as decisions about retirement finances and health care. However, lay beliefs about senior decision-making capacity are conflicting: One view sees older people as more knowledgeable; another sees them as suffering from deteriorating cognitive abilities. The complementary capabilities framework suggests that there is not only truth to both views, but proposes a way to help identify when each operates: Although, age-related cognitive declines are to some extent inevitable, the negative effects of these declines may be at least partially attenuated on tasks and in domains that are familiar and highly practiced. That is, the accumulated intellectual capital represented by crystallized intelligence may circumvent reduced capabilities due to diminished levels of fluid intelligence. Having greater experience and acquired knowledge from a lifetime of decision making may thereby provide older people with another way to make good decisions. Can we really afford to dismiss the value of experienced, domain-specific intelligence? Our senior judiciary may well have an opinion on the matter.

References

Agarwal, S., Driscoll, J., Gabaix, X., & Laibson, D. (2009). The age of reason: Financial decisions over the life-cycle with implications for regulation. *Brookings Papers on Economic Activity*, *21*(2), 164–177.

Anderson, J. (1976). *Language, memory, and thought*. Hillsdale, NJ: Erlbaum.

Anderson, J., & Reder, L. M. (1999). The fan effect: New results and new theories. *Journal of Experimental Psychology: General*, *128*(2), 186.

Appelt, K., Johnson, E., Knoll, M., & Westfall, J. (2011). Time to retire: Why Americans claim benefits early and how to encourage them to delay. In *Paper presented at the 2nd annual Boulder Summer Conference on consumer financial decision making, Boulder, CO.*

Beilock, S. L., Wierenga, S. A., & Carr, T. H. (2002). Expertise, attention, and memory in sensorimotor skill execution: Impact of novel task constraints on dual-task performance and episodic memory. *The Quarterly Journal of Experimental Psychology: Section A*, *55*(4), 1211–1240.

Berg, C. A., Meegan, S. P., & Klaczynski, P. (1999). Age and experiential differences in strategy generation and information requests for solving everyday problems. *International Journal of Behavioral Development*, *23*(3), 615–639.

Besedeš, T., Deck, C., Sarangi, S., & Shor, M. (2012). Age effects and heuristics in decision making. *Review of Economics and Statistics*, *94*(2), 580–596.

Bruine de Bruin, W., Parker, A. M., & Fischhoff, B. (2012). Explaining adult age differences in decision-making competence. *Journal of Behavioral Decision Making*, *25*(4), 352–360.

Brustkern, S.A., Denning, D.A., & Mayer, C.L. (2005). *Retirement income calculator.* US20060122924 A1. U.S. Patent Application.

Cattell, R. B. (1971). *Abilities: Their structure, growth, and action*. Boston: Houghton-Mifflin.

Cattell, R. B. (1987). *Intelligence: Its structure, growth and action*. Elsevier.

Chase, W. G., & Ericsson, K. A. (1981). Skilled memory. In J. R. Anderson (Ed.), *Cognitive skills and their acquisition* (pp. 141–189). Hillsdale, NJ: Erlbaum.

Chi, M. T., Glaser, R. E., & Farr, M. J. (1988). *The nature of expertise*. Hillsdale, NJ: Erlbaum.

Choi, J. J., Laibson, D., & Madrian, B. C. (2011). $100 bills on the sidewalk: Suboptimal investment in 401 (k) plans. *Review of Economics and Statistics*, *93*(3), 748–763.

Choi, J. J., Laibson, D., Madrian, B. C., & Metrick, A. (2002). Defined contribution pensions: Plan rules, participant choices, and the path of least resistance. *Tax policy and the economy* (Vol. 16, pp. 67–114). MIT Press.

Craik, F. I. M., & Salthouse, T. A. (2000). *The handbook of aging and cognition* (2nd ed.). Mahwah, NJ: Erlbaum.

Doane, S. M., Sohn, Y. W., & Jodlowski, M. T. (2004). Pilot ability to anticipate the consequences of flight actions as a function of expertise. *Human Factors: The Journal of the Human Factors and Ergonomics Society*, *46*(1), 92–103.

Ericsson, K. A., & Kintsch, W. (1995). Long-term working memory. *Psychological Review*, *102*(2), 211.

Ericsson, K. A., Prietula, M. J., & Cokely, E. T. (2007). The making of an expert. *Harvard Business Review*, *85*(7/8), 114.

Fernandes, D., Lynch Jr., J. G., & Netemeyer, R. G. (2014). Financial Literacy, financial education, and downstream financial behaviors. *Management Science*.

Frederick, S., Loewenstein, G., & O'Donoghue, T. (2002). Time discounting and time preference: A critical review. *Journal of Economic Literature*, *40*(2), 351–401.

Glaser, R. (1984). Education and thinking: The role of knowledge. *American Psychologist*, *39* (2), 93.

Gneezy, U., List, J. A., & Wu, G. (2006). The uncertainty effect: When a risky prospect is valued less than its worst possible outcome. *The Quarterly Journal of Economics*, *121*(4), 1283–1309.

Grossmann, I., Na, J., Varnum, M. E., Park, D. C., Kitayama, S., & Nisbett, R. E. (2010). Reasoning about social conflicts improves into old age. *Proceedings of the National Academy of Sciences*, *107*(16), 7246–7250.

Hansson, P., Rönnlund, M., Juslin, P., & Nilsson, L.-G. (2008). Adult age differences in the realism of confidence judgments: Overconfidence, format dependence, and cognitive predictors. *Psychology and Aging*, *23*(3), 531.

Healey, M. K., Ngo, K. J., & Hasher, L. (2014). Below-baseline suppression of competitors during interference resolution by younger but not older adults. *Psychological Science*, *25*(1), 145–151.

Hedden, T., & Park, D. (2001). Aging and interference in verbal working memory. *Psychology and Aging*, *16*(4), 666.

Horn, J. L., & Cattell, R. B. (1967). Age differences in fluid and crystallized intelligence. *Acta Psychologica*, *26*, 107–129.

Johnson, E. J., Gächter, S., & Herrmann, A. (2006). *Exploring the nature of loss aversion.* IZA(Discussion Papers).

Johnson, E. J., & Goldstein, D. (2003). Do defaults save lives? *Science, 302*, 1338–1339.

Johnson, E. J., Häubl, G., & Keinan, A. (2007). Aspects of endowment: A query theory of value construction. *Journal of Experimental Psychology: Learning, Memory, and Cognition, 33*(3), 461–474.

Johnson, E. J., Shu, S. B., Dellaert, B. G., Fox, C., Goldstein, D. G., Häubl, G., et al. (2012). Beyond nudges: Tools of a choice architecture. *Marketing Letters, 23*(2), 487–504.

Johnson-Laird, P. N., & Byrne, R. M. (1991). *Deduction*. Lawrence Erlbaum Associates, Inc.

Kim, S., & Hasher, L. (2005). The attraction effect in decision making: Superior performance by older adults. *The Quarterly Journal of Experimental Psychology Section A, 58*(1), 120–133.

Kovalchik, S., Camerer, C. F., Grether, D. M., Plott, C. R., & Allman, J. M. (2005). Aging and decision making: A comparison between neurologically healthy elderly and young individuals. *Journal of Economic Behavior & Organization, 58*(1), 79–94.

Lewis, C. H., & Anderson, J. (1976). Interference with real world knowledge. *Cognitive Psychology, 8*(3), 311–335.

Li, Y., Baldassi, M., Johnson, E. J., & Weber, E. U. (2013). Complementary cognitive capabilities, economic decision making, and aging. *Psychology and Aging, 28*(3), 595.

Li, Y., Gao, J., Enkavi, Z., Zaval, L., Weber, E. U., & Johnson, E. J. (2015). Sound credit scores despite cognitive aging. *Proceedings of the National Academy of Sciences, 112*(1), 65–69.

Li, S.-C., Lindenberger, U., Hommel, B., Aschersleben, G., Prinz, W., & Baltes, P. B. (2004). Transformations in the couplings among intellectual abilities and constituent cognitive processes across the life span. *Psychological Science, 15*(3), 155–163.

List, J. A. (2003). Does market experience eliminate market anomalies? *The Quarterly Journal of Economics, 118*(1), 41–71.

Lusardi, A., & Mitchell, O. S. (2007). Baby boomer retirement security: The roles of planning, financial literacy, and housing wealth. *Journal of Monetary Economics, 54*(1), 205–224.

Mata, R., Josef, A. K., Samanez-Larkin, G. R., & Hertwig, R. (2011). Age differences in risky choice: A meta-analysis. *Annals of the New York Academy of Sciences, 1235*(1), 18–29.

McArdle, J. J., Ferrer-Caja, E., Hamagami, F., & Woodcock, R. W. (2002). Comparative longitudinal structural analyses of the growth and decline of multiple intellectual abilities over the life span. *Developmental Psychology, 38*(1), 115–142.

McCloskey, M., & Bigler, K. (1980). Focused memory search in fact retrieval. *Memory & Cognition, 8*(3), 253–264.

McEvoy, G. M., & Cascio, W. F. (1989). Cumulative evidence of the relationship between employee age and job performance. *Journal of Applied Psychology, 74*(1), 11.

Meinz, E. J. (2000). Experience-based attenuation of age-related differences in music cognition tasks. *Psychology and Aging, 15*(2), 297.

Meyer, B. J., Talbot, A. P., & Ranalli, C. (2007). Why older adults make more immediate treatment decisions about cancer than younger adults. *Psychology and Aging, 22*(3), 505–524.

Miller, L. M. S., Cohen, J. A., & Wingfield, A. (2006). Contextual knowledge reduces demands on working memory during reading. *Memory & Cognition, 34*(6), 1355–1367.

Morrow, D. G., Miller, L. M. S., Ridolfo, H. E., Magnor, C., Fischer, U. M., Kokayeff, N. K., et al. (2008). Expertise and age differences in pilot decision making. *Aging, Neuropsychology, and Cognition, 16*(1), 33–55.

Muldoon, D., & Kopcke, R. W. (2008). *Are people claiming social security benefits later?* (Issue in Brief No. 8-7). Chestnut Hill, MA: Center for Retirement Research.

Myers, J. L., O'Brien, E. J., Balota, D. A., & Toyofuku, M. L. (1984). Memory search without interference: The role of integration. *Cognitive Psychology, 16*(2), 217–242.

Peters, E., & Bruine de Bruin, W. (2012). Aging and decision skills. In M. K. Dhami, A. Schlottmann, & M. Waldmann (Eds.), *Judgment and decision making as a skill: Learning, development, and evolution*. Cambridge University Press.

Peters, E., Hess, T. M., Auman, C., & Västfjäll, D. (2007). Adult age differences in dual information processes and their influence on judgments and decisions: A review. *Perspectives on Psychological Science, 2*, 1–23.

Qian, J., & Weber, E. U. (2008). The effect of age and gender in domain-specific risk taking. In *Paper presented at the annual meeting of the Society of Judgment and Decision Making*. Boston, MA.

Queen, T. L., Hess, T. M., Ennis, G. E., Dowd, K., & Grühn, D. (2012). Information search and decision making: Effects of age and complexity on strategy use. *Psychology and Aging, 27*(4), 817.

Radvansky, G. A., Spieler, D. H., & Zacks, R. T. (1993). Mental model organization. *Journal of Experimental Psychology: Learning, Memory, and Cognition, 19*(1), 95.

Rolison, J. J., Hanoch, Y., Wood, S., & Liu, P.-J. (2014). Risk-taking differences across the adult life span: A question of age and domain. *The Journals of Gerontology Series B: Psychological Sciences and Social Sciences, 69*(6), 870–880.

Rowley, J., & Slack, F. (2009). Conceptions of wisdom. *Journal of Information Science, 35*(1), 110–119.

Salthouse, T. A. (1992). Why do adult age differences increase with task complexity? *Developmental Psychology, 28*(5), 905–918.

Salthouse, T. A. (1994). The nature of the influence of speed on adult age differences in cognition. *Developmental Psychology, 30*(2), 240–259.

Salthouse, T. A. (1996). The processing-speed theory of adult age differences in cognition. *Psychological Review, 103*(3), 403–428.

Salthouse, T. A. (2004). What and when of cognitive aging. *Current Directions in Psychological Science, 13*(4), 140–144.

Salthouse, T. A. (2010). *Major issues in cognitive aging*. New York: Oxford University Press.

Salthouse, T. A. (2012). Consequences of age-related cognitive declines. *Annual Review of Psychology, 63*, 201.

Schaie, K. W. (1993). The Seattle longitudinal studies of adult intelligence. *Current Directions in Psychological Science, 2*(6), 171–175.

Schriver, A. T., Morrow, D. G., Wickens, C. D., & Talleur, D. A. (2008). Expertise differences in attentional strategies related to pilot decision making. *Human Factors: The Journal of the Human Factors and Ergonomics Society, 50*(6), 864–878.

Soederberg-Miller, L. M. (2009). Age differences in the effects of domain knowledge on reading efficiency. *Psychology and Aging, 24*(1), 63.

Spieler, D. H., Balota, D. A., & Faust, M. E. (1996). Stroop performance in healthy younger and older adults and in individuals with dementia of the Alzheimer's type. *Journal of Experimental Psychology: Human Perception and Performance, 22*(2), 461.

Strough, J., Karns, T. E., & Schlosnagle, L. (2011). Decision-making heuristics and biases across the life span. *Annals of the New York Academy of Sciences, 1235*(1), 57–74.

Strough, J., Mehta, C. M., McFall, J. P., & Schuller, K. L. (2008). Are older adults less subject to the sunk-cost fallacy than younger adults? *Psychological Science, 19*(7), 650–652.

Tentori, K., Osherson, D., Hasher, L., & May, C. (2001). Wisdom and aging: Irrational preferences in college students but not older adults. *Cognition, 81*(3), B87–B96.

Thaler, R. H., & Sunstein, C. R. (2008). *Nudge: Improving decisions about health, wealth, and happiness*. Yale University Press.

Thornton, W. J., & Dumke, H. A. (2005). Age differences in everyday problem-solving and decision-making effectiveness: A meta-analytic review. *Psychology and Aging, 20*(1), 85–99.

Van Overschelde, J. P., Rawson, K. A., Dunlosky, J., & Hunt, R. R. (2005). Distinctive processing underlies skilled memory. *Psychological Science, 16*(5), 358–361.

Wason, P. C. (1966). Reasoning. *New Horizons in Psychology, 1*, 135–151.

Weber, E. U., Johnson, E. J., Milch, K. F., Chang, H., Brodscholl, J. C., & Goldstein, D. G. (2007). Asymmetric discounting in intertemporal choice: A query-theory account. *Psychological Science, 18*(6), 516–523.

Yoon, C., Cole, C. A., & Lee, M. P. (2009). Consumer decision making and aging: Current knowledge and future directions. *Journal of Consumer Psychology, 19*(1), 2–16.

Zacks, R. T., Hasher, L., & Li, K. Z. H. (2000). Human memory. In F. I. M. Craik, & T. A. Salthouse (Eds.), *The handbook of aging and cognition* (2nd ed., pp. 293–357). Mahwah, NJ: Erlbaum.

Zacks, R. T., Radvansky, G., & Hasher, L. (1996). Studies of directed forgetting in older adults. *Journal of Experimental Psychology: Learning, Memory, and Cognition, 22*(1), 143–156.

CHAPTER

9

Aging, Emotion, and Decision Making

Joseph A. Mikels, Michael M. Shuster, Sydney T. Thai

Department of Psychology, DePaul University, Chicago, IL, USA

Notable discoveries in the psychology of aging correspond well to recent advances in the decision sciences. In particular, emotions have begun to figure prominently in decision making; and decision theory has begun to place greater emphasis on the dual contributions of both affective and analytic processes to judgments and decisions. Recent characterizations of human aging as involving divergent affective and deliberative trajectories map onto this distinction; in the face of declines in deliberative processes, older individuals show stability and potential gains in processes reliant on experiential and emotional processes. As such, the implications of these age-related divergent trajectories for decision making are vast—yet poorly understood. In particular, emotional processes may play a larger and more significant role in decision making as individuals age into the later parts of the life span. Thus, the interplay of affective and deliberative processes in decision making represents an important domain of inquiry, especially across the adult life span. Following a review of contemporary theory and findings regarding age differences in cognition and emotion, we review theoretical perspectives on the role of emotion in decision making. We then describe how age-related changes in emotion and cognition impact decision making across the adult life span—an approach that has only recently been incorporated into empirical investigations. Finally, we conclude with implications of extant findings and critical future research directions.

Aging and Decision Making
http://dx.doi.org/10.1016/B978-0-12-417148-0.00009-1

AGE-RELATED CHANGES IN COGNITION, EMOTION, AND MOTIVATION

To fully understand how emotions impact the decisions of older adults, it is imperative to first consider age-related changes in deliberative processing. Although some aspects of cognitive function remain stable or increase with age, deliberative-processing abilities (e.g., working memory, long-term memory, attention, reasoning) central to decision making generally decline with age (for comprehensive reviews, see Strough, Parker, & Bruine de Bruin, this volume; Zaval, Li, Johnson, & Weber, this volume). However, on tasks that require solving interpersonal problems, older people show greater flexibility than younger people, especially when problems are emotionally charged (Blanchard-Fields, Jahnke, & Camp, 1995). Findings such as these speak to the potential influence of emotion and motivation on cognitive performance. Interest in emotional influences on cognitive performance is all the more pertinent in light of emerging evidence that emotional functioning is well maintained or even improved with age.

Although emotional aging was initially characterized by deterioration (Banham, 1951), it has become increasingly clear that this is not the case. Emotion regulation and emotional experience in old age are as good if not better than they are in younger years. In general, older adults do not differ from younger adults in self-reports of emotional intensity or in emotionally expressive behavior (for a review, see Carstensen, Mikels, & Mather, 2006). However, older adults do report sustained or higher levels of positive affect and lower levels of negative affect relative to the young (Carstensen, Pasupathi, Mayr, & Nesselroade, 2000; Carstensen et al., 2011; Charles, Reynolds, & Gatz, 2001; Mroczek & Kolarz, 1998). Additionally, there are notable age differences for a few discrete negative emotions; relative to younger adults, older adults experience and display less disgust (Carstensen, Gottman, & Levenson, 1995; Kunzmann, Kupperbusch, & Levenson, 2005), less anger (Gross et al., 1997; Lawton, Kleban, & Dean, 1993), but potentially greater sadness (Alea, Bluck, & Semegon, 2004; Kunzmann & Grühn, 2005). With respect to regulation, older adults relative to younger adults report greater emotional control on self-report measures (Gross et al., 1997; Lawton et al., 1992), but also demonstrate an intact ability to regulate their emotions in laboratory tasks (see, e.g., Kunzmann et al., 2005). Importantly, these patterns coalesce to indicate that the emotion system is generally as functional as it is in younger adults.

Given the divergent trajectories of emotional and deliberative processes in the aging mind, there has been consideration of how preservations in emotional functioning may help assuage the cognitive difficulties that individuals have as they grow older. Findings indicate that there are emotional enhancements in information processing; older adults evidence superior memory for emotional relative to non-emotional information (e.g., Charles, Mather, & Carstensen, 2003; Fung & Carstensen, 2003) and show a preserved emotional memory enhancement effect (e.g., Kensinger, Brierley, Medford, Growdon, & Corkin, 2002). Importantly, this selective preservation of emotional processing is found even in working memory (Mikels, Larkin, Reuter-Lorenz, & Carstensen, 2005). Specifically, whereas age is negatively associated with working memory performance in virtually all content domains (see, e.g., Verhaeghen, Marcoen, & Goossens, 1993), Mikels et al. (2005) found that working memory for emotional information was selectively unimpaired. Insofar as working memory is the central cognitive system involved in the maintenance and manipulation of information (Baddeley, 1986), age-related changes in working memory have significant implications for decision making because increasingly complex decisions place high demands on processing capacity.

In addition to findings indicating a prioritization of emotional information, a surprising valence difference also has emerged: the positivity effect (for reviews, see Carstensen & Mikels, 2005; Carstensen et al., 2006; Mather & Carstensen, 2005). The positivity effect describes an age-related pattern in which a disproportionate preference for negative information in youth shifts across adulthood toward the positive. This phenomenon has been observed across numerous studies examining different processes from attention and memory to decision making (for reviews, see Reed & Carstensen, 2012; Reed, Chan, & Mikels, 2014). Though the reliability of the effect had been questioned, a recent meta-analysis of over 100 studies on memory and attention revealed a robust positivity effect (Reed et al., 2014). For instance, in studies of visual attention, eye-tracking methodologies have shown that older individuals have an increased preference toward positive stimuli and away from negative stimuli in contrast to their younger counterparts (Isaacowitz, Wadlinger, Goren, & Wilson, 2006). Also, older adults remember a higher proportion of positive emotional material relative to negative emotional material (Charles et al., 2003).

These age-related changes in emotion have been explained by different theoretical perspectives. One explanation is offered by a prominent lifespan theory of motivation, Socioemotional Selectivity Theory (SST; see Carstensen, 2006). The theory holds that younger adults are more likely to pursue information-seeking goals, whereas older adults are more likely to pursue emotionally meaningful goals and engage in emotion regulation. According to the theory, when future time horizons are broad—as is typical in youth—individuals focus on the future and in obtaining and acquiring resources, knowledge, and social connections. In contrast, when future time horizons narrow—as is typical in later life—individuals focus on the present moment and prioritize emotionally meaningful goals. In particular, older adults' regulation strategies are marked by optimization of positive affect and minimization of negative affect (for reviews, see Carstensen & Mikels, 2005; Carstensen et al., 2006; Mather & Carstensen, 2005).

It should be noted that other theoretical perspectives emphasize alternative but complementary mechanisms underlying these effects, such as declines in cognitive resources (Labouvie-Vief, 2003), selective use of preserved emotion regulation strategies (Urry & Gross, 2010), and the balance of emotion regulatory strengths versus physiological vulnerabilities (Charles, 2010), among others.

Given the focus of SST on motivation, predictions can be drawn from the theory regarding the emotional goals of older adults when making decisions. Extrapolating from SST, older adults may focus on emotional aspects of decisions to a greater extent and may be more influenced by positive emotions and less influenced by negative emotions. Alternatively, a recent goal-orientation perspective has been applied to the decision making of older adults (see, e.g., Depping & Freund, 2011; Depping & Freund, 2013). This perspective emphasizes that older adults have an increased motivation to avoid losses, relative to younger adults who are more focused on attaining gains. As many decisions involve consideration of losses and gains, a loss-prevention orientation among older adults would suggest that they respond differently to losses.

In order to aptly extend these age differences in emotion, cognition, and motivation to the decision domain, in the next section we will review broader theoretical perspectives on emotion and decision making. Then in the subsequent section, we will present empirical evidence on age differences in decision making that underscores the importance of considering the role of emotion—especially for the aging decision maker.

THEORETICAL PERSPECTIVES ON THE ROLE OF AFFECT IN JUDGMENT AND DECISION MAKING

As with much of psychology, descriptive decision research and theory have developed through consideration and examination of normative processes among younger adults. Most decision-making research—including most of that reviewed below—has been conducted on younger adults and may not generalize to older adults (see Strough, Karns, & Schlosnagle, 2011). Thus, expanding the scope of such work across the adult life span promises to shed new light on how decision processes may change as a function of age-related changes in emotion and cognition. Importantly, though, decision science has traditionally focused heavily on the cognitive, deliberative aspects of decision making. However, there has been burgeoning theoretical and empirical interest in understanding how emotions impact decision making. Specifically, when considering the role of affect in decision making, emotions can be integral, that is, centrally relevant to decisions, choice options, and/or outcomes, or incidental and unrelated to the choice at hand (see, e.g., Lerner & Keltner, 2001; Tiedens

& Linton, 2001). This distinction is critical to clearly delineating the role of emotion in decision making; *integral affect* can be used as an information-bearing heuristic to make a decision (see, e.g., Schwarz & Clore, 2007), whereas different *incidental affective states* can lead to greater reliance on either systematic or heuristic processing (e.g., Tiedens & Linton, 2001) and can lead to either increases or decreases in risk perception and behavior (e.g., Lerner & Keltner, 2001). We will first review theoretical perspectives that consider affect as an integral part of decision making, and then will consider perspectives that highlight an incidental role for emotions in the decision-making process.

Dual Process Models. The role of affect as an integral source of information in decision making can be aptly considered within the larger context of dual-process models that draw the distinction between two general processing streams: intuitive and deliberative (e.g., Epstein, 1994; Kahneman, 2003; Loewenstein, Weber, Hsee, & Welch, 2001; Reyna, 2004). The intuitive system (also referred to as system 1) is considered to be experiential and is generally characterized as quick, automatic, gist-based, and affective. In contrast, the deliberative system (also referred to as system 2) is considered to be generally slow, controlled, verbatim-based, and analytic in nature. Although the distinction between systems 1 and 2 is a useful heuristic, it is becoming increasingly clear that such an overarching dichotomy is oversimplified and cannot coherently accommodate all proposed distinctions (for a review, see Evans, 2008). The many criticisms of a broad dual-process theory of the mind underscore the inadequacy of an all-encompassing theory, thus requiring greater precision and the differentiation of multiple types of dual processes (Evans & Stanovich, 2013). For instance, whereas some dual process models include affect centrally within the intuitive system (see, e.g., Epstein, 1994), others do not include affect and consider the intuitive system to be entirely cognitive and implicit in nature (see Evans, 2008). As such, this chapter takes into account a dual-process model that includes affect as a central component: cognitive-experiential self-theory (CEST; Epstein, 1994).

Cognitive-Experiential Self-Theory. When individuals are faced with decisions, there are multiple sources of information to consider including "hot" and "cold" cognitions. The former stream of information is emotional in nature, whereas the latter involves "rational" and deliberative processes (see, e.g., Janis & Mann, 1977). According to CEST, behavior and decisions are guided by both affect-laden experiential and rational–analytic parallel systems (see Epstein, 1994). For instance, when purchasing a car, people can deliberate over the specifications that differentiate each model and/or consider their gut feelings. Critical to the current chapter, the experiential system is intuitive in nature and intimately—but not exclusively—associated with affect. In support of these specific dual processes, studies suggest that there may be separable working memory subsystems for emotional versus non-emotional information (Mikels et al., 2005). As working memory is centrally involved in decision-making processes (e.g., Del Missier et al., 2013), such separable subsystems may differentially support the deliberative and intuitive systems. Moreover, given age-related preservation of working memory processes for emotional versus non-emotional information (Mikels et al., 2005), the decisions of older adults may benefit from reliance on integral affect. Importantly, such benefits would arise when the two systems operate in an interactive and integrated manner; however, conflict can arise when these two sources of information urge the individual to pursue opposing actions.

When individuals are confronted with such conflict and rely on integral feelings that diverge from clear "rational" probabilities, they have been shown to make non-optimal decisions (Denes-Raj & Epstein, 1994). The ratio-bias phenomenon is a perfect example; people will often choose an option with a greater absolute number of desirable options over one with a smaller absolute number but better odds; e.g., 9 out of 100 versus 1 out of 10 (Alonso & Fernandez-Berrocal, 2003; Epstein & Pacini, 2000; Pacini & Epstein, 1999). CEST contends that greater experience with absolute numbers makes the non-optimal option feel better, though abstraction through rational processes would indicate otherwise. Findings regarding the ratio bias phenomenon dovetail with other research showing that reliance on the "intuitive" system can lead to flawed decisions via heuristics and biases (Gilovich, Griffin, & Kahneman, 2002). Insofar as older adults might rely more on affect in decision making, it is possible then that they would show a larger ratio bias and make more non-optimal choices.

The Framing Effect. Further evidence indicates that integral affect may indeed underlie decisions in one of the most robust biases in human decision making: the "framing effect." This effect refers to the observation that people will make different choices depending on how alternatives are described (Kahneman & Tversky, 2000). Specifically, when objectively equivalent options are described positively in terms of gains (e.g., you receive $100; you can either keep $40 or take a gamble with a 40% chance to keep it all), individuals show risk aversion (i.e., they choose to keep the $40); but when options are described negatively in terms of losses (e.g., you receive $100; you can either lose $60 or take a gamble with a 60% chance to lose it all), individuals show risk seeking (i.e., they chose to gamble). With respect to the role of affect in the framing effect, De Martino, Kumaran, Seymour, and Dolan (2006) examined the neural activation of participants completing a monetary gambling task. They found that when participants displayed framing-consistent behavior (i.e., risk seeking in a loss frame and risk avoidance in a gain frame), there was greater neural activity in the amygdala, a brain region associated with affective processes. Additionally, they found that when participants did not display framing, there was increased activity in the prefrontal cortex, a brain region associated with deliberative processes.

Although traditionally the framing effect has been explained as a cognitive phenomenon (see, e.g., Kahneman & Tversky, 2000; Reyna, 2004), these findings suggest that the framing effect is at least partially due to emotional reactions to the gain and loss frames. Behavioral findings provide additional insight into the role of integral affect in the framing effect (Cheung & Mikels, 2011). Participants completed a framing task that included affect probes to assess the extent to which they relied on emotion to make their decisions as well as how positive versus negative they felt about the decisions. Cheung and Mikels (2011) found that when young adults relied on emotion to make their decisions, they were more likely to choose the risky gamble option. Moreover, positive affect was a significant predictor of risk taking in the loss frames. These data delineate a precise role for integral affect—and specifically positive affect—in leading to biased decisions. Given the central role of emotion in the framing effect, it is likely that life-span differences in emotion would result in different patterns of performance between older and younger adults on framing tasks.

Such findings align with the views of some researchers, such as Forgas, Martin, and Clore (2001), who have concluded that reliance on affect generally in judgments and decisions is an "ineffective and dysfunctional strategy" (p. 104) that solely relies on mistaken inferences. However, others have suggested that affective processing and certain heuristics may benefit decision making (Gigerenzer, 2007). For instance, the feelings-as-information approach (Schwarz & Clore, 2007) suggests that when feelings are integral to a decision, they can be beneficial. Moreover, the potential benefits of the intuitive system have more broadly been highlighted (Kahneman, 2003; Slovic, Peters, Finucane, & MacGregor, 2005). For example, individuals who have a high level of skill or expertise within a given domain appear to rely to a greater extent on intuitive processes (see, e.g., Reyna & Lloyd, 2006).

The Affect Heuristic. Slovic and colleagues have developed a theoretical framework, the affect heuristic, that further elaborates the potentially beneficial role of integral affect in decision making, while also considering the role of risk perception. The affect heuristic delineates how decision options are "tagged" with varying amounts of positive and negative affect (see, e.g., Finucane, Alhakami, Slovic, & Johnson, 2000; Peters, Dieckmann, & Weller, 2011; Slovic et al., 2005). Slovic et al. (2002) contend that "using an overall, readily available affective impression can be far easier—more efficient—than weighing the pros and cons or retrieving from memory many relevant examples, especially when the required judgment or decision is complex or mental resources are limited" (p. 400). As a theoretical framework, the affect heuristic has been used to explain findings in judgment and decision making such as the ease or difficulty with which an attribute can be evaluated (e.g., Hsee, 1996), one's sensitivity to framed proportions (e.g., Hsee, 1998), probability estimations (Denes-Raj & Epstein, 1994), and so forth.

Additional findings indicate that under conditions of exceptionally high complexity, decision making greatly benefits from employing emotion-focused versus detail-focused approaches (Mikels, Maglio, Reed, & Kaplowitz, 2011). Thus, given age-related declines in deliberative processes, older adults may indeed benefit from using affect as a heuristic.

Regarding the differential role of positive and negative valence, the affect heuristic proposes links between positive affect and increased benefit perception, and between negative affect and increased risk perception (Slovic et al., 2005). Specifically, integral positive affect associated with an option is related to lower perceived risk and higher perceived benefit, whereas integral negative affect toward an option is related to higher perceived risk and lower perceived benefit. In support of these links, Alhakami and Slovic (1994) found that if affective evaluations for an activity were positive, then individuals judged its risks to be low and its benefits to be high. The opposite pattern was found if individuals had a negative evaluation of the activity. Thus, it is the balance of risk and benefit perception that is directly influenced by affective reactions, and together integral affect and risk judgments guide decisions. As a result of the age-related positivity effect, it is likely that older adults would place greater weight on benefits and less weight on risks.

Risk-As-Feelings Hypothesis. The affect heuristic suggests that emotion plays an informational role that contributes in tandem with cognition in order to facilitate decision making. The risk-as-feelings hypothesis (Loewenstein et al., 2001) differs from this account in terms of its explicit proposal that emotional reactions to risk can differ from the cognitive evaluations of the same risk. For instance, evaluations based on integral affect tend to be more polarized, less effortful, and less sensitive to numerical and probabilistic factors in comparison to deliberative evaluations. As such, cognitive evaluations can suggest one course of action, while emotions can suggest a completely contradictory one. An aim of the risk-as-feelings hypothesis is to predict when and how emotional and cognitive evaluations diverge. Emotional reactions to potential risks are evoked by factors such as how vividly the consequences of a choice can be imagined and the degree of personal experience with outcomes. In contrast, cognitive evaluations of risks depend on objective components of the situation (e.g., probabilities of outcomes).

A dramatic example of the crucial role of integral affect in risky decision making comes from the work of Damasio and colleagues (see, e.g., Damasio, 1994), who have documented that patients with damage to the ventromedial prefrontal cortex make severely flawed and non-optimal decisions in the Iowa Gambling Task (Bechara, Tranel, Damasio, & Damasio, 1996). In an extensive series of observations and studies, it has been demonstrated that the non-optimal decisions of these patients resulted from their inability to use anticipatory feelings and physiological markers to guide decisions despite preserved intellectual and deliberative abilities. Importantly and consistent with all of the theoretical perspectives, a concrete and specific distinction can be drawn between two dual processes: those that encode affective impressions versus those that encode the details into working memory.

Appraisal-Tendency Framework. Although it is important to consider how integral affect may be involved in decision making, incidental affect has also been shown to play a significant role. Lerner and Keltner's (2000) appraisal-tendency framework articulates how incidental emotions can change the way people appraise unrelated future events. Specifically, future events are appraised in a manner consistent with the appraisals associated with the specific incidental emotion. For instance, with respect to the framing effect, dispositional fear has been shown to be related to risk aversion, whereas dispositional anger was related to risk seeking—especially so in loss frames (Lerner & Keltner, 2001). Using the appraisal-tendency framework, appraisals of uncertainty associated with incidental fear lead to a bias favoring sure options, whereas appraisals of certainty associated with incidental anger lead to a bias favoring riskier gamble options. Further supporting these distinctions, Lerner, Gonzalez, Small, and Fischhoff (2003) found that increases in the experience of incidental fear led people to evaluate negative outcomes (e.g., terrorism risks) as more probable in comparison to individuals induced with incidental anger. In addition to framing, incidental discrete emotions have also been shown to influence another pervasive bias, the endowment effect, in which individuals offer disproportionally higher selling prices and lower buying prices for the same object. Specifically, incidental disgust eliminated the endowment effect, whereas incidental sadness resulted in a reverse endowment effect (Lerner, Small, & Loewenstein, 2004). Given age-related reductions in the experience of disgust and anger, such effects may be less prevalent later in the life span.

Though the appraisal tendency perspective underscores the importance of considering specific discrete emotions, there is also considerable evidence that general positive and negative affect can lead to different patterns of risk-seeking behavior. For instance, multiple studies have demonstrated that individuals induced with incidental positive moods view their probability of obtaining gains more optimistically (e.g., Johnson & Tversky, 1983; Mayer, Gaschke, Braverman, & Evans, 1992). Conversely, induced negative moods have been shown to lead to higher risk estimates for various undesirable events, such as causes of death, compared to induced positive moods (Johnson & Tversky, 1983). Here again, the age-related positivity effect may bias older adults toward positive outcomes with reduced consideration of risk.

When considering the role of affect in decision making, examining only positive and negative valence omits a key dimension of affect: arousal (Mano, 1994). Ariely and Loewenstein (2006) found that incidental arousal was related to an increase in the willingness to engage in hypothetical risky behaviors. In another study, Mano (1994) demonstrated that individuals in aroused states tended to take more risks as measured by their increased willingness to pay for lottery tickets but lower willingness to pay for insurance. There is also considerable research demonstrating that physiological markers of autonomic arousal (e.g., heart rate and skin conductance response) are elevated when individuals encounter risky decisions (for a review, see Lo & Repin, 2002).

In sum, these multiple perspectives all specify how emotions are importantly involved in decision making. Moreover, from a dual-process perspective, these affective contributions to decision-making stand in stark contrast to deliberative contributions. Given divergent age-related trajectories in deliberative versus affective processes, the role of emotion in decision making likely differs for older versus younger adults. As alluded to above, it is likely that emotional processing may be beneficial or harmful to the decision making of older adults in several ways. We will further elaborate these possibilities below and include pertinent findings, though empirical findings are at present somewhat limited.

DECISION MAKING ACROSS THE ADULT LIFE SPAN

In light of the age-related changes in cognition and emotion, it is perhaps not too surprising that older adults make decisions differently relative to their younger counterparts. Mirroring the focus on the cognitive aspects of decision making in the decision sciences, adult life-span studies too have predominantly focused on cognition. However, adult life-span research has begun to consider how emotions are involved in the decision making of older adults—though much work has yet to be done. We first consider the predominant focus on how aging impacts the cognitive aspects of decision making and then focus on other work in which emotion and emotion-related factors—such as risk, gains, and losses—are more strongly considered.

Age Differences in Deliberative Aspects of Decision Making. Considering the extensive declines in deliberative cognitive abilities, research has focused on how decision making is negatively impacted in later life. For instance, older adults prefer decision rules with lower cognitive processing demands (Johnson, 1990), seek and use less information prior to making decisions (for a review, see Löckenhoff & Carstensen, 2007), and prefer fewer options in numerous decision domains (Reed, Mikels, & Simon, 2008). Such characteristics of older adults' decision-making tendencies suggest that they may have difficulty making complex decisions (see Strough et al., this volume; Zaval et al., this volume).

Age Differences in Affective Aspects of Decision Making. Importantly, emotional processes may buttress the impact of declining deliberative abilities. As such, one possibility is that if older adults rely on their intact emotional abilities, perhaps this could be beneficial to their decision making. With respect to the influence of emotion, though, the distinction between integral and incidental affect is critical. We propose that under most circumstances, older adults will benefit when relying on their integral emotions. In contrast, when older adults are swayed by their incidental affect, their decisions may be negatively or positively impacted. Extant data support this supposition.

Regarding integral affect, one study examined different decision strategies in younger and older adults (Mikels, et al., 2010). In this study, decision strategies that involved holding the details of decisions in working memory and deliberating over the decisions improved the decision quality of younger adults but impaired that of older adults. In stark contrast, when participants were encouraged to hold in mind their integral emotional reactions to decision options and base their decisions on their feelings, the age differences disappeared and older adults made decisions of equally high quality compared to those of younger adults. Under the larger dual-process perspective of deliberative versus experiential/affective processing, other findings are consistent with this affective processing advantage, which indicates that experiential processes benefit the decision making of older adults (e.g., Bruine de Bruin, Parker, & Fischhoff, 2012; Queen & Hess, 2010; Strough, Mehta, McFall, & Schuller, 2008).

In related research, when older adults explicitly evaluate their choice options, they list a greater number of positive versus negative attributes relative to the young, which then leads to increased satisfaction with their ultimate choice (Kim, Healey, Goldstein, Hasher, & Wiprzycka, 2008). Thus, in the instance of attribute evaluation—which draws on integral affect—the age-related positivity effect benefits choice satisfaction. However, it is also important to note that older adults attend to and recall more positive versus negative information than younger adults (Löckenhoff & Carstensen, 2007; Mather, Knight, & McCaffrey, 2005), which could lead older adults to miss critical decision-relevant negative information and ultimately result in non-optimal decision outcomes.

In terms of health messages, the positivity effect has also been shown to further influence older adults, indicating that age differences in integral affect can influence decision making. In particular, many health-related messages use a particular type of framing, known as goal framing. Goal framing emphasizes either receiving a health benefit by performing a particular behavior or avoiding a negative consequence by performing the same behavior. One study examined impressions of, and memory for, positively and negatively framed health care messages that were presented in pamphlets to older and younger adults (Shamaskin, Mikels, & Reed, 2010).

Older adults relative to younger adults rated positive pamphlets as more informative than negative pamphlets and remembered a higher proportion of positive to negative messages. These findings demonstrate the age-related positivity effect in health care messages via the persuasive and lingering effects of positive messages. In a related study, relative to younger adults, older adults looked less at negative material about skin cancer but took more protective measures (Isaacowitz & Choi, 2012). Taken together, these findings suggest that integral positive emotional appeals are most effective for older adults in the health domain, and that the positivity effect may ultimately not be detrimental to older adults' health behaviors. Despite these findings that integral affect and experiential processing generally may be beneficial to the decisions of older adults, there is evidence that incidental affect can be both beneficial and detrimental to decision making in older adults.

Consistent with the benefits of the positivity effect on decision making, one study suggests that incidental positive affect was associated with better decisions for older adults. Carpenter, Peters, Västfjäll, and Isen (2013) found that older adults induced into a positive mood made more optimal decisions resulting in greater monetary earnings on a risky decision-making task. Further examining the role of incidental affect on changes in decision making across the adult life span, preliminary evidence indicates that positive and negative mood inductions differentially influence hypothetical risk seeking between older and younger adults (Chou, Lee, & Ho, 2007). Specifically, older adults were more willing to choose risky resolutions to hypothetical life-dilemmas after watching positive movie clips (relative to watching neutral or negative clips) than were younger adults. This study suggests that older adults may make different decisions relative to the young when under the influence of positive incidental affect.

Other studies suggest that incidental positive affect may be harmful to the decision making of older adults. For instance, von Helversen and Mata (2012) examined age differences in sequential decision making performance. Sequential decision-making tasks require individuals to either accept or reject an option while not allowing them to go back and accept a previously presented option. In order to succeed in such tasks, individuals must search through the optimal number of options first in order to create a threshold for selecting the option with the best value. Compared to younger adults, older adults set a lower threshold for accepting an option and thus performed worse on the task. Furthermore, fluid cognitive abilities (e.g., processing speed) were unrelated to performance, yet incidental positive affect was related to reduced search behavior prior to making a choice. These findings suggest that the higher levels of positive affect reported by older adults can lead them to search through fewer options and thus make poorer decisions. Similarly, a recent study found that incidental positive affect led older versus younger adults to make more non-optimal decisions on the above-mentioned ratio-bias task, in which intuition guides people toward a choice that feels better versus a choice that actually has a greater probability of winning (Mikels, Cheung, Cone, & Gilovich, 2013). Importantly, this age difference was not explained by age-related declines in deliberative abilities but by the greater incidental positive affect of the older adults.

Overall, it is clear that emotions impact the decision making of individuals across the adult life span. In general, it appears that older adults can harness their intact emotional abilities to benefit their complex decision-making. However, insofar as older adults are swayed by incidental positive affect, in certain instances it could benefit their decisions but in other instances prove problematic.

Aging, Emotion, and Risky Decisions Involving Gains and Losses. Studies examining different patterns of risky decision making between older and younger adults have examined the role of age-related changes in emotional processes to various extents. Using physiological measures of arousal, Denburg, Recknor, Bechara, and Tranel (2006) found that compared to their younger counterparts, older adults had lower galvanic skin responses (GSRs) to potential losses and higher GSRs to potential gains. In additional work, Bauer et al. (2013) found that older relative to younger adults have a hypersensitivity to reward regardless of the rate of loss.

Other research by Samanez-Larkin et al. (2007), however, indicates that whereas older and younger adults report similar subjective positive arousal when anticipating gains, older adults reported relatively lower negative arousal when anticipating losses. Furthermore, the findings from the self-report data mirrored patterns of older and younger adults' brain activity in reward processing areas. In related research on the framing effect, Mikels and Reed (2009) found that whereas both older and young adults displayed similar levels of risk aversion in gain frames, older adults did not display risk seeking in loss frames (cf. Peters et al., 2011, for a discussion of findings with different patterns of results). Although not all of the above studies had measures of performance or optimality, we can predict that the lower impact of potential losses found for older adults may contribute to their relatively poorer decision-making abilities, especially in tasks that require learning (see also, Mata, Josef, Samanez-Larkin, & Hertwig, 2011). For instance, Samanez-Larkin, Kuhnen, Yoo, and Knutson (2010) found that older adults made more risky and suboptimal decisions in an investment task in comparison to younger adults, and that this suboptimal performance was related to higher actual debt and less savings.

Another nuanced examination of the role of emotion in age differences in risky decision making was conducted by Mather et al. (2012). These researchers examined the certainty effect, in which an individual's decision between a sure and risky option depends on whether the decision is in the gain or loss domain. Specifically, people are theorized to be more risk averse in the domain of gains and are more risk seeking in the domain of losses due to an overweighing of certainty. Across a series of studies, Mather et al. (2012) found that older relative to younger adults had a greater preference for sure options in the domain of gains, while they were less willing to select sure options in the domain of losses. In this work, age was positively correlated with the proportion of positively valenced words used in explanations. Controlling for the positivity of the explanations (as opposed to numeracy or other cognitive measures) as a covariate eliminated the age difference in sure-loss avoidance. These findings indicate that relative to younger adults, older adults' greater focus on positive affect was related to their increased propensity to select options with at least some probability of a positive outcome. This research is consistent with the loss prevention perspective proposed by Depping and Freund (2011, 2013).

An additional account of age differences in risk taking proposes that loss aversion is present across the adult life span, but age differences in responses to gains are related to frontal lobe atrophy (Weller, Levin, & Denburg, 2011). However, other research indicates that older adults' risk taking is predicted by anticipated positive affect associated with a positive outcome, whereas younger adult risk taking is predicted by anticipated negative affect associated with a negative outcome (Chen & Ma, 2009). Thus, some findings suggest that older adults have higher sensitivity toward gains and rewards versus losses, whereas other work suggests greater sensitivity to losses. It will be critical for future research to investigate these patterns as these propensities may negatively impact the risky decisions of older adults, especially in the financial domain.

CONCLUSIONS AND FUTURE RESEARCH DIRECTIONS

Although the currently emerging patterns for the role of emotion in the decision making of older adults do not suggest a unified perspective, there are clear conclusions that can be extracted from the findings reviewed here. Primarily, it appears vitally important to consider how emotions impact decision making in later life. This premise is evident by amassing research showing that emotions explain age differences in decisions—above and beyond the influence of cognitive factors (Mather et al., 2012; Mikels et al., 2013; von Helversen & Mata, 2012). Specifically, several studies demonstrated that controlling for either incidental or integral emotions eliminated age differences in decision behavior. Such patterns suggest that decision researchers should continue to examine the contributions of incidental states and integral emotions to decision processes across the life span.

Importantly, though, the appraisal tendency framework highlights the important consideration of how different discrete emotions differentially impact decisions. Insofar as older adults experience less disgust and anger but potentially stronger instances of sadness, discrete emotions likely influence their decision making in different ways relative to the young (e.g., less risk seeking). Future research is needed to specify how discrete emotions may differentially influence older adults. Methodologically, researchers should increase their efforts to incorporate indirect measures of emotion in aging and decision research. For instance, facial electromyography has been used to measure the valence of emotional reactions (see, e.g., Larsen, Norris, & Cacioppo, 2003) and could be further incorporated into aging and decision research as a measure of integral feelings during choices. Additionally, it would also be beneficial for more studies to measure the GSRs of older and younger adults given the previously mentioned research on the role of arousal in decision making under risk.

It will also be critical to delineate when emotions are beneficial versus harmful to the decision making of older adults. We have highlighted the important distinction between integral and incidental affect in an attempt to differentiate when emotions may result in positive versus negative decision outcomes. In particular, we propose that in the face of their declining deliberative processes, older adults can benefit from using integral affect to make decisions under most circumstances. In light of CEST and dual-process models, such benefits should be most readily observed when deliberative and affective processes lead to similar as opposed to conflicting choices. In contrast, we maintain that incidental affect may mainly be detrimental to the decisions of older adults. Insofar as incidental affect is not directly relevant to a decision, older adults may often be led astray by their generally greater positivity. Future research directions considering such distinctions should be fruitful and would advance our understanding of when emotions are beneficial versus harmful to decision making across the adult life span.

Unfortunately, the extant literature on aging and risk taking is relatively inconclusive, with the suggestion that sometimes older relative to younger adults do not differ in risk taking, but sometimes they do. Critically, though, age differences in emotion are not always taken into consideration. Also, it appears likely that such age differences are contingent on the differential considerations of gains and losses. Research in this domain suggests that age-related changes in emotion likely underlie the complicated patterns observed in decisions involving risk. Systematically exploring how emotion may differentially influence risk taking with special attention to affective reactions to gains and losses will be informative.

Most importantly, the age differences in decision making reviewed here have critical implications for the health and financial domains.

Although research has begun to examine the role of emotion in such decisions, more research is necessary. For instance, as a result of the positivity effect, are health messages best conveyed with positive emotional tone focusing on gains and benefits? However, does a focus on benefits and gains lead older adults to make less optimal financial decisions?

The decision making of older adults is clearly influenced by emotion, and it is important to consider such influences. Though nascent, research in this domain has large societal implications and represents an exciting area for future research. By integrating the role of emotion in the decisions of older individuals with theoretical and methodological approaches, our understanding of decision making and aging will be more comprehensive, convergent, and balanced. Above all, however, this approach has the potential to enhance the lives of older individuals as they make decisions—which is to suggest that the societal impact and public policy applications are considerable.

Acknowledgments

Preparation of this chapter was supported by the Decision, Risk and Management Sciences program at the National Science Foundation, Research Grant SES-1139554 and National Institute on Aging Grant R01 AG043533-01 to the first author.

References

Alea, N., Bluck, S., & Semegon, A. B. (2004). Young and older adults' expression of emotional experience: Do autobiographical narratives tell a different story? *Journal of Adult Development, 11*(4), 235–250.

Alhakami, A. S., & Slovic, P. (1994). A psychological study of the inverse relationship between perceived risk and perceived benefit. *Risk Analysis, 14*(6), 1085–1096.

Alonso, D., & Fernandez-Berrocal, P. (2003). Irrational decisions: Attending to numbers rather than ratios. *Personality and Individual Differences, 35*(7), 1537–1547.

Ariely, D., & Loewenstein, G. (2006). The heat of the moment: The effect of sexual arousal on sexual decision making. *Journal of Behavioral Decision Making, 19*(2), 87–98.

Baddeley, A. D. (1986). *Working memory*. Oxford, UK: Clarendon Press.

Banham, K. M. (1951). Senescence and the emotions: A genetic theory. *The Pedagogical Seminary and Journal of Genetic Psychology, 78*(2), 175–183.

Bauer, A. S., Timpe, J. C., Edmonds, E. C., Bechara, A., Tranel, D., & Denburg, N. L. (2013). Myopia for the future or hypersensitivity to reward? Age-related changes in decision making on the Iowa Gambling Task. *Emotion, 13*(1), 19–24.

Bechara, A., Tranel, D., Damasio, H., & Damasio, A. R. (1996). Failure to respond autonomically to anticipated future outcomes following damage to prefrontal cortex. *Cerebral Cortex, 6*(2), 215–225.

Blanchard-Fields, F., Jahnke, H. C., & Camp, C. (1995). Age differences in problem-solving style: The role of emotional salience. *Psychology and Aging, 10*(2), 173–180.

Bruine de Bruin, W., Parker, A. M., & Fischhoff, B. (2012). Explaining adult age differences in decision-making competence. *Journal of Behavioral Decision Making, 25*(4), 352–360.

Carpenter, S. M., Peters, E., Västfjäll, D., & Isen, A. M. (2013). Positive feelings facilitate working memory and complex decision making among older adults. *Cognition & Emotion, 27*(1), 184–192.

Carstensen, L. L. (2006). The influence of a sense of time on human development. *Science, 312*, 1913–1915.

Carstensen, L. L., Gottman, J. M., & Levenson, R. W. (1995). Emotional behavior in long-term marriage. *Psychology and Aging, 10*(1), 140–149.

Carstensen, L. L., & Mikels, J. A. (2005). At the intersection of emotion and cognition: Aging and the positivity effect. *Current Directions in Psychological Science, 14*(3), 117–121.

Carstensen, L. L., Mikels, J. A., & Mather, M. (2006). Aging and the intersection of cognition, motivation and emotion. In J. Birren, & K. W. Schaie (Eds.), *Handbook of the psychology of aging* (6th ed., pp. 343–362). San Diego, CA: Academic Press.

Carstensen, L. L., Pasupathi, M., Mayr, U., & Nesselroade, J. R. (2000). Emotional experience in everyday life across the adult life span. *Journal of Personality and Social Psychology, 79*(4), 644–655.

Carstensen, L. L., Turan, B., Scheibe, S., Ram, N., Ersner-Hershfeld, H., Samanez-Larkin, G. R., et al. (2011). Emotional experience improves with age: Evidence based on over 10 years of experience sampling. *Psychology and Aging, 26*(1), 21–33.

Charles, S. T. (2010). Strength and vulnerability integration: A model of emotional well-being across adulthood. *Psychological Bulletin, 136*(6), 1068–1091.

Charles, S. T., Mather, M., & Carstensen, L. L. (2003). Aging and emotional memory: The forgettable nature of negative images for older adults. *Journal of Experimental Psychology: General, 132*(2), 310–324.

Charles, S. T., Reynolds, C. A., & Gatz, M. (2001). Age-related differences and change in positive and negative affect over 23 years. *Journal of Personality and Social Psychology, 80*(1), 136–151.

Chen, Y., & Ma, X. (2009). Age differences in risky decisions: The role of anticipated emotions. *Educational Gerontology, 35*(7), 575–586.

Cheung, E., & Mikels, J. A. (2011). I'm feeling lucky: The relationship between affect and risk-seeking in the framing effect. *Emotion, 11*(4), 852–859.

Chou, K., Lee, T. C., & Ho, A. Y. (2007). Does mood state change risk taking tendency in older adults? *Psychology and Aging, 22*(2), 310–318.

Damasio, A. R. (1994). *Descartes' error: Emotion, reason, and the human brain*. New York, NY: Avon Books.

De Martino, B., Kumaran, D., Seymour, B., & Dolan, R. J. (2006). Frames, biases, and rational decision-making in the human brain. *Science, 313*(5787), 684–687.

Del Missier, F., Mäntylä, T., Hansson, P., Bruine de Bruin, W., Parker, A. M., & Nilsson, L. (2013). The multifold relationship between memory and decision making: An individual-differences study. *Journal of Experimental Psychology: Learning, Memory, and Cognition, 39*(5), 1344–1364.

Denburg, N. L., Recknor, E. C., Bechara, A., & Tranel, D. (2006). Psychophysiological anticipation of positive outcomes promotes advantageous decision-making in normal older persons. *International Journal of Psychophysiology, 61*(1), 19–25.

Denes-Raj, V., & Epstein, S. (1994). Conflict between intuitive and rational processing: When people behave against their better judgment. *Journal of Personality and Social Psychology, 66*(5), 819–829.

Depping, M. K., & Freund, A. M. (2011). Normal aging and decision making: The role of motivation. *Human Development, 54*(6), 349–367.

Depping, M. K., & Freund, A. M. (2013). When choice matters: Task-dependent memory effects in older adulthood. *Psychology and Aging, 28*(4), 923–936.

Epstein, S. (1994). Integration of the cognitive and the psychodynamic unconscious. *American Psychologist, 49*(8), 709–724.

Epstein, S., & Pacini, R. (2000). The influence of visualization on intuitive and analytical information processing. *Imagination, Cognition and Personality, 20*(3), 195–216.

Evans, J. S. B.T. (2008). Dual-processing accounts of reasoning, judgment, and social cognition. *Annual Review of Psychology, 59*, 255–278.

Evans, J. T., & Stanovich, K. E. (2013). Dual-process theories of higher cognition: Advancing the debate. *Perspectives on Psychological Science*, *8*(3), 223–241.

Finucane, M. L., Alhakami, A., Slovic, P., & Johnson, S. M. (2000). The affect heuristic in judgments of risks and benefits. *Journal of Behavioral Decision Making*, *13*(1), 1–17.

Forgas, J. P., Martin, L. L., & Clore, G. L. (2001). The affect infusion model (AIM): An integrative theory of mood effects on cognition and judgments. In L. L. Martin, & G. L. Clore (Eds.), *Theories of mood and cognition: A user's guidebook* (pp. 99–134). Mahwah, NJ: Lawrence Erlbaum Associates.

Fung, H. H., & Carstensen, L. L. (2003). Sending memorable messages to the old: Age differences in preferences and memory for advertisements. *Journal of Personality & Social Psychology*, *85*(1), 163–178.

Gigerenzer, G. (2007). *Gut feelings: The intelligence of the unconscious*. New York, NY: Penguin.

Gilovich, T., Griffin, D., & Kahneman, D. (2002). *Heuristics and biases: The psychology of intuitive judgment*. New York, NY: Cambridge University Press.

Gross, J. J., Carstensen, L. L., Pasupathi, M., Tsai, J., Götestam Skorpen, C., & Hsu, A. Y. (1997). Emotion and aging: Experience, expression, and control. *Psychology and Aging*, *12*(4), 590–599.

von Helversen, B., & Mata, R. (2012). Losing a dime with a satisfied mind: Positive affect predicts less search in sequential decision making. *Psychology & Aging*, *27*(4), 825–839.

Hsee, C. K. (1996). The evaluability hypothesis: An explanation for preference reversals between joint and separate evaluations of alternatives. *Organizational Behavior and Human Decision Processes*, *67*(3), 247–257.

Hsee, C. K. (1998). Less is better: When low-value options are valued more highly than high-value options. *Journal of Behavioral Decision Making*, *11*(2), 107–121.

Isaacowitz, D. M., & Choi, Y. (2012). Looking, feeling, and doing: Are there age differences in attention, mood, and behavioral responses to skin cancer information? *Health Psychology*, *31*(5), 650–659.

Isaacowitz, D. M., Wadlinger, H. A., Goren, D., & Wilson, H. R. (2006). Selective preference in visual fixation away from negative images in old age? An eye-tracking study. *Psychology and Aging*, *21*(1), 40–48.

Janis, I. L., & Mann, L. (1977). *Decision making: A psychological analysis of conflict, choice, and commitment*. New York, NY: The Free Press.

Johnson, M. M. S. (1990). Age differences in decision making: A process methodology for examining strategic information processing. *Journal of Gerontology Psychological Sciences*, *45*(2), 75–78.

Johnson, E. J., & Tversky, A. (1983). Affect, generalization, and the perception of risk. *Journal of Personality and Social Psychology*, *45*(1), 20–31.

Kahneman, D. (2003). A perspective on judgment and choice: Mapping bounded rationality. *American Psychologist*, *58*(9), 697–720.

Kahneman, D., & Tversky, A. (2000). *Choices, values, and frames*. New York, NY: Cambridge University Press.

Kensinger, E. A., Brierley, B., Medford, N., Growdon, J. H., & Corkin, S. (2002). Effects of normal aging and Alzheimer's disease on emotional memory. *Emotion*, *2*(2), 118–134.

Kim, S., Healey, M. K., Goldstein, D., Hasher, L., & Wiprzycka, U. J. (2008). Age differences in choice satisfaction: A positivity effect in decision making. *Psychology and Aging*, *23*(1), 33–38.

Kunzmann, U., & Grühn, D. (2005). Age differences in emotional reactivity: The sample case of sadness. *Psychology and Aging*, *20*(1), 47.

Kunzmann, U., Kupperbusch, C. S., & Levenson, R. W. (2005). Behavioral inhibition and amplification during emotional arousal: A comparison of two age groups. *Psychology and Aging*, *20*(1), 144–158.

Labouvie-Vief, G. (2003). Dynamic integration affect, cognition, and the self in adulthood. *Current Directions in Psychological Science*, *12*(6), 201–206.

Larsen, J. T., Norris, C. J., & Cacioppo, J. T. (2003). Effects of positive and negative affect on electromyographic activity over zygomaticus major and corrugator supercilii. *Psychophysiology, 40*(5), 776–785.

Lawton, M. P., Kleban, M. H., & Dean, J. (1993). Affect and age: Cross-sectional comparisons of structure and prevalence. *Psychology and Aging, 8*(2), 165–175.

Lawton, M. P., Kleban, M. H., Rajagopal, D., & Dean, J. (1992). Dimensions of affective experience in three age groups. *Psychology and Aging, 7*(2), 171.

Lerner, J. S., Gonzalez, R. M., Small, D. A., & Fischhoff, B. (2003). Effects of fear and anger on perceived risks of terrorism. *Psychological Science, 14*(2), 144–150.

Lerner, J. S., & Keltner, D. (2000). Beyond valence: Toward a model of emotion-specific influences on judgement and choice. *Cognition & Emotion, 14*(4), 473–493.

Lerner, J. S., & Keltner, D. (2001). Fear, anger, and risk. *Journal of Personality and Social Psychology, 81*(1), 146–159.

Lerner, J. S., Small, D. A., & Loewenstein, G. (2004). Heart strings and purse strings: Carryover effects of emotions on economic decisions. *Psychological Science, 15*(5), 337–341.

Löckenhoff, C. E., & Carstensen, L. L. (2007). Aging, emotion, and health-related decision strategies: Motivational manipulations can reduce age differences. *Psychology and Aging, 22*(1), 134–146.

Loewenstein, G. F., Weber, E. U., Hsee, C. K., & Welch, N. (2001). Risk as feelings. *Psychological Bulletin, 127*(2), 267–286.

Lo, A. W., & Repin, D. V. (2002). The psychophysiology of real-time financial risk processing. *Journal of Cognitive Neuroscience, 14*(3), 323–339.

Mano, H. (1994). Risk-taking, framing effects, and affect. *Organizational Behavior and Human Decision Processes, 57*(1), 38–58.

Mata, R., Josef, A. K., Samanez-Larkin, G. R., & Hertwig, R. (2011). Age differences in risky choice: A meta-analysis. *Annals of the New York Academy of Sciences, 1235*(1), 18–29.

Mather, M., & Carstensen, L. L. (2005). Aging and motivated cognition: The positivity effect in attention and memory. *Trends in Cognitive Sciences, 9*(10), 496–502.

Mather, M., Knight, M., & McCaffrey, M. (2005). The allure of the alignable: Younger and older adults' false memories of choice features. *Journal of Experimental Psychology: General, 134*(1), 38–51.

Mather, M., Mazar, N., Gorlick, M. A., Lighthall, N. R., Burgeno, J., Schoeke, A., et al. (2012). Risk preferences and aging: The "certainty effect" in older adults' decision making. *Psychology and Aging, 27*(4), 801–816.

Mayer, J. D., Gaschke, Y. N., Braverman, D. L., & Evans, T. W. (1992). Mood-congruent judgment is a general effect. *Journal of Personality & Social Psychology, 63*(1), 119–132.

Mikels, J. A., Cheung, E., Cone, J., & Gilovich, T. (2013). The dark side of intuition: Aging and increases in nonoptimal intuitive decisions. *Emotion, 13*(2), 189–195.

Mikels, J. A., Larkin, G. R., Reuter-Lorenz, P. A., & Carstensen, L. L. (2005). Divergent trajectories in the aging mind: Changes in working memory for affective versus visual information with age. *Psychology and Aging, 20*(4), 542–553.

Mikels, J. A., Löckenhoff, C. E., Maglio, S. J., Carstensen, L. L., Goldstein, M. K., & Garber, A. (2010). Following your heart or your head: Focusing on emotions versus information differentially influences the decisions of younger and older adults. *Journal of Experimental Psychology: Applied, 16*(1), 87–95.

Mikels, J. A., Maglio, S. J., Reed, A. E., & Kaplowitz, L. J. (2011). Should I go with my gut? Investigating the benefits of emotion-focused decision making. *Emotion, 11*(4), 743–753.

Mikels, J. A., & Reed, A. E. (2009). Monetary losses do not loom large in later life: Age differences in the framing effect. *The Journals of Gerontology Series B, 64*(4), 457–460.

Mroczek, D. K., & Kolarz, C. M. (1998). The effect of age on positive and negative affect: A developmental perspective on happiness. *Journal of Personality and Social Psychology, 75*(5), 1333–1349.

Pacini, R., & Epstein, S. (1999). The interaction of three facets of concrete thinking in a game of chance. *Thinking & Reasoning*, *5*(4), 303–325.

Peters, E., Dieckmann, N. E., & Weller, J. (2011). Age differences in complex decision making. In K. Schaie, & S. L. Willis (Eds.), *Handbook of the psychology of aging* (7th ed., pp. 133–151). San Diego, CA: Elsevier Academic Press.

Queen, T. L., & Hess, T. M. (2010). Age differences in the effects of conscious and unconscious thought in decision making. *Psychology and Aging*, *25*(2), 251–261.

Reed, A. E., & Carstensen, L. L. (2012). The theory behind the age-related positivity effect. *Frontiers in Psychology*, *3*, 1–9.

Reed, A. E., Chan, L., & Mikels, J. A. (2014). Meta-analysis of the age-related positivity effect: Age differences in preferences for positive over negative information. *Psychology and Aging*, *29*(1), 1–15.

Reed, A. E., Mikels, J. A., & Simon, K. I. (2008). Older adults prefer less choice than young adults. *Psychology and Aging*, *23*(3), 671–675.

Reyna, V. F. (2004). How people make decisions that involve risk: A dual process approach. *Current Directions in Psychological Science*, *13*(2), 60–66.

Reyna, V. F., & Lloyd, F. J. (2006). Physician decision making and cardiac risk: Effects of knowledge, risk perception, risk tolerance, and fuzzy processing. *Journal of Experimental Psychology: Applied*, *12*(3), 179–195.

Samanez-Larkin, G. R., Gibbs, S. E. B., Khanna, K., Nielsen, L., Carstensen, L. L., & Knutson, B. (2007). Anticipation of monetary gain but not loss in healthy older adults. *Nature Neuroscience*, *10*(6), 787–791.

Samanez-Larkin, G. R., Kuhnen, C. M., Yoo, D. J., & Knutson, B. (2010). Variability in nucleus accumbens activity mediates age-related suboptimal financial risk taking. *The Journal of Neuroscience*, *30*(4), 1426–1434.

Schwarz, N., & Clore, G. L. (2007). Feelings and phenomenal experiences. In A. W. Kruglanski, & E. T. Higgins (Eds.), *Social psychology: Handbook of basic principles* (2nd ed., pp. 385–407). New York, NY: Guilford Press.

Shamaskin, A. M., Mikels, J. A., & Reed, A. E. (2010). Getting the message across: Age differences in the positive and negative framing of health care messages. *Psychology and Aging*, *25*(3), 746–751.

Slovic, P., Finucane, M., Peters, E., & MacGregor, D. (2002). The affect heuristic. In T. Gilovich, D. Griffin, & D. Kahneman (Eds.), *Heuristics and Biases: The Psychology of Intuitive Judgment* (pp. 397–420). New York: Cambridge University Press.

Slovic, P., Peters, E., Finucane, M. L., & MacGregor, D. G. (2005). Affect, risk, and decision making. *Health Psychology*, *24*(4S), S35–S40.

Strough, J., Karns, T. E., & Schlosnagle, L. (2011). Decision-making heuristics and biases across the life span. *Annals of the New York Academy of Sciences*, *1235*(1), 57–74.

Strough, J., Mehta, C. M., McFall, J. P., & Schuller, K. L. (2008). Are older adults less subject to the sunk-cost fallacy than younger adults? *Psychological Science*, *19*(7), 650–652.

Tiedens, L. Z., & Linton, S. (2001). Judgment under emotional certainty and uncertainty: The effects of specific emotions on information processing. *Journal of Personality and Social Psychology*, *81*(6), 973–988.

Urry, H. L., & Gross, J. J. (2010). Emotion regulation in older age. *Current Directions in Psychological Science*, *19*(6), 352–357.

Verhaeghen, P., Marcoen, A., & Goossens, L. (1993). Facts and fiction about memory aging: A quantitative integration of research findings. *Journal of Gerontology*, *48*(4), 157–171.

Weller, J. A., Levin, I. P., & Denburg, N. L. (2011). Trajectory of risky decision making for potential gains and losses from ages 5 to 85. *Journal of Behavioral Decision Making*, *24*(4), 331–344.

CHAPTER

10

A Prospect Theory-Based Evaluation of Dual-Process Influences on Aging and Decision Making: Support for a Contextual Perspective

Thomas M. Hess

Department of Psychology, North Carolina State University, Raleigh, NC, USA

Interest in the study of aging and decision making is rapidly growing for a number of different reasons. From a practical standpoint, effective decision making about finances, housing, and health in later life is likely to have significant consequences in terms of maintaining independence and decreasing the need for assistance from family, government, and other external supports. Decisions made by older adults in the areas of finance and health may be particularly consequential given that, relative to younger adults, they have less time and fewer opportunities to make up for poor decisions.

The study of decision making and aging is also interesting from a life-span developmental perspective. In contrast to traditional rational choice perspectives, in which decisions were thought to be based in logical analysis geared toward identifying a single best choice, decision making in real life typically involves the interplay between situational factors (e.g., task demands, task content, goal relevance) and individual characteristics (e.g., ability, experience, motivation) (e.g., Kahneman, 2003). Importantly, many influential individual attributes are related to age in adulthood, reflecting changes in factors such as health and underlying biological mechanisms, participation in age-graded social structures, accumulated knowledge—both general and domain-specific—and developmentally relevant goals. Implication of these multiple mechanisms

Aging and Decision Making
http://dx.doi.org/10.1016/B978-0-12-417148-0.00010-8

obviously complicates our task of understanding the relationship between aging and decision making, and it may also account for the absence of a coherent picture of age effects from existing empirical work. It does argue, however, for the adoption of a contextual perspective (Baltes, 1987) in examining adult age differences in decision processes. Such an approach is likely to lead to a more nuanced approach in research and theory, resulting in the identification of influential mechanisms and the boundary conditions associated with their operation.

In this chapter, I build on previous advocacy efforts for taking a contextual approach to understanding aging and decision making (Hess & Queen, 2014). I initially focus on dual-process perspectives on decision making, and some general expectations derived from our current understanding of the impact of aging on deliberative and affective processes. Using Prospect Theory (Kahneman & Tversky, 1979), I attempt to characterize these expectations within the context of probability weighting and value functions. I then review research that addresses predictions about the nature of age-related effects based on these functions, with the findings evaluated within the context of specific perspectives regarding the impact of aging on decision making. To foreshadow, extant research reveals few consistent, systematic trends, with much variation in the nature of age-related effects across studies examining similar phenomena. I conclude by arguing for consideration of a contextual perspective that takes into account interactions between an individual's life circumstances, ability, and motivation in studying aging and decision making.

DUAL-PROCESS PERSPECTIVES ON DECISION MAKING

A general approach characterizing much work on aging and decision making is based in what Hess and Blanchard-Fields (1996) have termed the cognitive aging perspective. A primary emphasis in this approach is on understanding how age-related declines in deliberative skills involving factors such as processing speed, working memory, executive control, and episodic memory skills impact the ability of older adults to make effective decisions. A general expectation from this perspective is that aging will be associated with decrements in decision making within many contexts, and indeed there is research suggesting that there is a relationship between age-related differences in ability and performance (e.g., Bruine de Bruin, Parker, & Fischhoff, 2012; Del Missier et al., 2013; Finucane, Mertz, Slovic, & Schmidt, 2005).

A layer of complexity is added, however, when changing deliberative skills are considered within the context of dual-process models of decision making (e.g., Epstein, 1994; Kahneman, 2003; Loewenstein, Weber, Hsee, & Welch, 2001). These models make a broad distinction between two sets of skills, which I will label as experiential (or affective) and deliberative.[1] Experiential processing is thought to be automatic, implicit, intuitive, associative, fast, and based primarily in affective responses. In contrast, deliberative processing is characterized as effortful, conscious, analytical, verbal (or symbolic), and slow. Both systems are thought to be operative in any given situation, although circumstances might dictate greater reliance on one system over the other. Many decisions can be made effectively based on experiential processes (e.g., somatic markers; Bechara & Damasio, 2005), which may draw upon past experience and associated affective responses. The deliberative system is thought to play a role in monitoring experiential outcomes, and is also likely to be operative in novel or complex situations (i.e., situations where experiential processing may not be effective; Kahneman, 2003). When considered with respect to aging, there are at least four different ways to characterize the changing nature of interaction of these two systems during adulthood in terms of understanding their impact on decision making.

Relative Preservation. One perspective is a straightforward extension of the cognitive aging view based in the presumed decline of deliberative functions and relative preservation of affective skills. We have previously termed this *affective resiliency* (Peters, Hess, Västfjäll, & Auman, 2007), and suggested that it should be manifested in terms of affective processes becoming more dominant in the decision-making process in later life. This may reflect less active monitoring of experiential processes or greater weighting of experiential products due to inefficiencies of deliberation. This perspective assumes not only that experiential processes remain relatively stable, but that they also operate in a similar fashion throughout adulthood.

Heightened Focus on Affect. A second perspective makes similar assumptions about age differences in the effectiveness of experiential and deliberative processes, but further assumes that affective processes are accentuated due to age-related shifts in the focus on such information. This *affective enhancement* perspective (Peters et al., 2007) can be viewed as an extension of Socioemotional Selectivity Theory (Carstensen, Isaacowitz, & Charles, 1999). Specifically, it is assumed that experiential processing increases in importance not only due to declining deliberative skills but also due to the heightened salience of chronic goals that increase the importance of, and focus on, affective content in promoting well-being.

Selective Focus on Affect. A modification of the preceding perspective is based on ideas drawn from the Selection, Optimization, and Compensation model (Baltes, 1997) and related propositions regarding shifts in goal orientation from a relative emphasis on gains in early adulthood to one focusing on loss prevention in later life (e.g., Freund & Ebner, 2005).

[1] These have also been referred to as System 1 and System 2 (e.g., Kahneman, 2003). I adopt the experiential-deliberative terminology here due to the descriptive nature of the labels.

Depping and Freund (2013) have argued that this should increase the salience of information relating to potential losses to older adults in decision-making situations. Given the specific focus of the loss-prevention goal orientation, this perspective can be characterized as involving *selective affective enhancement*. One might argue that Socioemotional Selectivity Theory would also be associated with selective enhancement given recent research suggesting a biased focus on positive information as a regulatory mechanism in older adulthood (Reed & Carstensen, 2012). At issue, however, is the fact the positive affective outcomes might be achieved in different ways. For example, an individual might focus on preserving gains and avoiding losses—which would be consistent with the previously described increased affective focus—or she might differentially focus on either one of these processes toward the same basic goal. Alternatively, Mata and Hertwig (2011) suggested that positivity might lead to greater utility—and thus risk-seeking—associated with gains, and less risk-seeking with losses relative to younger adults. This ambiguity in expected outcomes makes it somewhat difficult to formulate clear predictions and to interpret relevant research relating to Socioemotional Selectivity (e.g., Peters, Dieckmann, & Weller, 2011).

Selective Deployment of Resources. The fourth general perspective is based on our Selective Engagement Theory (Hess, 2014). Briefly, it is assumed that increased costs associated with deliberative cognitive activity in later life result in older adults becoming more selective in task engagement in order to conserve processing resources. This is manifested in terms of the self-relevance or personal meaningfulness of tasks becoming increasingly important in determining engagement of cognitive resources with increasing age (but especially in later life). This selective engagement perspective does not argue for stability of deliberative skills with age, but rather that these skills can often be effectively marshaled by older adults when necessary to support effective functioning. This suggests that age differences characterized by the *affective resiliency* perspective should be most evident in situations of low personal relevance. Although Selective Engagement Theory focuses on motivation, it is also not inconsistent with other motivational approaches to understanding age effects. It does, however, suggest that consistency of the situation with an individual's chronic goals is likely to be a determinant of the degree to which deliberative processes are engaged to support those goals.

DUAL-PROCESS INFLUENCES AND PROSPECT THEORY

One way to characterize the impact of age-related changes in experiential and deliberative processes within each of the aforementioned perspectives is through reference to Prospect Theory (Kahneman & Tversky, 1979).

This influential framework provides a counterweight to traditional economic theories, taking into account factors associated with the information-processing system that influence how individuals weight probabilities and attach value to specific outcomes in the decision-making process. These processes are described in terms of two specific functions: probability weighting and value. The impact of experiential and deliberative processing can be envisioned through these functions, resulting in relatively specific expectations regarding aging effects. Previous articles (Mata & Hertwig, 2011; Peters et al., 2007) have attempted to use Prospect Theory to make conjectures about the nature of aging effects. The present attempt expands upon these, however, by considering age differences across a broader framework of perspectives within the dual-process framework. In sections that follow, I discuss both the probability weighting and value functions in turn, along with dual-process and aging-related influences associated with each.

Probability Weighting

The probability-weighting function relates objective probability to subjective decision weights assigned to these same values (Kahneman & Tversky, 1979). For example, do the same absolute differences in probabilities between two outcomes have the same weight regardless of the value of the probabilities (e.g., is the difference between 0.05 and 0.10 viewed as similar to the difference between 0.45 and 0.50)? Assuming a totally rational or logical assignment of weights, this function would approximate a linear relationship, with decision weight increasing systematically with probability. In reality, however, this relationship has a curvilinear, reverse S-shaped form (Figure 1(A)). Thus, whereas there is a general increase in decision weights as probabilities increase, the departure from linearity suggests that not all probabilities are assigned similar weights. This function reflects at least three important characteristics.

First, there is an overweighting of small probabilities, as reflected in the steepness of the slope at the low probability end of the scale. In other words, people are more sensitive to small differences in probabilities, leading to greater investment in eliminating low probability outcomes. This results, for example, in individuals being willing to pay more to increase their odds of winning from 0.05 to 0.06 than from 0.40 to 0.41, even though the incremental impact on success is identical in each case (e.g., Gonzalez & Wu, 1999). Second, the curve is less steep in the middle, indicating less sensitivity to intermediate probabilities (as also reflected in the aforementioned example). Finally, the slope becomes steeper for high probabilities, once again reflecting greater sensitivity to small differences in probabilities. This reflects the fact that individuals are willing to pay more to achieve a "sure thing" (e.g., increasing the probability of winning from 0.99 to 1.0) than for a similar increment in the odds of winning at a lower probability (0.90–0.91). Another way of describing these effects is

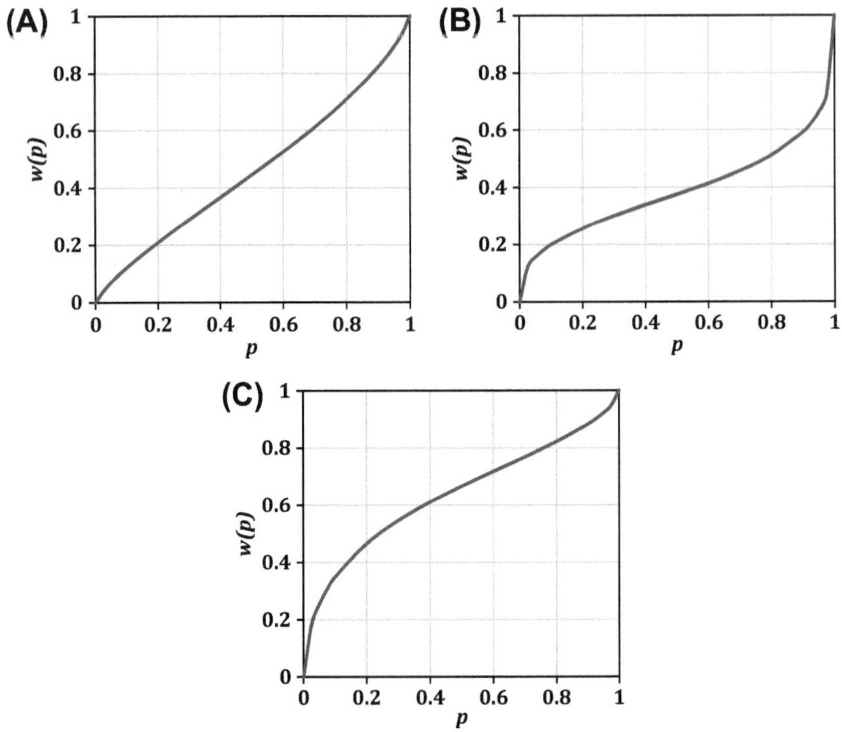

FIGURE 1 Probability weighting functions representing typical form (A), exaggerated impossibility and certainty effects involving overweighting of small probabilities and underweighting of high probabilities (B), and overall affective influence reflecting overall enhancement to midvalue probabilities (C).

that individuals tend to overweight low probabilities and underweight high probabilities. In the case of low probabilities, people will overweight small probabilities to avoid a certain loss—the *impossibility effect*—whereas individuals will underweight high probabilities when given the opportunity to achieve a certain gain—the *certainty effect*[2] (see Reyna & Brainerd, 1991 for a similar explanation for framing effects).

Dual-Process Influences. The impact of experiential processes can be seen in situations examining affective influences. In general, infusion of affect into the decision-making process increases the severity of departures of this curve from linearity. For example, Rottenstreich and Hsee (2001) found that individuals were more sensitive to probabilities when stimuli were affect-poor than when they were affect-rich. They suggested

[2] These two effects are often referred to collectively as relating to certainty. I have chosen to treat them in this fashion, however, since there are possible age-related influences that may affect one but not the other.

that the overweighting of small probabilities and underweighting of large probabilities may reflect hope associated with a shift from impossibility to possibility and fear associated with not obtaining a certain outcome. Thus, evidence of the operation of the experiential system is found in both the steepness of the initial slope of the curve at low probabilities as well as the degree of inflection of the function (i.e., severity of the stair-step nature of the curve; Figure 1(B)). Affect may also have its primary influence on the left-hand side of the curve (i.e., the degree of change from impossibility to possibility). This would be consistent with a perspective based in anticipatory emotions (e.g., savoring and dread; (Elster & Loewenstein, 1992), which would elevate weightings of affect-rich options at all levels of possibility (Figure 1(C)).

These different affective influences can be understood with reference to a commonly used (e.g., Gonzalez & Wu, 1999; Tversky & Fox, 1995) probability weighting function: $w(p) = \delta p^{\gamma} / \delta p^{\gamma} + (1-p)^{\gamma}$. Specifically, the weighting assigned to a specific probability (p) is affected by δ, which reflects the elevation of the function, and γ, which reflects the curvature. Thus, an affective focus consistent with the "hope and fear" account would have the greatest impact on γ, whereas δ would be associated with anticipatory emotions (Gonzalez & Wu, 1999; Mukherjee, 2011). Minimal affective influences would be associated with a relatively linear function.

Certainty and impossibility effects may be also related to the evaluability of individual pieces of information (e.g., specific probabilities), and the degree to which the situation encourages comparisons to specific reference information (Hsee & Zhang, 2010). For example, single evaluation (i.e., evaluating a choice or probability in isolation) is likely to result in individuals focusing on general categorical distinctions (e.g., a certain outcome vs an uncertain one) given the lack of a meaningful reference for more specific probabilities. Thus, in single evaluation, the difference between 95% and 100% is perceived as greater than that between 85% and 90% given that the former offers the possibility of a categorical judgment whereas the latter does not. In contrast, in joint evaluation—where pairs of probabilities might be presented together, thereby offering a meaningful reference point—individuals will be more sensitive to value. Thus, decision weights assigned to probabilities in these pairs will be similar, and the probability-weighting function will tend more toward linearity. These differences can be seen as reflecting the degree to which the task engages the deliberative system (e.g., by encouraging decision by calculation) versus the experiential system (e.g., basing judgments on global evaluations or feelings).

Characteristics of individuals might also lead to differences in what Hsee and Rottenstreich (2004) termed valuation by calculation versus valuation by feeling, even in cases where reference information is available (e.g., joint evaluation). For example, people who rate themselves as high in experiential reasoning exhibit a stronger impossibility effect (i.e., overweighting of small probabilities) than those low in experiential reasoning (Mukherjee, 2011). Ability is also likely to play a role in determining the shape of this function. For example, there is a growing body of research indicating that numeracy skills are positively associated with accuracy in interpretation of numbers such as percentages and probabilities (Peters, 2012). Thus, those high in numeracy—and perhaps cognitive ability in general—may engage more in valuation by calculation, resulting in a more systematic mapping of decision weights onto probabilities.

Aging Effects. Extrapolating from this to aging, we can make several predictions based on the previous perspectives of potential age differences. Consistent with the affective resiliency perspective, one would expect older adults to exhibit reduced magnitude sensitivity, resulting in increased impossibility and certainty effects (Figure 1(A) vs 1(B)). This effect may be particularly strong under conditions where integral affect—that is, affect that is relevant to the specific decision under consideration—associated with the task is low. Under such conditions, interpretation of probability would be highly dependent upon deliberative skills, whereas age differences associated with these skills might diminish somewhat in influence as affect became more integral to the task. Another way to phrase this is that older adults should be more likely to base decision weights on categorical distinctions as opposed to changes in magnitude. The affective enhancement perspective might predict a somewhat similar effect, with the general impact of affect on weight being enhanced. This might result in an even larger impossibility effect, but a reduced certainty effect as the overall weight assigned to mid-value probabilities would be increased (Figure 1(C)).

To what extent is there data consistent with these expectations? One way to examine this is by determining whether older adults' behavior is as sensitive to probabilistic information as that of younger adults. Research has generally shown that young and older adults respond to probabilistic information in a similar manner across a variety of tasks, at least when translation of such information is relatively straightforward. For example, a series of studies by Chasseigne and colleagues (Chasseigne, Grau, Mullet, & Cama, 1999; Chasseigne, Lafon, & Mullet, 2002; Chasseigne et al., 2004) examining probabilistic cue learning found that older adults exhibited levels of sensitivity to probability similar to those of the young, although some age deficits emerged under conditions involving higher levels of difficulty (e.g., use of multiple cues). Research using other types of tasks is consistent with this conclusion (e.g., Dror, Katona, & Mungur, 1998; Fisk, 2005; Okun & Elias, 1977; but see Deakin, Aitken, Robbins, & Sahakian, 2004).

Note, however, that age-related sensitivity to probabilistic information may be reduced when affective cues conflict with such information.

For example, Mutter and colleagues (Mutter & Pliske, 1994; Mutter, 2000) found that older adults are more susceptible to illusory correlation than are younger adults. That is, prior beliefs about the covariation of two variables interfered with processing of information regarding their actual covariation in a given situation. In situations involving online judgments (i.e., real-time processing) of covariation using stimuli without strong preexisting beliefs about covariation, age differences in processing information were significantly smaller than in those involving situations where judgments were memory-based (Mutter, 2000). Whereas this does suggest some problems in using probability information associated with declining deliberative skills in later life (see also Mutter & Williams, 2004), these findings also indicate that problems may be minimized "in the moment." Of importance, however, is the fact that this research suggests that when older adults have relevant experience in a domain, they might have a greater tendency to rely on experiential processes than younger adults even in situations where processing of probability information is possible. Note that this conclusion is somewhat inconsistent with the earlier conjecture that age differences in affective influences would be particularly strong in situations involving minimal affect. Instead, it implies that age differences may be greatest when strong affective cues compete with available probability cues. An important question then concerns whether such effects reflect a fundamental aspect of the aging information-processing system, or whether older adults might be able to overcome such experiential tendencies if sufficiently motivated.

Another way to examine age-related influences in probability weighting is by determining the extent to which there are systematic age differences in certainty and impossibility effects. If affective influences are greater in later life, then the strength of these effects should be positively associated with aging, resulting in older adults exhibiting relatively greater overweighting in the loss domain and underweighting in the gain domain. This would reflect the greater importance attached to (1) having the opportunity to avoid a loss as opposed to experiencing a certain loss—as reflected in greater risk-taking; and (2) obtaining a certain gain rather than simply having the possibility of obtaining one—as reflected in risk aversion.

Several studies have examined preferences for risky bets versus certain outcomes. In these studies, participants are typically presented with hypothetical situations in which they choose between an option involving either a certain win or loss versus one involving a probabilistic outcome (e.g., win $10 vs 0.8 chance of winning $15 or 0.2 chance of winning $0; lose $5 vs 0.6 chance of losing $10 or 0.4 chance of losing $0). Unfortunately, the results are somewhat inconsistent. Lauriola and Levin (2001) obtained evidence consistent with a general age-related increase in affective influence, with older adults exhibiting greater risk-taking for losses (i.e., enhanced impossibility effect) and greater risk aversion for gains (i.e., enhanced certainty effect) relative to younger adults. Similar results were obtained by Weller, Levin, and Denburg (2011), with the effects greatest when the risky choice was advantageous (i.e., greater expected value) relative to the certain choice. Boyle, Yu, Buchman, and Bennett (2012) examined performance in a large community-based sample of older adults and also found that increasing age was associated with stronger certainty effects; they did not, however, examine performance relating to losses. Mather et al. (2012) found a similar pattern to that of Lauriola and Levin (2001) when participants were exposed to sets of choice problems involving only losses or only gains (experiments 1–3). When participants made decisions about both types of problems, however, age differences were only observed within the loss domain (experiment 4), which also corresponds with the results of a meta-analysis conducted by Weber, Shafir, and Blaise (2004)—although the age range represented in their analysis was not reported.

The variation in results across studies and experiments suggest the manner in which the problems are presented may influence the nature of observed age effects. For example, when participants only saw either gain or loss problems, both Boyle et al. (2012) and Mather et al. (2012) observed age-related increases in both certainty and impossibility effects. Weller et al. (2011) obtained similar results using blocked presentation of loss and gain problems. In contrast, when participants saw both types of problems, Mather et al. (2012) observed only an age-related increase in certainty. Intermixing of the two types of problems may serve to accentuate differences between gains and losses, perhaps leading to the latter taking on increased salience. Problematic for this explanation, however, are the facts that (1) Lauriola and Levin (2001) also intermixed problems across trials and found age-related increases in both loss-aversion in gain problems and risk-taking in loss problems, and (2) Holliday (1988) found no age differences associated with certainty and impossibility when presenting problems in the same manner. Note that the tendency toward age differences in these effects being stronger in the loss than in the gain domain can be viewed as consistent with the *selective affective enhancement* perspective (e.g., minimizing losses; Depping & Freund, 2013). The variability across studies, however, suggests the possibility of yet-to-be-determined context-based moderators that influence the strength and form of obtained age functions.

Research on certainty and impossibility effects also provides an interesting counterpoint to the aforementioned research on sensitivity to probabilistic information. Specifically, the study of these effects suggests a degree of age-related insensitivity to such information. Mather et al. (2012) found, however, that this relative insensitivity disappeared when choices did not involve certainty. Thus, one interpretation of these observed effects is that certain outcomes are more affectively laden than other types of probabilities, and older adults are more likely to focus on this affective content. This may also reflect older adults being less likely to employ cognitive resources when more easily processed heuristic cues are available, a trend consistent with the previously discussed work of illusory correlation. When certain outcomes are not present, different-aged adults appear to be relatively similar in their attention to probabilistic information; when present, however, they may highlight a less cognitively demanding and more affectively engaging way to evaluate alternatives, with older adults minimizing drain on resources by using the presence of certainty as a cue for evaluation.

Based on the foregoing, we can conclude that, whereas there is some evidence for greater affective influence on probability weighting for older adults, the nature of this influence may vary with context. Thus, although older adults appear sensitive to probabilistic information, they may be less likely to use it if alternative, less demanding ways of processing information are available. The likelihood of relying on such information may also be dependent on motivational factors. For example, in the Holliday (1988) study—where no age differences were observed in the impact of certain outcomes—the problems were framed in terms of everyday situations (e.g., running a small business) as opposed to simple monetary outcomes. The former might be more likely to capture the interest of older adults, resulting in greater likelihood of engagement of cognitive resources and the elimination of age-related biases associated with experiential processes.[3] This interpretation of effects is consistent with the Selective Engagement perspective.

Interestingly, whereas the resulting age-related weighting biases introduced by the introduction of certain—as opposed to probabilistic—outcomes might reflect an increased focus on affective information or related factors (e.g., risk aversion) by older adults, they could just as easily be a simple reflection of cognitive demand. To distinguish between these age-related effects, it would be useful to examine personal attributes in relation to such outcomes. A related concern has to do with the nature of effects associated with hypothesized increases on emotional outcomes in later life, such as proposed by Socioemotional Selectivity Theory. Although the focus tends to be on positive affect, the manner in which positive affect is maximized is unclear (e.g., Isaacowitz & Blanchard-Fields, 2012).

[3] Everyday contexts may also allow participants to relate choices to past situations, resulting in perception of the problem as part of a series of choices over time (i.e., choice bracketing) as opposed to an isolated problem, which in turn influences level of risk aversion (Read, Loewenstein, & Rabin, 1999). Bracketing may allow older adults to base judgments on experience, resulting in fewer biases associated with interpretation of probabilities.

For example, older adults might focus on maximizing gains or minimizing losses. Indeed, research with young adults has shown that responses (e.g., risk-taking) to negative moods vary with type of mood (e.g., Raghunathan & Pham, 1999) and across studies examining the same mood (Cryder, Lerner, Gross, Dahl, & Ronald, 2008; Yuen & Lee, 2003), suggesting that the situation may influence the manner in which individuals attempt to regulate emotions through risk-seeking or risk-averse behaviors. The possibility that older adults might focus on minimizing losses is particularly problematic in distinguishing between different goal-based perspectives (e.g., Socioemotional Selectivity Theory vs Selection, Optimization, and Compensation). This again calls for a more systematic, but necessarily complex approach that focuses on interplays between the characteristics of the situation and of the individual. Of particular use would be measures specifically tied to goal orientation that could then be linked to behavioral outcomes.

Value

I now turn to a similar examination of the value function, which represents the personal value assigned to specific types of outcomes. As with the weighting function, if value is based in objective information about outcomes (e.g., expected value), then the resulting relationship should be linear in nature. The function itself is typically S-shaped, however, indicating the absence of a simple linear relationship between subjective values and objective magnitudes of outcomes (Figure 2(A)). There are several important characteristics of this function that have implications for evaluations of options and eventual decisions. First, outcomes are viewed in relation to a reference point that may vary across people and situations. Thus, for example, the outcome of gaining $100 would have more value to someone who is poor than to someone who is wealthy. Such differences would be expressed in variations in the steepness of the initial part of the curve relating value to outcomes, increasing more steeply with increments in outcomes for poor people than for wealthy people. Second, both gains and losses exhibit diminishing marginal value. Thus, the increase in value from $0 to $100 is seen as more consequential than the increase from $200 to $300. Finally, individuals tend to be loss averse, resulting in greater risk-taking when consequences are framed in terms of losses than when they are framed in terms of gains; that is, people tend to be willing to risk more to avoid a loss than they would to seek a gain. This is reflected in the value function being concave in the domain of gains, but convex in the loss domain.

Perceptions of risk are determined jointly by both the value and probability-weighting functions. For example, underweighting of probabilities in the moderate range between impossibility and certainty, along

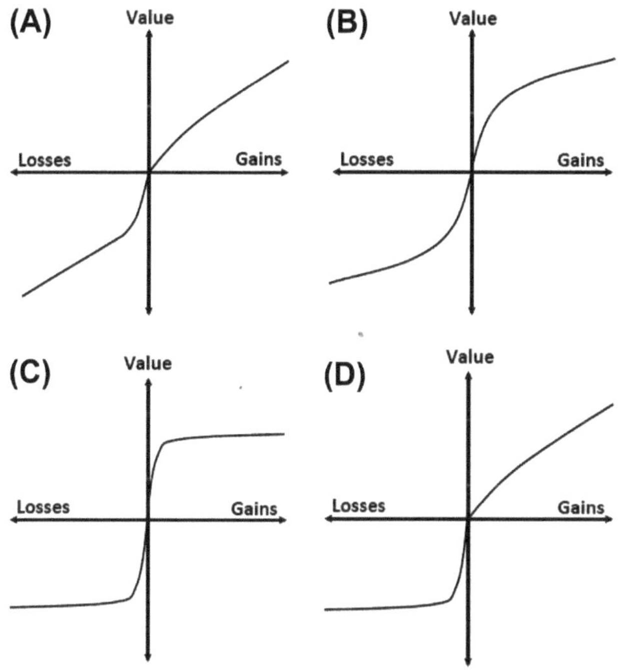

FIGURE 2 Value functions representing the typical Prospect Theory representation (A), reduced impact of scope or value due to poor deliberative skills (B), affective enhancement resulting in increased value assigned to small gains and losses (C), and selective enhancement of affect in the loss domain due to focus on loss prevention (D).

with diminishing marginal values in the gain domain result in undervaluing gambles in relation to certainty, leading to risk aversion. In contrast, in the domains of losses, this same undervaluing of probabilities reduces the weights given to risky prospects. This reduces their unattractiveness, thereby encouraging risk-seeking.

Dual-Process Influences. Affective influences on the value function can be seen in a number of ways. The most obvious effect is associated with insensitivity to magnitude or scope. When affect—either in terms of the nature of stimuli or processing—is introduced into the situation, individuals tend to pay more attention to the presence or absence of an event as opposed to the scope or value of the event. For example, in a famous study by Hsee and Rottenstreich (2004), college students were asked how much they would donate to save one or four newly discovered pandas. When information about the pandas was presented in a nonaffective fashion (i.e., a dot representing each animal), there was a linear relationship between number of pandas and donations, with the amount pledged to save four animals being approximately twice that pledged to save one. In contrast, when the information was presented in an affectively laden manner in the form of cute pictures of each panda, people were willing to donate more to save one panda, but less to save four pandas than those in the nonaffective condition. In addition, the donations in the affective condition did not increase with the number of animals. These results suggest that affect (1) leads to an increase in value of something as opposed to nothing and (2) reduces the impact of scope on value. In this same research, Hsee and Rottenstreich also demonstrated that focus on scope was increased when individuals were primed to engage in active deliberation, and decreased when they were primed to focus on feelings. One implication of this latter finding is that both deliberative ability and motivational tendencies will be positively associated with sensitivity to scope.

Hsee and Rottenstreich (2004) suggested that the impact of the experiential system can be captured by the function $V = A^{\alpha}S^{1-\alpha}$. V represents subjective value, which is determined by the interaction of the affective intensity of the target stimulus (A) and its scope (S). α is an affective focus coefficient, representing the degree to which affective processing is being emphasized. As this focus increases (i.e., α increases from 0 to 1), the concavity of the value function increases. In other words, subjective value becomes increasingly insensitive to scope. Notably, this equation highlights the fact that characteristics of both the situation (A) and the individual (α) will impact the degree to which affect influences subjective value (i.e., the affect associated with the stimuli and the degree to which the individual focuses on affective content).

Aging Effects. This formulation has interesting implications for not only understanding the decision-making process but also for determining the nature of age-related influences. Based on the first of the aforementioned aging perspectives (i.e., *affective resiliency*), age differences might come about due to declines in deliberative processes resulting in stronger influences of affective content on subjective value. This might result in inaccurate or vague information about scope (i.e., S), leading to the impact of integral affect associated with the decision task being amplified (i.e., stronger values of A). That is, scope decreases in importance due to lack of accurate information. (In this case, A and S can be used as stand-ins for the efficiency of processing associated with the experiential and deliberative systems, respectively.) This would result in a more-pronounced concavity in the value function in older adults than in younger adults; in other words, aging would be associated with greater insensitivity to scope (Figure 2(B)). The *affective enhancement* perspective would be more likely to be reflected in the α parameter, with the value of this parameter being larger in older than in younger adults. This would not only lead to insensitivity to scope in older adults, but to greater value assigned to small gains and losses (Figure 2(C)). For example, research in the Socioemotional Selectivity Theory tradition has argued for focus on positive information and minimization of negative affect, which might be reflected in larger α values when dealing with gain-related information, but smaller α values when dealing with losses. In the latter domain, sensitivity to scope would actually be increased. Alternatively, *selective enhancement* would be reflected in the relative focus on gains versus losses; a loss-prevention goal orientation should increase the affective focus on the loss domain (Figure 2(D)). Note in these situations, the shift in focus on experiential processing is related to motivational factors as opposed to inefficient deliberative skills.

Data relating to magnitude neglect can be found in the previously discussed research relating to processing of probability related information. Specifically, there is some evidence of magnitude neglect increasing with age, although there is also some tendency for this effect to be stronger when dealing with losses and when choices involve a risky versus certain outcome (e.g., Mather et al., 2012).

Aging might also be expected to be associated with greater framing effects. Such effects reflect a higher probability of risk-seeking behavior in situations where outcomes are depicted in terms of losses, whereas risk-averse behavior is more prevalent when dealing with gains, even though outcomes depicted with these situations are identical. For example, in a hypothetical scenario involving a fatal epidemic, people are more likely to choose a plan described as involving a 1/3 probability that no one would die and 2/3 probability that everyone would die than one described as involving a 1/3 probability that everyone would be saved and 2/3 probability that no one would be saved (Tversky & Kahneman, 1981). Different predictions would be made about the form of age differences based on different perspectives. For example, the *affective resiliency* and *affective enhancement* perspectives would predict an age-related increase in the strength of framing effects, whereas the *selective enhancement* perspective would predict age differences only in the loss domain. Several studies have been done to examine aging effects, but the results have been quite mixed. For example, studies have found no age differences (Mayhorn, Fisk, & Whittle, 2002; Rönnlund, Karlsson, Laggnäs, Larsson, & Lindstrom, 2005; Woodhead, Lynch, & Edelstein, 2011), greater framing effects in older adults (Bruine de Bruin, Parker, & Fischhof, 2007; Del Missier et al., 2013; Kim, Goldstein, Hasher, & Zacks, 2005; Thomas & Millar, 2012; Weller et al., 2011), and greater framing effects in younger adults (Mikels & Reed, 2009; Watanabe & Shibutani, 2010). In addition, Del Missier et al. (2013) found that older adults exhibited smaller framing effects than younger adults when working memory was controlled.

There may be several reasons for the discrepancies in findings across studies. One may have to do with the manner in which framing effects are assessed, with age differences being smaller when traditional measures based on frame effects on choice of the risky option are used as opposed to those based on consistency of choice across frames (Strough, Karns, & Schlosnagle, 2011). Motivational factors may also influence the degree to which age differences are observed. Although the stimuli were relatively similar across studies, there were differences in the actual content of the problems presented to participants. Personal relevance of the task may have influenced the extent to which individuals engaged deliberative skills, which have been demonstrated to be associated with reduced framing biases in younger adults (e.g., Del Missier, Mäntylä, & Bruine de Bruin, 2012). In addition, in line with Selective Engagement Theory, personal relevance has been shown to be a more important predictor of engagement in older than in younger adults (e.g., Hess, Queen, & Ennis, 2013). Specifically, in two studies where older adults were found to exhibit stronger framing effects than younger adults (Kim et al., 2005; Thomas & Millar, 2012), these age differences were eliminated when experimental procedures were employed to encourage engagement (e.g., requiring individuals to justify their choices). Thus, age differences in performance may depend upon factors associated with task engagement.

An examination of risk-averse versus risk-seeking responses across studies is also interesting, suggesting little consistency. For example, Mikels and Reed (2009) observed the typical pattern for responses across frames for younger adults, but found that older adults tended toward risk-aversion regardless of frame. In contrast, Weller et al. (2011) found the typical pattern in older adults, but general risk-seeking across frames in the young. This further contrasts with Mayhorn et al. (2002), who found the typical risk-aversion and risk-seeking reversal across positive and negative frames for both young and old. These findings point to possible person X situation effects, with the differences in patterns of risk-aversion and risk-seeking responses perhaps reflecting the extent to which the task context motivates devotion of resources to processing information in a manner consistent with personal or age-related chronic goals.

In a related vein, another possible source of age differences has to do with the reference point used to evaluate choices. Research using standard framing tasks assumes that the point of reference for making value judgments is relatively similar across participants. Such judgments may be reasonable when using homogeneous student samples, but are certainly questionable when comparing different-aged adults. A nice example of this can be seen in research by Winter and colleagues (Winter & Parker, 2007; Winter, Lawton, & Ruckdeschel, 2003; Winter, Moss, & Hoffman, 2009), who examined how health status influenced preferences for prolonging life in older adults. Using the *x*-axis in the value function to represent gain versus loss defined in terms of perfect health versus death, these researchers assumed that healthier people would be less likely to discriminate between different states of disability than less healthy individuals. This was based in the assumption that the point of reference for healthy people would be shifted farther to the right of the negative endpoint of death. Due to the nature of diminishing marginal values, the difference between death and various states of incapacity (e.g., confined to a bed/chair in one's home vs confused and confined to a nursing home) would then be viewed as less significant for these individuals than for someone in frail health, whose point of reference was shifted farther to the left of the health continuum. Their results supported this Prospect Theory perspective, demonstrating that frail people expressed greater desire to prolong life in these incapacitated states and made greater value distinctions between various states of incapacity than did healthy people. Notably, frail individuals actually exhibited greater sensitivity to magnitude within the loss domain than did healthy individuals. It is likely that similar types of reference point distinctions based in health status, financial status, future time perspective and other age-related factors may account for some of the variation observed across studies with respect to framing effects.

Taken together with the aforementioned studies, the work on framing argues for taking a more contextual approach to understanding aging and decision making, in that simple age-related declines in deliberative skills provide a relatively weak perspective for predicting age differences in framing effects. A similar point can be made with respect to motivational perspectives. Instead, it is important to consider the decision-making context, represented in terms of the interaction between the individual and the situation, in interpreting age effects. A nice illustration of contextual influences comes from the study by Woodhead et al. (2011), who examined the type of information used in relation to severity of framing biases. Based on qualitative responses, they distinguished between participants who based their decisions about cancer treatment on personally generated information (e.g., a friend's experience) versus the information provided in the test scenarios (e.g., probabilities). They found that older adults were more likely than younger adults to base their decisions on personal information, and that reliance on such information was associated with reduced framing effects. Notably, these effects were independent of accuracy of information reported about the scenarios. These results suggest a preference for experiential processing in this situation by older adults that is not necessarily based in declining deliberative skills. Of interest would be exploration of the extent to which availability of relevant experiential information influences use of such information. For example, older adults are likely to have more experience with cancer treatment through friends and relatives than are younger adults, perhaps biasing experiential influences. It would be interesting to conduct a similar study employing stimuli that might be more age-neutral or biased toward younger adults' experience to see if domain moderates these effects.

CONCLUSIONS

This attempt to examine aging effects in decision-making processes through an integration of dual-process models with constructs drawn from prospect theory has been instructive in several ways. It illustrates the benefits of using a well-grounded descriptive theory to inform predictions about age effects. Using general views of the interaction of experiential and deliberative processes across the life span, relatively clear differences in expectations regarding how different-aged adults assign decision weights and evaluate outcomes could be identified across the different views of aging effects. This allowed relevant empirical data to be evaluated against these expectations. Use of the Prospect Theory framework also identified some difficulties that might occur in clearly identifying expected outcomes across frameworks. For example, from the Socioemotional Selectivity perspective, it is not clear how chronic goals in later life associated with optimizing affective outcomes would influence assignments of subjective value within loss and gain domains (i.e., how would the shape of the value function be affected?). This complicates the evaluation of hypotheses about age effects, and argues for greater specificity in identification of mechanisms underlying age differences in performance.

Based on the present review, there are several general conclusions that can be made about aging. Of primary importance is the observation that context matters in evaluating potential age effects.

The Importance of Context

The first observation that can be made is that existing data do not clearly conform to any of the four proposed general age-related perspectives characterizing the interaction between experiential and deliberative processes. For each of these perspectives, there were findings that were both consistent and inconsistent. Part of this variability may relate to the aforementioned problems associated with specification of theory-based mechanisms underlying age effects, along with the fact that most of the research reviewed was not designed to specifically evaluate the predictions constructed from the present analysis. The one general conclusion that might be drawn about aging and dual-process mechanisms is that experiential influences do appear to be stronger—although not consistently so—in later life. That is, older adults appear to rely more on experiential processes than do younger adults in constructing preferences. Complicating this, however, is the fact that the experiential influences were not always consistent, and age differences were not always present. Thus, for example, older adults are more likely than younger adults to ignore probability or magnitude information when more easily processed affective (e.g., certainty-based categorical cues (e.g., Mather et al., 2012)) or experience-based content (e.g., Woodhead et al., 2011) is available.

Unfortunately, the form of these experiential influences—when observed—was not always consistent across studies. Thus, for example, the greater certainty/impossibility effects observed in later life were sometimes consistent with a general elevation of affective influences (e.g., Weller et al., 2011) and other times with a more focused impact in the loss domain (e.g., Mather et al., 2012).

In this regard, it should also be noted that the presence of stronger affective influences in older adults was not always accompanied by decrements in deliberative skills. Thus, for example, in the research by Mather et al. (2012), young and old were equally sensitive to probability information in the absence of choices involving certainty. This perhaps suggests that some effects have to do more with minimizing use of cognitively demanding resources by older adults when other cues are available for making evaluations.

A second conclusion that can be derived from the reviewed research is that context matters. Specifically, interactions between the characteristics of the aging decision maker and the task are likely to determine the nature of the observed age effects. Much of the variability across studies might be accounted for by differences in the types of tasks and stimulus materials used to assess performance. This may impact the manner in which choices are conceptualized by different-aged individuals who may vary in terms of personal characteristics (e.g., perceptions of the future, health status, ability) and life circumstances (e.g., income, financial need, living circumstances). The research by Winter and colleagues (e.g., Winter & Parker, 2007; Winter et al., 2009) represents a nice case in point, whereby health status was associated with differences in reference points used to make judgments about prolonging life. As reference points change, a specific outcome might change in value as well in terms of it being perceived as a loss or gain. This could affect the extent to which aging might be found to be associated with greater loss aversion or risk aversion. Thus, some of the variability across studies may reflect different outcomes being perceived in qualitatively different ways by young and older adults, which in turn influences the values assigned to those outcomes.

The relevance of the task to the individual may also be an important determinant of age differences in evaluations processes. Consistent with the selective engagement framework (Hess, 2014), task relevance may impact the relative influence of experiential versus deliberative processes on performance. Age differences in processing of information reliant on active deliberation (e.g., probabilities) may be reduced in personally meaningful situations versus more generic contexts (e.g., compare the results of Holliday, 1988 to those of Weller et al., 2011). The extent to which processing is subsequently guided by chronic goals may also depend on perceived relevance of the task to personal goals, with subsequent engagement of deliberative processes guiding processes in a goal-consistent manner (see also Strough et al., 2011, for a related perspective). For example, when older adults are presented with a series of choices that highlight both gain- and loss-related information, activation of goals associated with loss prevention (e.g., Depping & Freund, 2013) might result in differential focus of processing on problems involving the latter, resulting in very different patterns of responses than those observed when problems in each domain are considered separately (e.g., Mather et al., 2012).

Age differences in the nature of dual-process influences might also arise due to the availability of relevant knowledge. For example, older adults may rely more on experiential processing in situations that are personally relevant and in which they have personal experience. The Woodhead et al. (2011) study again provides a case in point, where the nature of the observed framing effects was not based in accuracy of representation of problem information, but rather the extent to which individuals based their judgments on personal experience. This may suggest that older adults—as well as younger adults—with domain-specific experience will fall back on such information not just because it is less-resource consuming to do so, but due to beliefs regarding its relevance to the problem at hand.

The apparent context specificity of age effects suggests that the search for general trends associated with aging (e.g., increased risk aversion) might be somewhat misguided, or at least would need to be conceived of within a broader framework that takes into account the meaningfulness of the situation to the individual. People of all ages are likely to evaluate specific decision-making tasks within the context of relevant chronic and situational goals (Hess & Queen, 2014; Strough et al., 2011). For example, risk aversion, which might be tied to factors such as financial concerns interacting with one's position in the life span, may indeed be more prevalent in later life. It is likely to only be observed, however, under situations tapping into these concerns. There may be little reason to expect that risk aversion associated with finance would generalize to, for example, earning points in a laboratory setting.

Caveats

Two important caveats should be mentioned at this point. First, our examination of the impact of the experiential and deliberative processes was focused on situations that can be characterized as involving *decision by description*. In such situations, individuals are informed of the parameters defining the problem space, and then make a decision based on this information. Typically, no feedback is given about the actual outcomes associated with their response. Thus, the present focus can best be described as characterizing age differences in dual-process mechanisms at the front end of the decision-making process, as individuals evaluate choices and construct preferences based on their processing of available information and anticipatory affective responses to this information. It is quite likely that age differences in the impact of experiential processes will be observed following feedback about the outcomes of a bet (e.g., how much money was won). In such situations evaluating *decisions by experience*, additional factors influencing affective responses and their impact on performance are likely to come into play. These sorts of effects are explored in other chapters in this volume (e.g., Mikels, Shuster, & Thai).

A second related concern has to do with using prospect theory to guide the evaluation of research results. As Mata and Hertwig (2011) pointed out, the focus of prospect theory is on expected utility, which may take into account anticipatory affect, but does not necessarily account for affect associated with experienced outcomes. Responses to such outcomes are particularly important to motivational accounts of age differences in decision making. This obviously builds on the aforementioned concerns associated with focusing on decision by description. Mata and Hertwig also note that Prospect Theory assumes that values are assigned based on stable preferences, which does not characterize much decision making in real life. This concern actually fits in well with the current focus on the importance of context. I would argue, however, that use of ideas drawn from the probability-weighting and value functions can still be useful in characterizing age differences in performance across contexts and in evaluating associated data.

Acknowledgements

Writing of this chapter was supported by NIA grant AG05552.

References

Baltes, P. B. (1987). Theoretical propositions of life-span developmental psychology: On the dynamics between growth and decline. *Developmental Psychology, 23*, 611–626.

Baltes, P. B. (1997). On the incomplete architecture of human ontogeny: Selection, optimization, and compensation as foundation of developmental theory. *American Psychologist, 52*, 366–380.

Bechara, A., & Damasio, A. R. (2005). The somatic marker hypothesis: A neural theory of economic decision. *Game and Economic Behavior, 52*, 336–372.

Boyle, P. A., Yu, L., Buchman, A. S., & Bennett, D. A. (2012). Risk aversion is associated with decision making among community-based older persons. *Frontiers in Psychology, 3*, 205.

Bruine de Bruin, W., Parker, A. M., & Fischhoff, B. (2007). Individual differences in adult decision-making competence. *Journal of Personality and Social Psychology, 92*, 938–956.

Bruine de Bruin, W., Parker, A. M., & Fischhoff, B. (2012). Explaining adult age differences in decision-making competence. *Journal of Behavioral Decision Making, 25*, 352–360.

Carstensen, L. L., Isaacowitz, D. M., & Charles, S. T. (1999). Taking time seriously: A theory of socioemotional selectivity. *American Psychologist, 54*, 165–181.

Chasseigne, G., Grau, S., Mullet, E., & Cama, V. (1999). How well do elderly people cope with uncertainty in a learning task? *Acta Psychologica, 103*, 229–238.

Chasseigne, G., Lafon, P., & Mullet, E. (2002). Aging and rule learning: The case of the multiplicative law. *The American Journal of Psychology, 115*, 315–330.

Chasseigne, G., Ligneau, C., Grau, S., Le, G. A., Roque, M., & Mullet, E. (2004). Aging and probabilistic learning in single- and multiple-cue tasks. *Experimental Aging Research, 30*, 23–45.

Cryder, C. E., Lerner, J. S., Gross, J. J., Dahl, R. E., & Ronald, E. (2008). Misery is not miserly: Sad and self-focused individuals spend more. *Psychological Science, 19*, 525–530.

Deakin, J., Aitken, M., Robbins, T., & Sahakian, B. J. (2004). Risk taking during decision-making in normal volunteers: Changes with age. *Journal of the International Neuropsychological Society, 10*, 590–598.

Del Missier, F., Mäntylä, T., & Bruine de Bruin, W. (2012). Decision-making competence, executive functioning, and general cognitive abilities. *Journal of Behavioral Decision Making, 25*, 331–351.

Del Missier, F., Mäntylä, T., Hansson, P., Bruine de Bruin, W., Parker, A. M., & Nilsson, L.-G. (2013). The multifold relationship between memory and decision making: An individual-differences study. *Journal of Experimental Psychology: Learning, Memory, and Cognition, 39*, 1344–1364.

Depping, M. K., & Freund, A. M. (2013). When choice matters: Task-dependent memory effects in older adulthood. *Psychology and Aging, 28*, 923–936.

Dror, I. E., Katona, M., & Mungur, K. (1998). Age differences in decision making: To take a risk or not? *Gerontology, 44*, 67–71.

Elster, J., & Loewenstein, G. (1992). Utility from memory and anticipation. In J. Elster, & G. Loewenstein (Eds.), *Choice over time* (pp. 213–234). New York: Russell Sage Foundation.

Epstein, S. (1994). Integration of the cognitive and the psychodynamic unconscious. *American Psychologist, 49*, 709–724.

Finucane, M. L., Mertz, C. K., Slovic, P., & Schmidt, E. S. (2005). Task complexity and older adults' decision-making competence. *Psychology and Aging, 20*, 71–84.

Fisk, J. E. (2005). Age and probabilistic reasoning: biases in conjunctive, disjunctive, and Bayesian judgments in early and late adulthood. *Journal of Behavioral Decision Making, 18*, 55–82.

Freund, A. M., & Ebner, N. C. (2005). The aging self: Shifting from promoting gains to balancing losses. In W. Greve, K. Rothermund, & D. Wentura (Eds.), *The adaptive self: Personal continuity and intentional self-development* (pp. 185–202). Ashland, OH: Hogrefe & Huber Publishers.

Gonzalez, R., & Wu, G. (1999). On the shape of the probability weighting function. *Cognitive Psychology, 38*, 129–166.

Hess, T. M. (2014). Selective engagement of cognitive resources: Motivational influences on older adults' cognitive functioning. *Perspectives on Psychological Science, 9*.

Hess, T. M., & Blanchard-Fields, F. (1996). Issues in the study of cognitive change in adulthood. In F. Blanchard-Fields, & T. M. Hess (Eds.), *Perspectives on cognitive change in adulthood and aging* (pp. 3–24). New York: McGraw-Hill.

Hess, T. M., & Queen, T. L. (2014). Aging influences on judgment and decision processes: Interactions between ability and experience. In P. Verhaeghen & C. Hertzog (Eds.), *The Oxford handbook of emotion, social cognition, and problem solving in adulthood* (pp. 238–255). New York: Oxford University Press.

Hess, T. M., Queen, T. L., & Ennis, G. E. (2013). Age and self-relevance effects on information search during decision making. *Journals of Gerontology Series B: Psychological Sciences and Social Sciences, 68*, 703–711.

Hsee, C. K., & Rottenstreich, Y. (2004). Music, pandas, and muggers: On the affective psychology of value. *Journal of Experimental Psychology: General, 133*, 23–30.

Hsee, C. K., & Zhang, J. (2010). General evaluability theory. *Perspectives on Psychological Science, 5*, 343–355.

Holliday, S. G. (1988). Risky-choice behavior: A life-span analysis. *International Journal of Aging & Human Development, 27*, 25–33.

Isaacowitz, D. M., & Blanchard-Fields, F. (2012). Linking process and outcome in the study of emotion and aging. *Perspectives on Psychological Science, 7*, 3–17.

Kahneman, D. A. (2003). A perspective on judgment and choice: Mapping bounded rationality. *American Psychologist, 58*, 697–720.

Kahneman, D., & Tversky, A. (1979). Prospect theory: An analysis of decision under risk. *Econometrica, 47*, 263–291.

Kim, S., Goldstein, D., Hasher, L., & Zacks, R. T. (2005). Framing effects in younger and older adults. *The Journals of Gerontology, Series B: Psychological Sciences and Social Sciences, 60B*, 215–218.

Lauriola, M., & Levin, I. P. (2001). Personality traits and risky decision-making in a controlled experimental task: An exploratory study. *Personality and Individual Differences, 31*, 215–226.

Loewenstein, G. F., Weber, E. U., Hsee, C. K., & Welch, E. S. (2001). Risk as feelings. *Psychological Bulletin, 127*, 267–286.

Mata, R., & Hertwig, R. (2011). How to model age-related motivational reorientations in risky choice. *Human Development, 54*, 368–375.

Mather, M., Mazar, N., Gorlick, M. A., Lighthall, N. R., Burgeno, J., Schoeke, A., et al. (2012). Risk preferences and aging: the "certainty effect" in older adults' decision making. *Psychology and Aging, 27*, 801–816.

Mayhorn, C. B., Fisk, A. D., & Whittle, J. D. (2002). Decisions, decision: Analysis of age, cohort, and time of testing on framing risky decision options. *Human Factors, 44*, 515–521.

Mikels, J. A., & Reed, A. E. (2009). Monetary losses do not loom large in later life: Age differences in the framing effect. *The Journals of Gerontology, Series B: Psychological Sciences and Social Sciences, 64B*, 457–460.

Mutter, S. A. (2000). Illusory correlation and group impression formation in young and older adults. *The Journals of Gerontology, Series B: Psychological Sciences and Social Sciences, 55B*, 224–237.

Mutter, S. A., & Pliske, R. M. (1994). Aging and illusory correlation in judgments of co-occurrence. *Psychology and Aging, 9*, 53–63.

Mutter, S. A., & Williams, T. W. (2004). Aging and the detection of contingency in causal learning. *Psychology and Aging, 19*, 13–26.

Mukherjee, K. (2011). Thinking styles and risky decision-making: Further exploration of the affect–probability weighting link. *Journal of Behavioral Decision Making, 24*, 443–455.

Okun, M. A., & Elias, C. S. (1977). Cautiousness in adulthood as a function of age and payoff structure. *Journal of Gerontology, 32*, 451–455.

Peters, E. (2012). Beyond comprehension: The role of numeracy in judgment and decisions. *Current Directions in Psychological Science, 21*, 31–35.

Peters, E., Dieckmann, N. E., & Weller, J. (2011). Age differences in complex decision making. In K. W. Schaie, & S. L. Willis (Eds.), *Handbook of the psychology of aging* (7th ed., pp. 133–151). San Diego, CA: Elsevier Academic Press.

Peters, E., Hess, T. M., Västfjäll, D., & Auman, C. (2007). Adult age differences in dual information processes: Implications for the role of affective and deliberative processes in older adults' decision making. *Perspectives on Psychological Science, 2*, 1–23.

Raghunathan, R., & Pham, M. (1999). All negative moods are not equal: Motivational influences of anxiety and sadness on decision making. *Organizational Behavior and Human Decision Processes, 79*, 56–77.

Read, D., Loewenstein, G., & Rabin, M. (1999). Choice bracketing. *Journal of Risk and Uncertainty, 19*, 171–197.

Reed, A. E., & Carstensen, L. L. (2012). The theory behind the age-related positivity effect. *Frontiers in Psychology, 3* Article 339.

Reyna, V. F., & Brainerd, C. J. (1991). Fuzzy-trace theory and framing effects in choice: Gist extraction, truncation, and conversion. *Journal of Behavioral Decision Making, 4*, 249–262.

Rönnlund, M., Karlsson, E., Laggnäs, E., Larsson, L., & Lindstrom, T. (2005). Risky decision making across three arenas of choice: Are younger and older adults differently susceptible to framing effects? *Journal of General Psychology, 132*, 81–93.

Rottenstreich, Y., & Hsee, C. (2001). Money, kisses, and electric shocks: on the affective psychology of risk. *Psychological Science, 12*, 185–190.

Strough, J., Karns, T. E., & Schlosnagle, L. (2011). Decision-making heuristics and biases across the life span. *Annals of the New York Academy of Sciences, 1235*, 57–74.

Thomas, A. K., & Millar, P. R. (2012). Reducing the framing effect in older and younger adults by encouraging analytic processing. *The Journals of Gerontology: Series B: Psychological Sciences and Social Sciences, 67B*, 139–149.

Tversky, A., & Kahneman, D. (1981). The framing of decisions and the psychology of choice. *Science, 211*, 453–458.

Tversky, A., & Fox, C. R. (1995). Weighing risk and uncertainty. *Psychological Review, 102*, 269–283.

Watanabe, S., & Shibutani, H. (2010). Aging and decision making: Differences in susceptibility to the risky-choice framing effect between older and younger adults in Japan. *Japanese Psychological Research, 52*, 163–174.

Weber, E. U., Shafir, S., & Blaise, A.-R. (2004). Predicting risk sensitivity in humans and lower animals: risk as variance or coefficient of variation. *Psychological Review, 111*, 430–455.

Weller, J. A., Levin, I. P., & Denburg, N. (2011). Trajectory of risky decision making for potential gains and losses from ages 5 to 85. *Journal of Behavioral Decision Making, 24*, 331–344.

Winter, L., Lawton, M. P., & Ruckdeschel, K. (2003). Preferences for prolonging life: A prospect theory approach. *International Journal on Aging and Human Development, 56*, 155–170.

Winter, L., Moss, M. S., & Hoffman, C. (2009). Affective forecasting and advance care planning: anticipating quality of life in future health statuses. *Journal of Health Psychology, 14*, 447–456.

Winter, L., & Parker, B. (2007). Current health and preferences for life-prolonging treatments: An application of prospect theory to end of-life decision making. *Social Science & Medicine, 65*, 1695–1707.

Woodhead, E. L., Lynch, E. B., & Edelstein, B. A. (2011). Decisional strategy determines whether frame influences treatment preferences for medical decisions. *Psychology and Aging, 26*, 285–294.

Yuen, K. S. L., & Lee, T. M. C. (2003). Could mood state affect risk-taking decisions? *Journal of Affective Disorders, 75*, 11–18.

CHAPTER

11

Age Differences in Time Perception and Their Implications for Decision Making Across the Life Span

Corinna E. Löckenhoff, Joshua L. Rutt

Department of Human Development, College of Human Ecology, Cornell University, Ithaca, NY, USA

Every decision we make—from mundane choices about everyday activities to the selection of long-term career paths—is situated in a temporal context (Klapproth, 2008). On the one hand, decisions are aimed at controlling what will happen to us and the world around us in the days, months, and years to come. On the other hand, decisions are firmly rooted in the past and draw on previous experiences to inform present preferences. Individual decisions differ in the duration of possible outcomes (e.g., signing up for a weekend workshop versus a 4-year program of study) and the point in the future at which an outcome is realized (e.g., making plans for next weekend versus next summer's vacation). Some important life choices (ranging from family planning to financial investments) focus on the timing of a given outcome rather than the outcome itself (Berns, Laibson, & Loewenstein, 2007; Frederick, Loewenstein, & O'Donoghue, 2002), and some harrowing end-of-life decisions involve trade-offs between quality of life and remaining lifetime (Chapman, 2003; Lee, Leipzig, & Walter, 2013).

The ability to monitor time, reconstruct the past, and anticipate future events can be considered as a universal human characteristic (Brown, 1991; Carstensen, 2006). Drawing on this capacity, most of us are well equipped to navigate the temporal trade-offs inherent in our choices. Nonetheless, people vary in how they think about time, how far they look ahead, and how

http://dx.doi.org/10.1016/B978-0-12-417148-0.00011-X

far they delve into the past, and these factors may influence decision making (Klapproth, 2008). Chronological age in particular has been found to be significantly associated with time perceptions and temporal construals, and the present chapter considers the implications of such effects for various aspects of the decision process across the adult life span (Löckenhoff, 2011).

Time intersects with decision making on multiple levels. In this chapter, we selectively focus on age-related shifts in mental representations of time and global time horizons, which have been a growing area of interest in life-span developmental research (for a discussion of age differences in processing speed and internal clocks, see Block, Zakay, & Hancock, 1998; Löckenhoff, 2011; McAuley, Jones, Holub, Johnston, & Miller, 2006). We begin this chapter by reviewing the literature on adult age differences in mental representations of time, and proceed to discuss potential mechanisms behind such effects. We then consider implications for various aspects of decision making and conclude with a discussion of practical implications and future directions.

AGE DIFFERENCES IN GLOBAL TIME HORIZONS AND MENTAL REPRESENTATIONS OF TIME

Perceptions of time can be considered along multiple dimensions including temporal extension into the future and the past, qualitative and affective characteristics, and accuracy relative to objective markers. Age differences have been observed in many of these dimensions, although effect sizes vary and some aspects have been researched more thoroughly than others.

Temporal Extension

Perhaps the most obvious age effects in temporal representations are seen with regard to one's perceived position in the life span. Most people show little hesitation when asked to mark their current location on a horizontal line ranging from "birth" to "death," suggesting that they keep close track of their path through life and—by extension—their relative distance from birth or closeness to death (Cottle & Pleck, 1969; Hancock, 2010). Not surprisingly, perceived position in life is strongly associated with chronological age, although compared to younger adults, older adults are more likely to underestimate their current position in life relative to their actuarial life expectancy (Hancock, 2010; Kleinspehn-Ammerlahn, Kotter-Grühn, & Smith, 2008). Convergent findings come from studies using questionnaire-based measures to assess global time horizons. Compared to younger adults, older adults experience time and future opportunities as limited, and this age-related sense that "time is running out"

(Carstensen & Lang, 1996) holds true across different cultures (Fung, Lai, & Ng, 2001; Lang & Carstensen, 2002).

A complementary line of research examined age differences in the past and future extension of autobiographical thought (for a review, see Schacter, Gaesser, & Addis, 2013). Typical paradigms ask participants to produce a series of specific past events (sometimes prompted by a cue word) and to indicate at what point in time each event occurred. Matching data are collected for probable and specific future events (Schacter, Addis, & Buckner, 2007; Schacter et al., 2013; Spreng & Levine, 2006). Across adult age groups, the temporal distance of future events was found to follow a power function, with a clustering of events in the near present. However, older as compared to younger adults show a steeper slope and report fewer events in the more distant future than their younger counterparts. The distribution of recalled events follows a similar power function, but in contrast to future events, age is associated with a more shallow slope such that older adults recall more distant events than younger adults (Addis, Musicaro, Pan, & Schacter, 2010; Addis, Wong, & Schacter, 2008; Gaesser, Sacchetti, Addis, & Schacter, 2011; Schacter et al., 2013; Spreng & Levine, 2006). In other words, autobiographical thought is clustered around the present, but consistent with research on age differences in global horizons, older adults' thoughts extend farther into the past but not as far into the future.

Qualitative Characteristics

In addition to age differences in the quantitative extension of past and future thought, there is evidence for shifts in qualitative characteristics. The idea that time passes more quickly with age, for instance, is widespread in popular culture but hard to demonstrate experimentally (Friedman, 2013). A systematic meta-analysis of age differences in duration judgments for short-term intervals (i.e., seconds and minutes; Block et al., 1998) found that older adults' judgments were more variable than those of younger adults, but there was no main effect of age on perceived duration. Research examining longer-term intervals is very rare, and the few available studies suggest that compared to younger adults, older adults report that the most recent decade has passed more quickly. In contrast, no age differences are found for shorter time intervals involving months and years (Friedman & Janssen, 2010; Janssen, Naka, & Friedman, 2013; Wittmann & Lehnhoff, 2005).

Indirect evidence for age differences in the speed of time comes from research examining the mapping of subjective to objective time. Zauberman and colleagues (Kim & Zauberman, 2009; Zauberman, Kim, Malkoc, & Bettman, 2009) examined the subjective length of various objective time intervals (ranging from months to years) as rated on a scale from "very short" to "very long."

Evidence from student samples suggests that subjective time perceptions are more compressed (relative to objective time) as the length of the time interval increases (Kim & Zauberman, 2009; Zauberman et al., 2009). In other words, people appear to place greater emphasis on the immediate present and exhibit diminishing sensitivity for increasingly distant intervals. Preliminary data collected by our laboratory (Rutt & Löckenhoff, 2013) suggests that this subjective compression of time is greater with advanced age, indicating that the future may appear closer to older adults, which would be consistent with an age-related acceleration of time.

Compared to younger adults, older adults' mental representations of past and future also tend to be less detailed and more general. Episodic memory for the details of specific past events shows pronounced age-related decrements (for a review, see Old & Naveh-Benjamin, 2008). More specifically, older adults recall a smaller proportion of "internal" details (perceptions and thoughts relevant to the specific event) and a larger proportion of "external" details (semantic knowledge and details related to other events; Levine, Svoboda, Hay, Winocur, & Moscovitch, 2002). Research extending these findings to the future has yielded convergent patterns, with older adults providing greater semantic content but fewer episodic details for imagined future events (Addis et al., 2010; Cole, Morrison, & Conway, 2013; Gaesser et al., 2011; Schacter et al., 2013). Moreover, older adults show specific difficulties generating detailed descriptions of future events, as opposed to atemporal events (Rendell et al., 2012), and confuse past and future events more easily (Gallo, Korthauer, McDonough, Teshale, & Johnson, 2011; McDonough & Gallo, 2013) suggesting limitations in autonoetic consciousness (i.e., the ability for mental time travel).

Finally, there are systematic age differences in the affective valence of temporal construals. Even younger people tend to recall their past with a positive slant, but this effect is more pronounced with increasing age. Similar patterns are found for spontaneously recalled autobiographical events (Schlagman, Kliegel, Schulz, & Kvavilashvili, 2009), memories retrieved in response to cue words (Comblain, D'Argembeau, & Van der Linden, 2005; Ros & Latorre, 2010; Tomaszczyk & Fernandes, 2012), and the recall of past self-evaluations—even when the recency of the memory is held constant (Kennedy, Mather, & Carstensen, 2004; Ready, Weinberger, & Jones, 2007). More recently, this line of research has been extended to imagined future events indicating that, compared to their younger counterparts, older adults generate more positive future events in response to both neutral and emotional cue words (Gallo et al., 2011).

In summary, whereas support for an age-related acceleration of subjective time perceptions is fairly limited, robust evidence suggests that older adults construe their future and past in less detail but in more positive terms than their younger counterparts.

Accuracy of Future Thought

Although the specific characteristics of temporal construals differ by age, this does not necessarily imply age-related decrements in the accuracy of future thought. Such effects are best documented with regard to affective forecasting, the ability to correctly predict one's future emotions. In laboratory settings, no age differences were found in the prediction of sadness responses to emotional photographs (Pearman, Andreoletti, & Isaacowitz, 2010). Also, when asked to predict their future emotional reactions to monetary gains and losses, older adults were found to be as accurate as younger adults in predicting the valence of their future responses and more accurate in predicting arousal levels (Nielsen, Knutson, & Carstensen, 2008). Further, while younger adults show "future anhedonia," a systematic tendency to underestimate the intensity of their future emotional responses (Kassam, Gilbert, Boston, & Wilson, 2008), this effect is not found in older adults (Löckenhoff, O'Donoghue, & Dunning, 2011).

Age-related stability or improvements in affective forecasting extend to real-world scenarios. In a study examining predictions about emotional responses to election outcomes, age was positively associated with accuracy, especially among those who considered the election results as favorable (Scheibe, Mata, & Carstensen, 2010). Also, older adults were found to be better than younger adults at predicting their future life satisfaction over the course of years and decades (Lachman, Röcke, Rosnick, & Ryff, 2008; Lang, Weiss, Gerstorf, & Wagner, 2013). Taken together, these findings suggest that the ability to predict one's future emotions and internal states is well preserved with age. In contrast, there is little research on age differences in the accuracy of prediction for meaningful future outcomes (beyond the limits of sequential laboratory paradigms where "predictions" primarily capture age differences in learning and memory), and this constitutes an important gap in the research record (for a promising approach to studying accuracy in autobiographical anticipation, see Spreng & Levine, 2013).

In summary, systematic age differences are found in both quantitative and qualitative aspects of time perceptions, whereas the ability to predict one's affective responses to future events appears to remain stable or possibly improve with age. To evaluate potential implications for decision making we now consider the underlying mechanisms that drive such effects.

MECHANISMS

Actuarial Life Expectancy and Prior Experience

Some aspects of age differences in time perceptions can of course be traced back to actuarial life expectancy. Jeanne Calment, the person with the longest confirmed life span, was asked on her 120th birthday what kind of future she envisioned, and famously joked "a very short one" (Guinness Book of World Records, 2014). Such age-related limitations in remaining life expectancy offer an obvious explanation for age differences in global time horizons and the sense that time is "running out" (Carstensen, 2006). Similarly, age-related reductions in the temporal extension of future thought (e.g., Spreng & Levine, 2006) likely reflect older adults' realistic assessment that they may not be around to experience events in the more distant future.

However, chronological age is not only associated with time left to live but also with time already lived. As a result, the ratio of a given time interval relative to the time a person has already experienced decreases with age (Fraisse, 1963): For a young adult, 1 year represents one-twentieth of their life span, but for an octogenarian, this ratio shrinks to one-eightieth, and some have suggested that this may account for age-related increases in the subjective speed of time (Friedman & Janssen, 2010; Lemlich, 1975; Wittmann & Lehnhoff, 2005). In addition, older adults' longer life spans provide them with a larger repository of past experiences, which may affect mental representations of time in a number of ways. First, older adults are more likely to have "seen it all," resulting in a lower number of novel and memorable events in everyday life and an increasing reliance on routines and habits (Fraisse, 1963; James, 1890). This may not only create the illusion that time is passing more quickly (since nothing new is happening; Bruss & Rüschendorf, 2010), but could also contribute to age-related extensions in past autobiographical thought (Spreng & Levine, 2006): Older adults not only have more decades to look back on, but they may also have to think farther back to arrive at a memorable event.

Cognition

Whereas remaining life expectancy and past experience are inherently linked with chronological age, other age-associated variables may affect mental representations of time as well. In particular, age is associated with systematic changes in cognition that may influence temporal construals in a number of ways (Salthouse & Davis, 2006; Verhaeghen & Salthouse, 1997). Reductions in processing speed and attentional resources (Salthouse, 1996) were found to be associated with age differences in the subjective speed of time and the estimation of short-term intervals, although the exact mechanisms remain to be explored (Baudouin, Vanneste, & Isingrini, 2004; Block et al., 1998). Age-related limitations in working memory, in turn, may affect both duration judgments (Pan & Luo, 2012; Roy, Grondin, & Roy, 2012; Woehrle & Magliano, 2012) and the ability to perform detailed mental simulations of specific future events (Addis et al., 2010; Cole et al., 2013; Gabbard, Lee, & Caçola, 2013; Hill & Emery, 2013). Executive functioning also decreases with age and may specifically limit older adults' future planning skills (Sanders & Schmitter-Edgecombe, 2012; Sorel & Pennequin, 2008; de Paula, Neves, Levy, Nassif, & Malloy-Diniz, 2012).

The interplay between age-related cognitive changes and mental representations of time has been most closely examined in the context of the constructive episodic simulation hypothesis (Schacter & Addis, 2008; Schacter et al., 2013), which proposes that remembering past events and imagining future events draws on similar processing resources, and that episodic memory serves as a repository of stored information that can be reconfigured for simulating future events. Empirical data generally support this hypothesis documenting that the episodic recall of past events and the simulation of future events are closely associated and rely on similar neural mechanisms (Addis et al., 2010; Schacter et al., 2007; Schacter et al., 2013). However, these effects cannot explain the full range of age differences in temporal construals, and additional factors are likely to play a role. For one, semantic world knowledge and long-term autobiographical memory are comparatively well preserved with age (Salthouse & Davis, 2006). Thus, older adults may not have to recombine past events into detailed simulations of the future, but may be able to directly draw conclusions from comparable experiences in their past. Moreover, it has been argued that older adults' tendency toward abstract and metaphorical processing (as opposed to younger adults' verbatim processing style) reflects a motivated and intentional emphasis on generalizable meaning rather than decrements in cognitive resources (Adams, Smith, Nyquist, & Perlmutter, 1997).

Motivation and Emotion

In support of motivational explanations, there is broad evidence for age-related shifts in emotional experience and goal priorities (Scheibe & Carstensen, 2010). In particular, older adults prioritize emotionally salient stimuli, and the processing of such stimuli is comparatively spared from age-related cognitive decline (Charles & Carstensen, 2010; Samanez-Larkin & Carstensen, 2011; Scheibe & Carstensen, 2010). Furthermore, older adults are found to selectively direct their attention and processing resources toward positive and away from negative material, a phenomenon known as the age-related positivity effect (Mather & Carstensen, 2005; Mikels, Reed, Hardy, & Löckenhoff, 2014; Reed & Carstensen, 2012). These processes can not only account for the age-related shift toward affect-rich and positively slanted representations of future events (Gallo et al., 2011), but growing evidence suggests that they may themselves be driven by age-related shifts in global time horizons. Specifically, Socioemotional Selectivity Theory (Carstensen, 2006; Carstensen et al., 1999) posits that with age, people become aware that their future is limited, and adjust their goal priorities accordingly: Younger adults' open-ended time horizons are thought to emphasize future-oriented goals aimed at information acquisition and the development of new relationships, whereas older adults' increasingly limited time horizons are thought to promote present-oriented goals aimed at emotionally meaningful experiences shared with close social partners (Scheibe & Carstensen, 2010). Consistent with this theory, empirical evidence suggests that age differences in emotional processing are more closely associated with shifting time horizons (Mather & Knight, 2005; Mikels et al., 2014; Reed & Carstensen, 2012) than with neural degradation (Cacioppo, Berntson, Bechara, Tranel, & Hawkley, 2011) and limitations in cognitive resources (Labouvie-Vief, Grühn, & Studer, 2010).

To sum up, age differences in mental representations of time are likely driven by a combination of mechanisms, and while some of these factors are inextricably linked with chronological age (e.g., remaining life expectancy, past experience), others may vary considerably among individual older adults (e.g., cognitive functioning and motivational priorities). Keeping this in mind, we now consider how age differences in time perception and temporal construal may manifest themselves in various aspects of decision making.

IMPLICATIONS FOR DECISION MAKING

Intertemporal Choice

The most obvious implications of age differences in time horizons and temporal construals pertain to so-called "intertemporal choices" that require individuals to decide about the timing of a given outcome, rather than the outcome per se (Berns et al., 2007). In a typical scenario, participants are asked to choose between a more favorable, delayed outcome and a less favorable outcome that is available immediately. When faced with such trade-offs, most people show a disproportionate emphasis on immediate outcomes and a tendency to devalue more delayed outcomes, a phenomenon known as "temporal discounting" (Frederick et al., 2002).

Age differences in time horizons and perceptions may affect temporal discounting in several ways. On the one hand, research on younger adults suggests that discounting is reduced when future events are seen as subjectively close (Kim & Zauberman, 2009) and emotionally salient (Kassam et al., 2008). To the extent that older adults experience time as more compressed (Rutt & Löckenhoff, 2013) and fast-paced than younger adults (Wittmann & Lehnhoff, 2005), they are likely to perceive future outcomes as more proximal, which would imply reduced temporal discounting. Further, older adults' well-preserved affective forecasting skills (Scheibe et al., 2010) allow them to vividly anticipate future experiences, which may reduce discounting as well. On the other hand, age-related limitations in future horizons (Carstensen, 2006) could also place a limit on how far older adults are willing to postpone delayed outcomes, given that they may not be around to experience them, pointing toward an age-related increase in temporal discounting.

To date, empirical research on age differences in temporal discounting has focused primarily on monetary gains (often hypothetical in nature) that are realized within a few years. In general, these studies suggest that, compared to younger adults, older adults are less likely to discount future outcomes (Green, Fry, & Myerson, 1994; Halfmann, Hedgcock, & Denburg, 2013; Jimura et al., 2011; Löckenhoff et al., 2011; Whelan & McHugh, 2009). However, these effects are not found in all studies (Harrison, Lau, & Williams, 2002; Read & Read, 2004), and they do not extend to the discounting of monetary losses (Halfmann et al., 2013; Löckenhoff et al., 2011), primary rewards (i.e., liquids: Jimura et al., 2011), and emotional experiences (Löckenhoff, Reed, & Maresca, 2012). Also, little is known about underlying mechanisms, although there is some initial evidence that both affective forecasting (Löckenhoff et al., 2011) and cognition (Halfmann et al., 2013) may play a role.

Recently, research has been extended beyond the standard discounting paradigm to examine preferences for temporal sequences of events. Many real-life choices require decision makers to sort a given set of events or outcomes into a preferred temporal order (e.g., arranging tasks during the workday, managing chronic health conditions, allocating financial resources over time). When faced with such choices, younger adults tend to prefer "increasing" sequences in which the most positive events are saved for last (Frederick et al., 2002; Loewenstein & Prelec, 1993). In contrast, the single study examining age differences in such effects found that when asked to view a series of positive, negative, and neutral images (Löckenhoff et al., 2012), younger adults preferred increasing sequences whereas older adults preferred "flat" sequences in which images of different valence were evenly interspersed. Age differences in global time horizons accounted for the effects, which is consistent with prior findings indicating that limitations in time horizons are associated with a tendency to experience and pursue mixed emotional experiences (Carstensen, 2006; Ersner-Hershfield, Mikels, Sullivan, & Carstensen, 2008).

In addition, there are illusory forms of intertemporal choice where decision-makers respond as if future outcomes depended on past commitments even though there is no actual association. A prime example is the sunk-cost fallacy, which involves the irrational tendency to "throw good money after bad" (van Putten, Zeelenberg, & van Dijk, 2010) or—in more general terms—to commit additional future resources to an option into which one has already invested (i.e., sunk costs in terms of money, time, or effort) as compared to an option where no prior investments have been made (Arkes & Ayton, 1999). Research consistently suggests that older adults are less likely to be swayed by sunk costs than their younger counterparts (Bruine de Bruin, Parker, & Fischhoff, 2007; Strough, Karns, & Schlosnagle, 2011; Strough, Mehta, McFall, & Schuller, 2008), and there are some hints that an age-related tendency to focus on the present moment (as opposed to the past or future) may contribute to this effect: Research on college students suggests that those who focus on either the past or the future (as opposed to the present) are more likely to escalate investments after sunk costs (Karlsson, Juliusson, Grankvist, & Garling, 2002; van Putten et al., 2010). Moreover, statistically controlling thoughts about past investments accounted for age differences in sunk-cost effects (Strough, Schlosnagle, & DiDonato, 2011), and experimentally restricting global time horizons was found to reduce the sunk-cost fallacy in younger adults (Strough, Schlosnagle, Karns, Lemaster, & Pichayayothin, 2014).

Decision Outcomes

Age differences in time horizons may also influence relative preferences for decision outcomes depending on the extent to which they support present- versus future-oriented goals. Based on Socioemotional Selectivity Theory (Carstensen, 2006; Carstensen et al., 1999), one would expect that age-related limitations in global time horizons make older adults more likely to prefer outcomes that optimize immediate emotional well-being over long-term benefits.

The most comprehensive support for this view comes from research on interpersonal choices. Specifically, older as compared to younger adults show a preference for encounters with close social partners (i.e., immediately rewarding and emotionally meaningful interactions) over encounters with new acquaintances (i.e., potential for future learning or expanded social networks; Fung, Carstensen, & Lutz, 1999). Consistent with the proposition that limitations in time horizons, not age per se, are driving these effects, experimental manipulations of participants' time perspectives (e.g., imagining an upcoming geographical move; Fung & Carstensen, 2004) and societal triggers of limited time horizons (e.g., political turnovers, Fung & Carstensen, 2006; Fung et al., 1999) precipitate similar changes in social partner preferences as advanced chronological age.

Comparable effects are seen in the work domain. In occupational settings, future-oriented goals can be mapped onto a preference for growth (e.g., training opportunities) and extrinsic motivators (e.g., financial rewards), whereas present-oriented goals are linked to social and intrinsic motivators (e.g., social embeddedness, organizational commitment; Kooij, De Lange, Jansen, Kanfer, & Dikkers, 2011). Consistent with age-related limitations in time horizons, older employees were found to show a relative preference for affectively salient goals (e.g., generativity, social commitment) whereas younger employees prioritized status, pay, and potential for growth (Kooij et al., 2011; Zacher & Frese, 2011; Zacher, Degner, Seevaldt, Frese, & Ludde, 2009). Moreover, future time horizons were found to statistically account for age differences in work-related motivations (Kooij, de Lange, Jansen, & Dikkers, 2013). Conceivably, limited time horizons may also prompt employees to completely disengage from the work domain and reorient toward goals with higher personal meaning. In support of this idea, more limited time horizons were found to predict the decision to retire (Griffin, Hesketh, & Loh, 2012).

Further evidence for an influence of global time horizons on age differences in decision preferences comes from the health domain, where older patients are found to be more likely to dismiss treatments that require some time and effort to become effective. For instance, older adults and individuals with more limited time horizons were found to show lower compliance with a prescribed exercise regimen (Ziegelmann, Lippke, & Schwarzer, 2006) as well as lower medication adherence and weight management behaviors when diagnosed with diabetes (Hall, Fong, & Cheng, 2012; Sansbury, Dasgupta, Guthrie, & Ward, 2014). Time horizons also play a role in end-of-life scenarios that require trade-offs between quality of life and lengthening life at all costs. In a sample of older adults, those with more extended time horizons reported stronger preference for various life-prolonging treatments while those with shorter horizons resorted to comfort care (Allen, Hilgeman, & Allen, 2011).

Decision Processing and Strategies

Even if potential outcomes do not systematically vary in timing, temporal horizons and mental representations of time may influence how decision-related information is acquired and processed (for a review, see Löckenhoff, 2011). Specifically, following Socioemotional Selectivity Theory, it has been argued that limited time horizons are associated with a focus on strategies that downregulate negative responses to the decision process and prioritize emotionally salient and positively valenced material (Luce, 2005; Mather & Carstensen, 2005). Open-ended time horizons, in contrast, are thought to engender an emphasis on information seeking and exhaustive processing to optimize long-term outcomes (Löckenhoff & Carstensen, 2004).

Consistent with these predictions, pre-decisional information seeking is negatively associated with age across a variety of decision scenarios, both in the laboratory (for a review, see Mata & Nunes, 2010) and in more realistic settings (Streufert, Pogash, Piasecki, & Post, 1990; Turk Charles, Meyerowitz, & Gatz, 1997). Compared to younger adults, older adults also limit their exposure to decision-related information by making their choices more quickly (e.g., Meyer & Pollard, 2004; Zwahr, Park, & Shifren, 1999) and considering a smaller range of options (for a review, see Reed, Mikels, & Löckenhoff, 2013).

In part, age differences in pre-decisional information seeking can be attributed to deficits in information acquisition and processing capacity (Bruine de Bruin et al., 2007; Finucane et al., 2002; Mata & Nunes, 2010; Salthouse & Davis, 2006). However, rather than showing uniform decrements with age, information-seeking in older adults is selectively reduced for negatively valenced and non-emotional material but not for positive material (for a review, see Mikels et al., 2014). In decision contexts, age-related positivity effects have been demonstrated for information-seeking in tabular decision arrays (Löckenhoff & Carstensen, 2007; Löckenhoff & Carstensen, 2008; Mather, Knight, & McCaffrey, 2005), verbal descriptions of decision options (Kim, Healey, Goldstein, Hasher, & Wiprzycka, 2008), as well as relative sensitivity to positive as compared to negative instructional frames (Shamaskin, Mikels, & Reed, 2010) and gain as compared to loss cues (Mikels & Reed, 2009; Samanez-Larkin et al., 2007). Consistent with Socioemotional Selectivity Theory, age differences in positivity during pre-decisional information seeking were shown to be associated with global time horizons (rather than cognitive decline) and eliminated when instructional manipulations selectively emphasized information-seeking goals (Löckenhoff & Carstensen, 2007).

Compared to younger adults, older adults also rely to a greater extent on existing cognitive frameworks (Gilinsky & Judd, 1994), prior experience, and general background knowledge during decision making (Gould, 1999; Stephens & Johnson, 2000), and they tend to employ affect-rich and gist-based problem-solving styles (Blanchard-Fields, 2007; Mienaltowski, 2011; Peters, 2010; Peters, Hess, Västfjäll, & Auman, 2007). These findings are not only consistent with the age-related prioritization of emotion-regulatory goals, but also map onto the relatively greater emphasis on past experiences in the temporal extension of older adults' mental representations of time (Schacter et al., 2013), as well as their tendency to depict the future in terms of general meaning as opposed to specific details (Adams et al., 1997). However, formal evaluations of the relative contribution of time perceptions to age differences in analytic versus experience-based decision styles have yet to be conducted.

Finally, age was found to be associated with a tendency to postpone or delay decisions (e.g., Chen, Ma, & Pethtel, 2011; Finucane et al., 2002). At first glance, it may appear paradoxical that older adults prefer to make their choices later rather than sooner, given that they have a more limited future to plan for and given that—once they have fully engaged in the decision process—they tend to make their choices more quickly (e.g., Zwahr et al., 1999).

The most likely explanation is that decision postponement helps older adults to avoid negative decision-related emotions (Luce, 2005) that may interfere with their pursuit of emotional well-being in the present moment. This may also explain why advanced age is associated with a tendency to delegate choices to others (Curley, Eraker, & Yates, 1984;

Finucane et al., 2002). Consistent with an emotion-regulatory explanation, older adults who deferred difficult choices in an experimental scenario reported lower negative emotions than those who did not defer their choices (Chen et al., 2011).

FUTURE DIRECTIONS AND PRACTICAL IMPLICATIONS

Taken together, the evidence presented in this chapter supports the idea that age-related shifts in time horizons and temporal construals contribute to age differences in decision preferences, strategies, and outcomes. At the same time, there are many open questions that remain to be addressed. Most importantly, although the patterns of findings are generally consistent with a role of time perceptions in decision making, only a small portion of the extant research explicitly tests such hypotheses by including relevant covariates, and even fewer studies provide evidence for a causal role of time horizons by manipulating them experimentally (e.g., Strough et al., 2014; Fung et al., 1999; Rutt & Löckenhoff, in press). Future research should also examine the mutual relationship among different aspects of temporal horizons and perceptions and explore their relative association with cognitive functioning, motivational priorities, and affective responses. Recent evidence from our laboratory (Rutt & Löckenhoff, in press) suggests that subjective position in the life span is closely linked to questionnaire measures of global time horizons, but only weakly associated with other aspects of time perception (e.g., temporal extension of autobiographical thought). Since existing decision-making studies rarely examine more than one aspect at a time, possible interactions among different subcomponents remain to be explored. Limited future horizons, for instance, might have a stronger impact on decision making when subjective speed of time is high. Another shortcoming of prior research is its overwhelming focus on laboratory scenarios and hypothetical outcomes, which are not likely to elicit strong emotional responses and are therefore ill-suited to explore affective components of temporal representations. Future research should also move beyond the current emphasis on monetary outcomes (which are fungible and could conceivably benefit a person's future heirs) to examine primary, personally relevant rewards that have to be consumed or experienced at a specific moment (e.g., Jimura et al., 2011). Last but not least, we need to examine a wider range of time intervals mapping both the near (days to weeks) and distant future (years to decades). This would allow for the exploration of systematic shifts in decision behavior at the point when potential outcomes extend beyond an individuals' actuarial life expectancy.

Apart from theoretical questions about specific pathways and mechanisms, the potential influence of time horizons on decision making raises questions about practical implications for optimizing decision making across the life span. Subjectively, older adults report higher choice satisfaction than younger adults (Kim et al., 2008) and show reduced evidence of post-decisional regret (Brassen, Gamer, Peters, Gluth, & Buchel, 2012). However, such findings are likely skewed by an age-related positivity effect in choice-supportive recall (Löckenhoff & Carstensen, 2007, 2008; Mather & Johnson, 2000; although see Queen & Hess, 2010) and may not reflect objective decision quality.

With regard to global time horizons, there is cause for concern if there is a mismatch between perceived and actual time horizons. In medical settings, for instance, older adults who overestimate their remaining life expectancy may engage in treatments and screening programs even though the expected lag time to benefit exceeds their remaining life expectancy (Lee et al., 2013). In turn, underestimating one's remaining time left in life may be just as detrimental if it prevents adherence to health-promoting interventions and promising treatment approaches (Hudak et al., 2002). Further complications may arise during joint decision-making scenarios when patients, physicians, and relatives operate under different time horizons as they weigh in on possible treatments. A recent qualitative study documents such dynamics in the context of pain management choices, and implicates discrepancies in time horizons among patients and their providers as an important source of conflict (Löckenhoff et al., 2013).

Finally, although older adults' tendency toward experience-rich and affect-based strategies can be interpreted as a sign of a mature and efficient decision-making style (Reyna & Brainerd, 2011), there are some contexts where the encoding of specific details and an accurate anticipation of future events is critical for good choices. This is not only true for financial decisions, where comparing percentages and reading the small print may reveal important caveats (Mikels, Cheung, Cone, & Gilovich, 2013), but also for many health-related choices that confront older decision-makers with complex and novel information. The successful self-management of chronic pain, for example, depends upon patients' ability to track variations in their symptoms in response to specific activities and treatment approaches (Du et al., 2011). In this respect, episodic encoding of past experiences and detailed simulation of future events are likely to retain their relevance across the life span.

Ultimately, a better understanding of the potential pitfalls and benefits of age-related shifts in time horizons opens promising new avenues for decision-making interventions. Other than chronological age and cognitive decrements, time horizons are amenable to be nudged (Thaler & Sunstein, 2008) through instructional manipulations (Löckenhoff & Carstensen, 2007) or perspective taking (Löckenhoff & Carstensen, 2008) to align more accurately with reality and promote more adaptive decisions across the life span.

Acknowledgment

The writing of this chapter was supported in part by NIA grant 1R21AG043741 awarded to Corinna Löckenhoff.

References

Adams, C., Smith, M. C., Nyquist, L., & Perlmutter, M. (1997). Adult age-group differences in recall for the literal and interpretive meanings of narrative text. *The Journals of Gerontology: Series B: Psychological Sciences and Social Sciences, 52B*(4), P187–P195.

Addis, D. R., Musicaro, R., Pan, L., & Schacter, D. L. (2010). Episodic simulation of past and future events in older adults: Evidence from an experimental recombination task. *Psychology and Aging, 25*(2), 369–376.

Addis, D. R., Wong, A. T., & Schacter, D. L. (2008). Age-related changes in the episodic simulation of future events. *Psychological Science, 19*(1), 33–41.

Allen, J. Y., Hilgeman, M. M., & Allen, R. S. (2011). Prospective end-of-life treatment decisions and perceived vulnerability: Future time left to live and memory self-efficacy. *Aging & Mental Health, 15*(1), 122–131.

Arkes, H. R., & Ayton, P. (1999). The sunk cost and concorde effects: Are humans less rational than lower animals? *Psychological Bulletin, 125*(5), 591–600.

Baudouin, A., Vanneste, S., & Isingrini, M. (2004). Age-related cognitive slowing: The role of spontaneous tempo and processing speed. *Experimental Aging Research, 30*(3), 225–239.

Berns, G. S., Laibson, D., & Loewenstein, G. (2007). Intertemporal choice - toward an integrative framework. *Trends in Cognitive Sciences, 11*(11), 482–488.

Blanchard-Fields, F. (2007). Everyday problem solving and emotion: An adult developmental perspective. *Current Directions in Psychological Science, 16*(1), 26–31.

Block, R. A., Zakay, D., & Hancock, P. A. (1998). Human aging and duration judgments: A meta-analytic review. *Psychology and Aging, 13*(4), 584–596.

Brassen, S., Gamer, M., Peters, J., Gluth, S., & Buchel, C. (2012). Don't look back in anger! Responsiveness to missed chances in successful and nonsuccessful aging. *Science, 336*(6081), 612–614.

Brown, D. E. (1991). *Human universals*. New York: McGraw-Hill.

Bruine de Bruin, W., Parker, A. M., & Fischhoff, B. (2007). Individual differences in adult decision-making competence. *Journal of Personality and Social Psychology, 92*(5), 938–956.

Bruss, F. T., & Rüschendorf, L. (2010). On the perception of time. *Gerontology, 56*(4), 361–370.

Cacioppo, J. T., Berntson, G. G., Bechara, A., Tranel, D., & Hawkley, L. C. (2011). Could an aging brain contribute to subjective well-being? The value added by a social neuroscience perspective. In A. Todorov, S. T. Fiske, & D. A. Prentice (Eds.), *Social neuroscience: Toward understanding the underpinnings of the social mind* (pp. 249–262). New York, NY: Oxford University Press.

Carstensen, L. L. (2006). The influence of a sense of time on human development. *Science, 312*(5782), 1913–1915.

Carstensen, L. L., Isaacowitz, D., & Charles, S. T. (1999). Taking time seriously: A theory of socioemotional selectivity. *American Psychologist, 54*, 165–181. [PMID: 10199217].

Carstensen, L. L., & Lang, F. R. (1996). *Future time perspective scale*. Stanford, CA: Stanford University.

Chapman, G. B. (2003). Time discounting of health outcomes. In G. Loewenstein, D. Read, & R. Baumeister (Eds.), *Time and decision: Economic and psychology perspectives on intertemporal choice*. New York: Russel Sage Foundation.

Charles, S. T., & Carstensen, L. L. (2010). Social and emotional aging. *Annual Review of Psychology, 61*, 383–409.

Chen, Y. W., Ma, X. D., & Pethtel, O. (2011). Age differences in trade-off decisions: Older adults prefer choice deferral. *Psychology and Aging, 26*(2), 269–273.

Cole, S. N., Morrison, C. M., & Conway, M. A. (2013). Episodic future thinking: Linking neuropsychological performance with episodic detail in young and old adults. *The Quarterly Journal of Experimental Psychology, 66*(9), 1687–1706.

Comblain, C., D'Argembeau, A., & Van der Linden, M. (2005). Phenomenal characteristics of autobiographical memories for emotional and neutral events in older and younger adults. *Experimental Aging Research, 31*(2), 173–189.

Cottle, T. J., & Pleck, J. H. (1969). Linear estimations of temporal extension: The effect of age, sex, and social class. *Journal of Projective Techniques & Personality Assessment, 33*(1), 81–93.

Curley, S. P., Eraker, S. A., & Yates, J. F. (1984). An investigation of patients' reactions to therapeutic uncertainty. *Medical Decision Making, 4*(4), 501–511.

Du, S., Yuan, C., Xiao, X., Chu, J., Qiu, Y., & Qian, H. (2011). Self-management programs for chronic musculoskeletal pain conditions: A systematic review and meta-analysis. *Patient Education and Counseling, 85*(3), e299–e310.

Ersner-Hershfield, H., Mikels, J. A., Sullivan, S. J., & Carstensen, L. L. (2008). Poignancy: Mixed emotional experience in the face of meaningful endings. *Journal of Personality and Social Psychology, 94*(1), 158–167.

Finucane, M. L., Slovic, P., Hibbard, J. H., Peters, E., Mertz, C. K., & MacGregor, D. G. (2002). Aging and decision-making competence: An analysis of comprehension and consistency skills in older versus younger adults considering health-plan options. *Journal of Behavioral Decision Making, 15*(2), 141–164.

Fraisse, P. (1963). *The psychology of time*. Westport, CT: Greenwood Press.

Frederick, S., Loewenstein, G., & O'Donoghue, T. (2002). Time discounting and time preference: A critical review. *Journal of Economic Literature, 40*(2), 351–401.

Friedman, R. A. (2013). *Fast time and the aging mind*. New York Times.

Friedman, W. J., & Janssen, S. M. J. (2010). Aging and the speed of time. *Acta Psychologica, 134*(2), 130–141.

Fung, H. H., & Carstensen, L. L. (2004). Motivational changes in response to blocked goals and foreshortened time: testing alternatives to socioemotional selectivity theory. *Psychology and Aging, 19*(1), 68–78.

Fung, H. H., & Carstensen, L. L. (2006). Goals change when life's fragility is primed: Lessons learned from older adults, the September 11 attacks and sars. *Social Cognition, 24*(3), 248–278.

Fung, H. H., Carstensen, L. L., & Lutz, A. M. (1999). Influence of time on social preferences: implications for life-span development. *Psychology and Aging, 14*(4), 595–604.

Fung, H. H., Lai, P., & Ng, R. (2001). Age differences in social preferences among Taiwanese and mainland Chinese: The role of perceived time. *Psychology and Aging, 16*(2), 351–356.

Gabbard, C., Lee, J., & Caçola, P. (2013). Role of working memory in transformation of visual and motor representations for use in mental simulation. *Cognitive Neuroscience, 4*(3–4), 210–216.

Gaesser, B., Sacchetti, D. C., Addis, D. R., & Schacter, D. L. (2011). Characterizing age-related changes in remembering the past and imagining the future. *Psychology and Aging, 26*(1), 80–84.

Gallo, D. A., Korthauer, L. E., McDonough, I. M., Teshale, S., & Johnson, E. L. (2011). Age-related positivity effects and autobiographical memory detail: Evidence from a past/future source memory task. *Memory, 19*(6), 641–652.

Gilinsky, A. S., & Judd, B. B. (1994). Working memory and bias in reasoning across the life span. *Psychology and Aging, 9*(3), 356–371.

Gould, O. N. (1999). Cognition and affect in medication adherence. In D. C. Park, R. W. Morrell, & K. Shifren (Eds.), *Processing of medical information in aging patients: Cognitive and human factors perspectives* (pp. 167–183). Mahwah, NJ: Lawrence Erlbaum Associates Publishers.

Green, L., Fry, A. F., & Myerson, J. (1994). Discounting of delayed rewards - a life-span comparison. *Psychological Science, 5*(1), 33–36.

Griffin, B., Hesketh, B., & Loh, V. (2012). The influence of subjective life expectancy on retirement transition and planning: A longitudinal study. *Journal of Vocational Behavior, 81*(2), 129–137.

Guinness book of World Records. (2014). *Oldest Person*. Retrieved February 26, 2014, from http://www.guinnessworldrecords.com/records-5000/oldest-person/.

Halfmann, K., Hedgcock, W., & Denburg, N. L. (2013). Age-related differences in discounting future gains and losses. *Journal of Neuroscience, Psychology, and Economics*, *6*(1), 42–54.

Hall, P. A., Fong, G. T., & Cheng, A. Y. (2012). Time perspective and weight management behaviors in newly diagnosed type 2 diabetes: A mediational analysis. *Journal of Behavioral Medicine*, *35*(6), 569–580.

Hancock, P. A. (2010). The effect of age and sex on the perception of time in life. *The American Journal of Psychology*, *123*(1), 1–13.

Harrison, G. W., Lau, M. I., & Williams, M. B. (2002). Estimating individual discount rates in Denmark: A field experiment. *American Economic Review*, *92*(5), 1606–1617.

Hill, P. F., & Emery, L. J. (2013). Episodic future thought: contributions from working memory. *Consciousness and Cognition: An International Journal*, *22*(3), 677–683.

Hudak, P. L., Clark, J. P., Hawker, G. A., Coyte, P. C., Mahomed, N. N., Kreder, H. J., et al. (2002). "You're perfect for the procedure! Why don't you want it?" Elderly arthritis patients' unwillingness to consider total joint arthroplasty surgery: a qualitative study. *Medical Decision Making*, *22*(3), 272–278.

James, W. (1890). *The principles of psychology* (Vol. 1). New York: Henry Holt and Co.

Janssen, S. M. J., Naka, M., & Friedman, W. J. (2013). Why does life appear to speed up as people get older? *Time & Society*, *22*(2), 274–290.

Jimura, K., Myerson, J., Hilgard, J., Keighley, J., Braver, T. S., & Green, L. (2011). Domain independence and stability in young and older adults' discounting of delayed rewards. *Behavioural Processes*, *87*(3), 253–259.

Karlsson, N., Juliusson, A., Grankvist, G., & Garling, T. (2002). Impact of decision goal on escalation. *Acta Psychologica*, *111*(3), 309–322.

Kassam, K. S., Gilbert, D. T., Boston, A., & Wilson, T. D. (2008). Future anhedonia and time discounting. *Journal of Experimental Social Psychology*, *44*(6), 1533–1537.

Kennedy, Q., Mather, M., & Carstensen, L. L. (2004). The role of motivation in the age-related positivity effect in autobiographical memory. *Psychological Science*, *15*(3), 208–214.

Kim, B. K., & Zauberman, G. (2009). Perception of anticipatory time in temporal discounting. *Journal of Neuroscience, Psychology, and Economics*, *2*(2), 91–101.

Kim, S., Healey, M. K., Goldstein, D., Hasher, L., & Wiprzycka, U. J. (2008). Age differences in choice satisfaction: A positivity effect in decision making. *Psychology and Aging*, *23*(1), 33–38.

Klapproth, F. (2008). Time and decision making in humans. *Cognitive Affective & Behavioral Neuroscience*, *8*(4), 509–524.

Kleinspehn-Ammerlahn, A., Kotter-Grühn, D., & Smith, J. (2008). Self-perceptions of aging: Do subjective age and satisfaction with aging change during old age? *The Journals of Gerontology: Series B: Psychological Sciences and Social Sciences*, *63B*(6), P377–P385.

Kooij, D., De Lange, A. H., Jansen, P. G. W., Kanfer, R., & Dikkers, J. S. E. (2011). Age and work-related motives: Results of a meta-analysis. *Journal of Organizational Behavior*, *32*(2), 197–225.

Kooij, D. T. A.M., de Lange, A. H., Jansen, P. G. W., & Dikkers, J. S. E. (2013). Beyond chronological age: Examining perceived future time and subjective health as age-related mediators in relation to work-related motivations and well-being. *Work & Stress*, *27*(1), 88–105.

Labouvie-Vief, G., Grühn, D., & Studer, J. (2010). Dynamic integration of emotion and cognition: Equilibirium regulation in development and aging. In M. E. Lamb, A. M. Freund, & R. M. Lerner (Eds.), *The handbook of life-span development social and emotional development: Vol. 2*. (pp. 79–115). Hoboken, NJ: John Wiley & Sons Inc.

Lachman, M. E., Röcke, C., Rosnick, C., & Ryff, C. D. (2008). Realism and illusion in Americans' temporal views of their life satisfaction: Age differences in reconstructing the past and anticipating the future. *Psychological Science*, *19*(9), 889–897.

Lang, F. R., & Carstensen, L. L. (2002). Time counts: Future time perspective, goals, and social relationships. *Psychology and Aging*, *17*(1), 125–139.

Lang, F. R., Weiss, D., Gerstorf, D., & Wagner, G. G. (2013). Forecasting life satisfaction across adulthood: Benefits of seeing a dark future? *Psychology and Aging, 28*(1), 249–261.

Lee, S. J., Leipzig, R. M., & Walter, L. C. (2013). Incorporating lag time to benefit into prevention decisions for older adults. *Jama-Journal of the American Medical Association, 310*(24), 2609–2610.

Lemlich, R. (1975). Subjective acceleration of time with aging. *Perceptual and Motor Skills, 41*, 235–238.

Levine, B., Svoboda, E., Hay, J. F., Winocur, G., & Moscovitch, M. (2002). Aging and autobiographical memory: Dissociating episodic from semantic retrieval. *Psychology and Aging, 17*(4), 677–689.

Löckenhoff, C. E. (2011). Age, time, and decision making: From processing speed to global time horizons. *Annals of the New York Academy of Sciences, 1235*, 44–56.

Löckenhoff, C. E., & Carstensen, L. L. (2004). Socioemotional selectivity theory, aging, and health: The increasingly delicate balance between regulating emotions and making tough choices. *Journal of Personality, 72*(6), 1395–1424.

Löckenhoff, C. E., & Carstensen, L. L. (2007). Aging, emotion, and health-related decision strategies: Motivational manipulations can reduce age differences. *Psychology and Aging, 22*(1), 134–146.

Löckenhoff, C. E., & Carstensen, L. L. (2008). Decision strategies in health care choices for self and others: Older but not younger adults make adjustments for the age of the decision target. *Journals of Gerontology: Series B: Psychological Sciences and Social Sciences, 63*(2), P106–P109.

Löckenhoff, C. E., Laucks, S., Port, A. D., Tung, J., Wethington, E., & Reid, M. C. (2013). Temporal horizons in pain management: A focus group study of physicians, physical therapists, and middle-aged and older adult patients. *Gerontologist, 53*(5), 850–860.

Löckenhoff, C. E., O'Donoghue, T., & Dunning, D. (2011). Age differences in temporal discounting: The role of dispositional affect and anticipated emotions. *Psychology and Aging, 26*(2), 274–284.

Löckenhoff, C. E., Reed, A. E., & Maresca, S. N. (2012). Who saves the best for last? Age differences in preferences for affective sequences. *Psychology and Aging, 27*(4), 840–848.

Loewenstein, G. F., & Prelec, D. (1993). Preferences for sequences of outcomes. *Psychological Review, 100*(1), 91–108.

Luce, M. F. (2005). Decision making as coping. *Health Psychology, 24*(4), S23–S28.

Mata, R., & Nunes, L. (2010). When less is enough: Cognitive aging, information search, and decision quality in consumer choice. *Psychology and Aging, 25*(2), 289–298.

Mather, M., & Carstensen, L. L. (2005). Aging and motivated cognition: The positivity effect in attention and memory. *Trends in Cognitive Sciences, 9*(10), 496–502.

Mather, M., & Johnson, M. K. (2000). Choice-supportive source monitoring: Do our decisions seem better to us as we age? *Psychology and Aging, 15*(4), 596–606.

Mather, M., & Knight, M. (2005). Goal-directed memory: The role of cognitive control in older adults' emotional memory. *Psychology and Aging, 20*(4), 554–570.

Mather, M., Knight, M., & McCaffrey, M. (2005). The allure of the alignable: Younger and older adults' false memories of choice features. *Journal of Experimental Psychology-General, 134*(1), 38–51.

McAuley, J. D., Jones, M. R., Holub, S., Johnston, H. M., & Miller, N. S. (2006). The time of our lives: Life span development of timing and event tracking. *Journal of Experimental Psychology: General, 135*(3), 348–367.

McDonough, I. M., & Gallo, D. A. (2013). Impaired retrieval monitoring for past and future autobiographical events in older adults. *Psychology and Aging, 28*(2), 457–466.

Meyer, B. J. F., & Pollard, C. A. (2004). Why do older adults make faster decisions about treatments for breast cancer. In *Paper presented at the Cognitive Aging Conference*.

Mienaltowski, A. (2011). Everyday problem solving across the adult life span: Solution diversity and efficacy. In G. R. SamanezLarkin (Ed.), *Decision making over the life span* (Vol. 1235) (pp. 75–85), Hoboken, NJ: Wiley-Blackwell.

Mikels, J. A., Cheung, E., Cone, J., & Gilovich, T. (2013). The dark side of intuition: Aging and increases in nonoptimal intuitive decisions. *Emotion*, *13*(2), 189–195.

Mikels, J. A., & Reed, A. E. (2009). Monetary losses do not loom large in later life: Age differences in the framing effect. *Journals of Gerontology: Series B: Psychological Sciences and Social Sciences*, *64*(4), 457–460.

Mikels, J. A., Reed, A. E., Hardy, L. N., & Löckenhoff, C. E. (2014). Positive emotions across the adult life span. In M. Tugade, M. N. Shiota, & L. Kirby (Eds.), *Handbook of positive emotions* (pp. 256–272). New York: Guilford Press.

Nielsen, L., Knutson, B., & Carstensen, L. L. (2008). Affect dynamics, affective forecasting, and aging. *Emotion*, *8*(3), 318–330.

Old, S. R., & Naveh-Benjamin, M. (2008). Differential effects of age on item and associative measures of memory: a meta-analysis. *Psychology and Aging*, *23*(1), 104–118.

Pan, Y., & Luo, Q.-Y. (2012). Working memory modulates the perception of time. *Psychonomic Bulletin & Review*, *19*(1), 46–51.

de Paula, J. J., Neves, F., Levy, Â., Nassif, E., & Malloy-Diniz, L. F. (2012). Assessing planning skills and executive functions in the elderly: Preliminary normative data for the Tower of London Test. *Arquivos de Neuro-Psiquiatria*, *70*(10), 826–830.

Pearman, A., Andreoletti, C., & Isaacowitz, D. M. (2010). Sadness prediction and response: Effects of age and agreeableness. *Aging & Mental Health*, *14*(3), 355–363.

Peters, E. (2010). Aging-related changes in decision making. In A. Drolet, N. Schwarz, & C. Yoon (Eds.), *The aging consumer: Perspectives from psychology and economics* (pp. 75–101). New York, NY: Routledge/Taylor & Francis Group.

Peters, E., Hess, T. M., Västfjäll, D., & Auman, C. (2007). Adult age differences in dual information processes: Implications for the role of affective and deliberative processes in older adults' decision making. *Perspectives on Psychological Science*, *2*(1), 1–23.

van Putten, M., Zeelenberg, M., & van Dijk, E. (2010). Who throws good money after bad? Action vs state orientation moderates the sunk cost fallacy. *Judgment and Decision Making*, *5*(1), 33–36.

Queen, T. L., & Hess, T. M. (2010). Age differences in the effects of conscious and unconscious thought in decision making. *Psychology and Aging*, *25*(2), 251–261.

Read, D., & Read, N. L. (2004). Time discounting over the lifespan. *Organizational Behavior and Human Decision Processes*, *94*(1), 22–32.

Ready, R. E., Weinberger, M. I., & Jones, K. M. (2007). How happy have you felt lately? Two diary studies of emotion recall in older and younger adults. *Cognition and Emotion*, *21*(4), 728–757.

Reed, A. E., & Carstensen, L. L. (2012). The theory behind the age-related positivity effect. *Frontiers in Psychology*, *3*, 339.

Reed, A. E., Mikels, J., & Löckenhoff, C. E. (2013). Preferences for choice across adulthood: Age trajectories and potential mechanisms. *Psychology and Aging*, *23*, 625–632.

Rendell, P. G., Bailey, P. E., Henry, J. D., Phillips, L. H., Gaskin, S., & Kliegel, M. (2012). Older adults have greater difficulty imagining future rather than atemporal experiences. *Psychology and Aging*, *27*(4), 1089–1098.

Reyna, V. F., & Brainerd, C. J. (2011). Dual processes in decision making and developmental neuroscience: A fuzzy-trace model. *Developmental Review*, *31*(2–3), 180–206.

Ros, L., & Latorre, J. M. (2010). Gender and age differences in the recall of affective autobiographical memories using the autobiographical memory test. *Personality and Individual Differences*, *49*(8), 950–954.

Roy, M., Grondin, S., & Roy, M.-A. (2012). Time perception disorders are related to working memory impairment in schizophrenia. *Psychiatry Research*, *200*(2–3), 159–166.

Rutt, J. L., & Löckenhoff, C. E. (2013). Time keeps on slipping? Age differences in the subjective compression of future time. In *Paper presented at the annual meeting of the Society for Personality and Social Psychology, New Orleans, LA*.

Rutt, J.L., & Löckenhoff, C.E. (in press). Age patterns in multiple aspects of time perception: The role of covariates. *Experimental Aging Research*.

Salthouse, T. A. (1996). The processing-speed theory of adult age differences in cognition. *Psychological Review, 103*(3), 403–428.

Salthouse, T. A., & Davis, H. P. (2006). Organization of cognitive abilities and neuropsychological variables across the lifespan. *Developmental Review, 26*(1), 31–54.

Samanez-Larkin, G. R., & Carstensen, L. (2011). Socioemotional functioning and the aging brain. In J. Decety, & J. T. Cacioppo (Eds.), *The Oxford handbook of social neuroscience* (pp. 507–521). New York: Oxford University Press.

Samanez-Larkin, G. R., Gibbs, S. E. B., Khanna, K., Nielsen, L., Carstensen, L. L., & Knutson, B. (2007). Anticipation of monetary gain but not loss in healthy older adults. *Nature Neuroscience, 10*, 787–791.

Sanders, C., & Schmitter-Edgecombe, M. (2012). Identifying the nature of impairment in planning ability with normal aging. *Journal of Clinical and Experimental Neuropsychology, 34*(7), 724–737.

Sansbury, B., Dasgupta, A., Guthrie, L., & Ward, M. (2014). Time perspective and medication adherence among individuals with hypertension or diabetes mellitus. *Patient Education and Counseling, 95*(1), 104–110.

Schacter, D. L., & Addis, D. R. (2008). The cognitive neuroscience of constructive memory: Remembering the past and imagining the future. In J. Driver, P. Haggard, & T. Shallice (Eds.), *Mental processes in the human brain* (pp. 27–47). New York, NY: Oxford University Press.

Schacter, D. L., Addis, D. R., & Buckner, R. L. (2007). Remembering the past to imagine the future: The prospective brain. *Nature Reviews Neuroscience, 8*(9), 657–661.

Schacter, D. L., Gaesser, B., & Addis, D. R. (2013). Remembering the past and imagining the future in the elderly. *Gerontology, 59*(2), 143–151.

Scheibe, S., & Carstensen, L. L. (2010). Emotional aging: Recent findings and future trends. *Journals of Gerontology: Series B: Psychological Sciences and Social Sciences, 65*(2), 135–144.

Scheibe, S., Mata, R., & Carstensen, L. L. (2010). Age differences in affective forecasting and experienced emotion surrounding the 2008 US presidential election. *Cognition and Emotion, 25*(6), 1029–1044.

Schlagman, S., Kliegel, M., Schulz, J., & Kvavilashvili, L. (2009). Differential effects of age on involuntary and voluntary autobiographical memory. *Psychology and Aging, 24*(2), 397–411.

Shamaskin, A. M., Mikels, J. A., & Reed, A. E. (2010). Getting the message across: Age differences in the positive and negative framing of health care messages. *Psychology and Aging, 25*(3), 746–751.

Sorel, O., & Pennequin, V. (2008). Aging of the planning process: The role of executive functioning. *Brain and Cognition, 66*(2), 196–201.

Spreng, R. N., & Levine, B. (2006). The temporal distribution of past and future autobiographical events across the lifespan. *Memory & Cognition, 34*(8), 1644–1651.

Spreng, R. N., & Levine, B. (2013). Doing what we imagine: Completion rates and frequency attributes of imagined future events one year after prospection. *Memory, 21*(4), 458–466.

Stephens, E. C., & Johnson, M. M. S. (2000). Dr. Mom and other influences on younger and older adults' OTC medication purchases. *Journal of Applied Gerontology, 19*(4), 441–459.

Streufert, S., Pogash, R., Piasecki, M., & Post, G. M. (1990). Age and management team performance. *Psychology and Aging, 5*(4), 551–559.

Strough, J., Karns, T. E., & Schlosnagle, L. (2011). Decision-making heuristics and biases across the life span. In G. R. Samanez-Larkin (Ed.), *Decision making over the life span* (Vol. 1235) (pp. 57–74), Hoboken, NJ: Wiley-Blackwell.

Strough, J., Mehta, C. M., McFall, J. P., & Schuller, K. L. (2008). Are older adults less subject to the sunk-cost fallacy than younger adults? *Psychological Science, 19*(7), 650–652.

Strough, J., Schlosnagle, L., & DiDonato, L. (2011). Understanding decisions about sunk costs from older and younger adults' perspectives. *Journals of Gerontology: Series B: Psychological Sciences and Social Sciences, 66*(6), 681–686.

Strough, J., Schlosnagle, L., Karns, T., Lemaster, P., & Pichayayothin, N. (2014). No time to waste: Restricting life-span temporal horizons decreases the sunk-cost fallacy. *Journal of Behavioral Decision Making*, *27*(1), 78–94.

Thaler, R. H., & Sunstein, C. R. (2008). *Nudge: Improving decisions about health, wealth, and happiness*. New Haven, CT: Yale University Press.

Tomaszczyk, J. C., & Fernandes, M. A. (2012). A positivity effect in autobiographical memory, but not phonemic fluency, in older adults. *Aging, Neuropsychology, and Cognition*, *19*(6), 699–722.

Turk Charles, S., Meyerowitz, B. E., & Gatz, M. (1997). Age differences in information-seeking among cancer patients. *International Journal of Aging & Human Development*, *45*(2), 85–98.

Verhaeghen, P., & Salthouse, T. A. (1997). Meta-analyses of age–cognition relations in adulthood: Estimates of linear and nonlinear age effects and structural models. *Psychological Bulletin*, *122*(3), 231–249.

Whelan, R., & McHugh, L. A. (2009). Temporal discounting of hypothetical monetary rewards by adolescents, adults, and older adults. *Psychological Record*, *59*(2), 247–258.

Wittmann, M., & Lehnhoff, S. (2005). Age effects in perception of time. *Psychological Reports*, *97*(3), 921–935.

Woehrle, J. L., & Magliano, J. P. (2012). Time flies faster if a person has a high working-memory capacity. *Acta Psychologica*, *139*(2), 314–319.

Zacher, H., Degner, M., Seevaldt, R., Frese, M., & Ludde, J. (2009). What do younger and older workers want to accomplish? Age-related differences in content and characteristics of occupational goals. *Zeitschrift Fur Personalpsychologie*, *8*(4), 191–200.

Zacher, H., & Frese, M. (2011). Maintaining a focus on opportunities at work: The interplay between age, job complexity, and the use of selection, optimization, and compensation strategies. *Journal of Organizational Behavior*, *32*(2), 291–318.

Zauberman, G., Kim, B. K., Malkoc, S. A., & Bettman, J. R. (2009). Discounting time and time discounting: Subjective time perception and intertemporal preferences. *Journal of Marketing Research*, *46*(4), 543–556.

Ziegelmann, J. P., Lippke, S., & Schwarzer, R. (2006). Subjective residual life expectancy in health self-regulation. *The Journals of Gerontology: Series B: Psychological Sciences and Social Sciences*, *61B*(4), P195–P201.

Zwahr, M. D., Park, D. C., & Shifren, K. (1999). Judgments about estrogen replacement therapy: The role of age, cognitive abilities, and beliefs. *Psychology and Aging*, *14*(2), 179–191.

CHAPTER

12

Understanding Life-Span Developmental Changes in Decision-Making Competence

JoNell Strough[1], *Andrew M. Parker*[2], *Wändi Bruine de Bruin*[3, 4]

[1]Department of Psychology, West Virginia University, Morgantown, WV, USA; [2]RAND Corporation, Pittsburgh, PA, USA; [3]University of Leeds, West Yorkshire, England; [4]Carnegie Mellon University, Pittsburgh, PA, USA

OVERVIEW

Decision-making competence is likely to be critical for making decisions emerging in later life, such as those pertaining to spending down wealth, health insurance, and end-of-life planning. This chapter reviews research on age-related differences in decision-making competence. We begin by defining decision-making competence. We trace evolving views of the relative roles of deliberation and affect for decision-making competence within the behavioral decision-making literature. Next, we review how decision-making competence is influenced by deliberative, affective, and experience-based skills and the changing interplay of these skills with age. We then propose a conceptual model of decision making that uses insights from life-span theory to emphasize the importance of considering motivation when making predictions about decision-making skills that may decline, be maintained, or even improve across adulthood. We review research relevant to our predictions. Finally, we discuss challenges to understanding decision-making competence and aging, and offer suggestions for future research.

Aging and Decision Making
http://dx.doi.org/10.1016/B978-0-12-417148-0.00012-1

DEFINING DECISION-MAKING COMPETENCE

Behavioral decision research involves normative, descriptive, and prescriptive approaches. *Normative* theories define "good" decisions as ones that are most likely to provide the decision maker with desired outcomes (Edwards, 1954; Yates, 1990). *Descriptive* accounts investigate how people's actual decisions deviate from normative standards, thus identifying biases and errors. *Prescriptive* approaches aim to help people make better decisions by overcoming biases and errors.

Normative theories outline four processes essential for good decision making (Edwards, 1954; Raiffa, 1968): *belief assessment*—for each option, judging the likelihood of specific outcomes if it is chosen; *value assessment*—judging how well outcomes meet one's goals; *integration*—combining beliefs and values into coherent decisions, and *metacognition*—understanding of the strengths and limits of one's abilities. Evaluations of these processes typically focus on *accuracy* or correspondence with external criteria and *consistency* with other beliefs, rather than decision outcomes (Keren & Bruine de Bruin, 2003). Because decision outcomes are affected by chance, good decision processes may sometimes yield undesired decision outcomes. However, across a large number of decisions, better decision processes should lead to better decision outcomes.

To measure the quality of the main decision processes identified by normative decision theories, we adapted six tasks from the behavioral decision-making literature to create the Adult Decision-Making Competence (A-DMC) battery (Bruin de Bruine, Parker, & Fischhoff, 2007). Performance on these tasks has been linked to real-world decision outcomes in age-diverse samples (Bruine de Bruin et al., 2007; Parker & Fischhoff, 2005). For each task, decision processes are judged for accuracy or for consistency (see Table 1). *Consistency in risk perception* examines consistency in paired risk judgments (e.g., judged likelihood of dying next year should be less than or equal to judged likelihood of dying within next 5 years). *Resistance to sunk costs* assesses how well choices follow the normative rule to ignore prior investments that remain lost independent of how one proceeds (Arkes & Blumer, 1985). *Resistance to framing* measures resistance to irrelevant changes in question wording (e.g., whether ground beef is "20% fat" or "80% lean;" Levin & Gaeth, 1988b). *Recognizing social norms* (Jacobs, Greenwald, & Osgood, 1995) first asks for judgments of whether negative behaviors (e.g., settling an argument with your fists) are sometimes OK, and later asks "how many out of 100 people your age would say that it is sometimes OK." The latter measures judged social norms, which are compared for accuracy to actual social norms seen in mean responses to the first questions. *Applying decision rules* assesses accuracy of use of specific decision rules for hypothetical choices (i.e., between Blu-ray players) varying on relevant features (e.g., sound quality). *Under/*

TABLE 1 Six Components of Decision-Making Competence (DMC)

DMC Component	Description of Performance Score	General Decision-Making Skill	Criterion	Correlation with Age[a]
Consistency in risk perception	Risk judgments are consistent with probability theory	Belief assessment	Consistency	−0.05
Resistance to sunk costs	Willingness to consider only future consequences when making choices	Value assessment	Accuracy	0.26[c]
Resistance to framing	Consistency in choice across equivalent, positively, and negatively worded questions	Value assessment, integration	Consistency	−0.20[b]
Recognizing social norms	Judged social norms correlate with actual social norms	Belief assessment, value assessment	Accuracy	0.05
Applying decision rules	Accurately applying specified decision rules in choices among options with multiple attributes	Integration	Accuracy	−0.18[b]
Under/ overconfidence	Correspondence between confidence in knowledge and actual knowledge	Belief assessment, metacognition	Accuracy	0.09

[a] *From the study reported in Bruine de Bruin, Parker, & Fischhoff (2012) involving a community sample of 360 respondents, age 18–88 years.*
[b] *Two-sided p-value* < 0.01.
[c] $p < 0.001$.

overconfidence reflects appropriate confidence in one's knowledge. After a series of true/false questions (e.g., "Alcohol causes dehydration"), we ask for confidence assessments, from 50% (just guessing) to 100% (absolutely sure). The score is the absolute difference between mean confidence and percent correct (Yates, 1990).

Most behavioral decision research is based on college students (Peters & Bruine de Bruin, 2012; Strough, Karns, & Schlosnagle, 2011). However, initial findings from research using the A-DMC measure (see Figure 1) and other behavioral decision tasks with age-diverse samples (reviewed later), suggest that specific decision skills may decline, be maintained, or even improve with age, highlighting the need to understand mechanisms contributing to decision-making competence across the life span. As background, we discuss the evolution of thinking about the relative roles of deliberation and affect in decision-making competence.

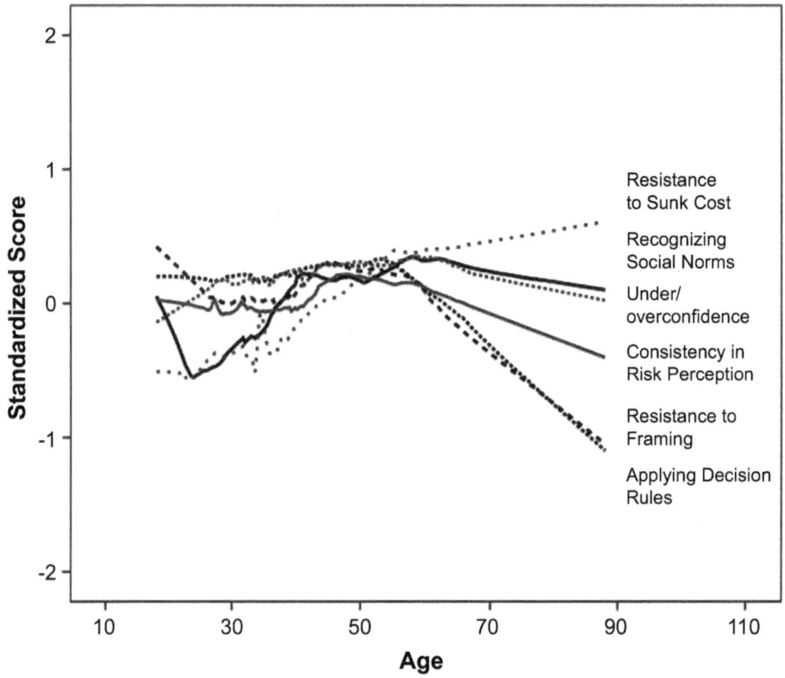

FIGURE 1 Age-spectrum trends in A-DMC component tasks in a convenience community sample, LOESS fit-line estimation. Data come from a cross-sectional sample, as first reported in Bruine de Bruin et al. (2007).

DELIBERATION, AFFECT, AND DECISION-MAKING COMPETENCE

Deliberation. Due to origins in economics, early normative decision theories viewed good decisions as requiring deliberation to choose the option that maximizes utility or value (Edwards, 1954). As the field evolved, descriptive theories recognized that decisions are made with limited cognitive resources. For example, simple rules such as "satisficing," or choosing a "good enough" option, reduce cognitive effort (Simon, 1956). This recognition spurred interest in heuristics or "shortcuts" that conserve cognitive resources (Tversky & Kahneman, 1974). Although such shortcuts can be effective, they sometimes produce systematic deviations from normative standards (Kahneman, Slovic, & Tversky, 1982).

Affect. Following from the idea that affective reactions often occur first in information processing (Zajonc, 1980), early decision research investigated how induced affect shaped judgments (e.g., Johnson & Tversky, 1983) and how anticipated affective consequences of decisions influenced preferences (e.g., Isen, Nygren, & Ashby, 1988). Later work recognized that incidental affect unrelated to the decision may undermine decision quality (e.g., Loewenstein, Weber, Hsee, & Welch, 2001). Along these lines, the idea that people rely on their feelings as a shortcut to make decisions, or use an "affect heuristic," was advanced (Slovic, Finucane, Peters, & MacGregor, 2002). The idea that affect facilitates analytical decision making has received less attention (cf. Damasio, 1994).

Dual-Process Models. Dual-process models describe the interplay of deliberation and affect in terms of two different systems (for reviews, see Evans, 2008; Mikels, Shuster, & Thai, this volume; Osman, 2004). Most dual-process models assume that the affective/experiential system is a source of systematic biases and errors, whereas the deliberative/analytic system results in unbiased, objective decisions (e.g., Kahneman, 2003). One function of the deliberative mode is to monitor and, as needed, edit "snap decisions" from the affective/experiential mode (Kahneman, 2003). Others suggest that decisions from the affective/experiential system are often "good enough" (Gigerenzer, 2008) or even superior, such as when essential meaning or "gist" is quickly extracted or rules are automatically applied (Reyna, 2004; Yates & Patalano, 1999). Hence, in some dual-process models there has been a shift away from conceptualizing good decision making solely as a deliberative process.

AGING AND DECISION-MAKING COMPETENCE

Building from dual-process models, much initial research on aging and decision making focused on the interplay of deliberative/analytical and affective/experiential systems in older adults' decision-making competence (e.g., Peters, Hess, Västfjäll, & Auman, 2007). Age-related declines in cognitive capacity may undermine deliberative decision making and fuel greater reliance on affect (e.g., Hanoch, Wood, & Rice, 2007; Peters et al., 2007). Such a shift may allow older people to compensate for age-related cognitive declines, or even improve performance (e.g., Peters & Bruine de Bruin, 2012; Strough, Karns et al., 2011). In the following section, we review research that links age-related changes in deliberative, affective, and experiential skills to declines, maintenance, and improvements in decision-making competence.

Deliberation and Age. Initial work on aging and decision-making competence showed that cognitive declines adversely affect older adults' performance on cognitively demanding decision tasks (Finucane, Mertz, Slovic, & Schmidt, 2005). Age-related declines in fluid intelligence (e.g., Salthouse, 2004), processing speed (Salthouse, 1996), and short-term, working, and long-term memory (e.g., Park, Lautenschlager, Hedden, Davidson & Smith, 2002) are well-documented. These skills have been described as the "mechanics" of cognition (Baltes, Lindenberger, & Staudinger, 2006).

Age differences in performance on several A-DMC tasks (Bruine de Bruin et al., 2007) have been linked to age-related cognitive declines. Fluid intelligence mediates the association between older age and worse performance on resistance to framing and applying decision rules (Bruine de Bruine, Parker, & Fischhoff, 2012). Working memory mediates the association between older age and worse performance on under/overconfidence, whereas episodic memory mediates age differences in recognizing social norms (Del Missier et al., 2013). Fluid intelligence, working memory, and episodic memory are also related to older adults' poorer performance on a variety of other behavioral decision-making tasks (e.g., Bernstein, Erdfelder, Meltzhoff, Perria, & Loftus, 2011; Finucane & Gullion, 2010; Henninger, Madden, & Huettel, 2010; Hess, Queen, & Patterson, 2012; Mata, Schooler, & Rieskamp, 2007; Wood et al., 2011). Hence, age-related declines in "cognitive mechanics" are clearly important for understanding why some aspects of decision-making competence decline with age (see also Del Missier, Mäntylä, & Nilsson, this volume).

Affect and Age. Researchers have begun to consider the role of affect in decision-making competence across the life span. Improvement in affect regulation with age is increasingly well-documented (e.g., Blanchard-Fields, 2007; Charles & Carstensen, 2010). Positive emotional experience increases until about age 70, when it begins to level off and decline among those 80 years and older (e.g., Carstensen et al., 2011). These age-related changes have been posited both to facilitate and to undermine decision-making competence (e.g., Mikels et al., this volume).

Adding affective, evaluative information to numerical information influences older adults' preferences for hypothetical health care plans (Peters, Dieckmann, Västjfäll, Mertz, & Slovic, 2009). Dispositional affect and anticipated affect are better predictors of age differences in discounting of gains and losses than are basic cognitive abilities (Löckenhoff, O'Donoghue, & Dunning, 2011). Older adults pay more attention than younger adults to affective cues when learning which deck of cards yields the highest payoff (Bauer et al., 2013; Wood, Busemeyer, Koling, Cox, & Davis, 2005). Inducing positive affect improves older adults' learning of which card decks result in gains versus losses (Carpenter, Peters, Västjfäll, & Isen, 2013). However, positive affect can have negative consequences such as when older adults fail to attend to odds of winning and instead focus on number of chances to win (Mikels, Cheung, Cone, & Gilovich, 2012). These latter studies show how "incidental affect" unrelated to the decision itself can influence older adults' decisions.

Cuing affective versus deliberative processing influences older adults' decisions. Older adults make higher-quality decisions when affective processing is cued than when deliberative processing is cued; the opposite is true for younger adults (Mikels et al., 2010). However, another study shows that cuing deliberative processing similarly influences older and younger adults' choices about gambles with different expected values (Thomas & Millar, 2012). Differences in findings across studies may reflect that the optimal decision-making mode for a given task influences how well older adults perform. When decision quality requires processing information valence, older adults' performance may benefit from relying on affective skills that improve with age. However, when decision quality requires deliberation based on expected value, older adults' performance will be harmed by age-related cognitive declines (see Weller, Levin, & Denburg, 2011). Yet, more research is needed to understand the interplay between cognitive and affective skills in decision-making competence across the life span.

Experience and Age. Research investigating aging and decision-making competence has focused relatively little on experience, but it has been hypothesized that with age and experience people learn better decision-making strategies. Crystallized intelligence or experience-based practical knowledge improves with age (Baltes et al., 2006; Park et al., 2002; Salthouse, 2004), and may be relevant to decision making. Initial findings suggest that performance on the A-DMC tasks improves with age-related life experience—although age-related declines in fluid cognition may suppress those effects in cognitively demanding decision tasks (Bruine de Bruin et al., 2012). Presumably as a result of life experience, older adults also express more consistent preferences, even when younger adults have more domain-specific knowledge (i.e., extra credit for course work; Kim & Hasher, 2005). Furthermore, older adults' greater general life experience is thought to explain why they perform similarly to younger adults on tasks that tap application of normative economic principles (i.e., temporal discounting tasks, financial literacy, debt literacy) despite their declining fluid intelligence (Li, Baldassi, Johnson, & Weber, 2013).

In addition to general life experience, domain-specific experience may give older adults an advantage over younger adults. Older adults' greater consumer experience may explain why their preferences for shopping discount cards were more consistent than younger adults' preferences (Tentori, Osherson, Hasher, & May, 2001). Social experience is thought to explain age differences in social judgments (Hess, Osowski, & Leclerc,

2005). Training in economics reduces the sunk-cost bias (Larrick, Morgan, & Nisbett, 1990; cf. Arkes & Blumer, 1985), and experts are less subject to the sunk-cost bias than nonexperts (Fennema & Perkins, 2008). However, in these studies, age and expertise were confounded. Moreover, experts may not always avoid decision biases (Reyna, Chick, Corbin, & Hsia, 2014; Shafir & LeBoeuf, 2002). Thus, the extent and conditions under which experience facilitates decision-making competence in later adulthood remain unclear.

MOTIVATIONAL MODEL OF AGING AND DECISION-MAKING COMPETENCE

To predict how individual differences in deliberative, affective, and experiential skills may lead to declines, maintenance, or improvement in decision-making competence across the life-span, we have developed a conceptual model that accords a key role to motivation (see Figure 2; see also Strough, Karns et al., 2011). First, our model views decision making as a contextually embedded process. Our conceptualization of context includes aspects of the immediate situation (e.g., decision topic, whether the decision is made alone or with others), and the larger

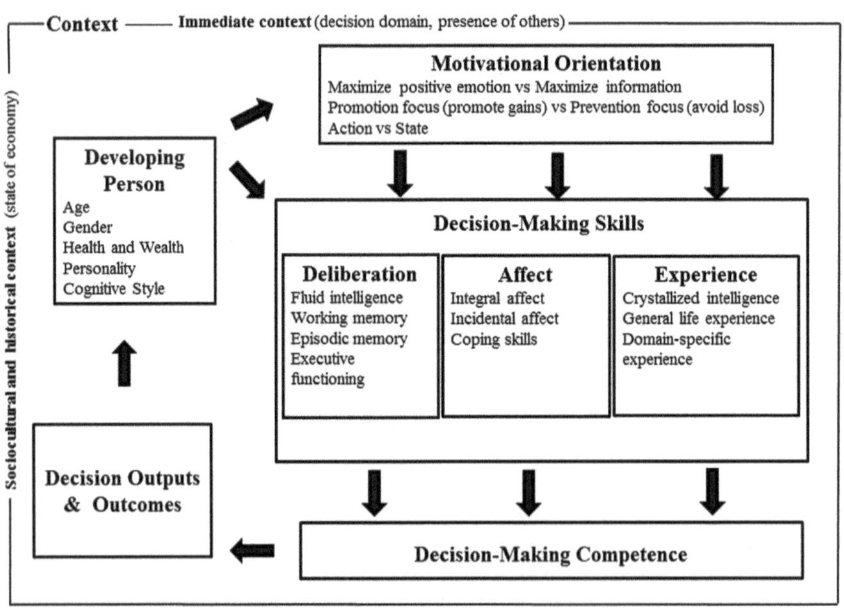

FIGURE 2 Process model of decision-making competence across the life span. Elements of the process depicted are meant to be representative examples, not an exhaustive list.

sociocultural historical context (e.g., the state of the economy, cultural attitudes about aging). Second, our model posits that individual characteristics such as age, personality, and cognitive style are important antecedents that affect the decision-making process (see also Bruine de Bruin, Parker, & Fischhoff, in press). Third, our model emphasizes that people are motivated by concerns reflecting both their personal characteristics and features of the decision context (see also Berg & Strough, 2011; Strough & Keener, 2014). Finally, a distinguishing feature of our model is that it recognizes developmental changes in deliberative, affective, and experiential skills, as well as developmental changes in the motivation to use those skills when making decisions.

Our model is based on conceptualizations of motivation taken from dual-process theories of decision making and from life-span theories of how motivation may change with age. First, dual-process theorists posit that motivation influences the thinking mode applied to the decision (Kahneman, 2003). Personally relevant decisions motivate use of the cognitively taxing deliberative mode. When lacking such motivation, people rely on the experiential/affective mode. Other theories of motivation used in the behavioral decision-making literature distinguish motivation to promote gains ("promotion-focused") from motivation to avoid losses ("prevention-focused"; e.g., Crowe & Higgins, 1997; Molden & Hui, 2011). "Action" versus "state" orientation, a person's tendency to initiate and follow through with intentions versus engage in unproductive thoughts (Diefendorff, Hall, Lord, & Strean, 2000), has also been investigated (e.g., van Putten, Zeelenberg, & van Dijk, 2010). A limitation of these approaches is that they do not address how motivation changes with age.

Second, life-span theories address age-related changes in motivation and can be extended to understand age differences in decision making. For example, Carstensen's (2006) Socioemotional Selectivity Theory outlines how motivation to maximize positive emotion versus seek information changes with age as a function of life-span temporal horizons. Expansive time horizons in early adulthood motivate seeking new experiences and information. In later adulthood, shortened time horizons due to awareness of life's finitude motivate maximizing positive emotions in the "here and now." In the following section, we show how taking motivation into account facilitates a better understanding of aspects of decision-making competence that may decline, be maintained, or even improve across adulthood.

Motivation and Affect. Two lines of research provide initial insights about motivation and age differences in decision-making competence. The first focuses on "resistance to framing," (one component task of the A-DMC measure; Bruine de Bruin et al., 2007) which, as noted earlier, refers to the ability to be unaffected by whether options are described in positive or negative terms (Levin & Gaeth, 1988a). Studies with college-age samples show violations of the normative principle that responses should be consistent across frames (see Kuhberger, 1998, for a review), which has been attributed to greater attention to losses than to gains (Tversky & Kahneman, 1981; cf., Reyna, 2004). It has been suggested that, if older adults' motivation to maximize positive emotion dampens attention to loss, they may be less subject to framing errors (e.g., Mikels & Reed, 2009). However, studies investigating age differences in framing errors yield inconsistent results (for reviews, see Mata, Josef, Samanez-Larkin, & Hertwig, 2011; Peters, Dieckman, & Weller, 2011; Strough, Karns et al., 2011).

Second, research on "resistance to sunk cost" (another A-DMC task, Bruine de Bruin et al., 2007) examines the ability to discontinue commitments that are no longer the most optimal choice, despite prior investments that have been made and lost (Arkes & Blumer, 1985). People often violate the normative rule of ignoring irretrievable losses due to loss aversion and concerns about waste (Arkes & Blumer, 1985).

Older adults' motivation to maximize positive emotion and the strategies they use to facilitate positive affect (e.g., Charles & Carstensen, 2010) may give them an advantage over younger adults when dealing with sunk costs. We have found that older adults are better able than younger adults to resist sunk costs, even after taking into account fluid intelligence and education—suggesting that other skills play a role (Bruine de Bruin et al., 2012; Strough, Mehta, McFall, & Schuller, 2008). Older adults' decisions about sunk costs are less motivated by past losses than those of younger adults (Strough, Schlosnagle, & DiDonato, 2011). Moreover, instead of engaging in unproductive rumination about irretrievable past losses, older adults choose to use action-oriented coping strategies (Bruine de Bruin, Strough, & Parker, 2014). Similarly, among people younger than 50, those who are motivated to promote gains ("promotion focus") are better at ignoring sunk costs compared to those who are motivated to prevent loss ("prevention focus"; Molden & Hui, 2011). College students with an "action" orientation are less subject to the sunk-cost bias compared to those with a "state" orientation, presumably because those with a state orientation ruminate about past losses (van Putten et al., 2010). Together, these studies point to the importance of age-related changes in motivation for understanding decision-making competence, and suggest that coping strategies may lead to age-related improvements in performance in one aspect of decision-making competence.

Notably, although motivation to maximize positive emotion may be, on average, more characteristic of older adults than younger adults, individual differences exist (e.g., van Putten et al., 2010). And, as our model posits, motivation shifts depending on the context. Such shifts are not limited to decisions about sunk costs. In line with the idea that older adults are motivated to maximize positive emotions, in one study when asked to choose a physician and a health plan, adults 62 and older reviewed more positive than negative health-care information compared to adults aged 22–39 (Löckenhoff & Carstensen, 2007). However, this age difference was eliminated when participants were motivated to focus on information-gathering goals (see also Depping & Freund, 2013). The sunk-cost bias decreases when younger adults' usually expansive life-span temporal horizons are experimentally restricted to create a motivational orientation that mimics that of older adults (Strough, Schlosnagle, Karns, Lemaster, & Pichayayothin, 2014). These findings illustrate how contextual demands may modify age-typical motivational orientations to influence decisions.

Motivation and Deliberation. Research reviewed earlier has established that age-related declines in deliberative skills are important for understanding why older adults perform worse on cognitively demanding behavioral decision tasks. However, motivation may affect whether or not older adults apply their deliberative skills. Recent research shows that older adults may be less motivated to think about numbers, and this helps to explain why age is associated with lower scores on cognitively demanding measures of numeracy (Bruine de Bruin, McNair, Taylor, Summers, & Strough, 2014).

Hess and Queen (2014) offer the selective engagement hypothesis to explain how motivation influences age differences in cognitively effortful decisions. Because cognitive processing has greater costs for older adults than younger adults (i.e., requires more effort, is more likely to induce fatigue), older adults selectively allocate their cognitive resources and only do so when self-relevance is high (Ennis, Hess, & Smith, 2013). Indeed, adults 64 and older were more likely to use a satisficing strategy (requiring less cognitive effort) to search information when self-relevance was low, but were more likely to use a systematic search strategy (requiring more effort) when self-relevance was high; younger adults' (21–41 years) search strategies were less influenced by self-relevance (Hess, Queen, & Ennis, 2013). Research on self-relevance suggests how the decision context may shape older adults' motivation to apply deliberative skills.

Motivation and Experience. A small number of studies begin to suggest how motivation may influence experiential processing among older adults and lead to either good or bad consequences. When presented with hypothetical decisions about medical treatments, older adults tend to rely on personal experience instead of data about short- and long-term rates of survival and mortality (Woodhead, Lynch, & Edelstein, 2011). Interestingly, relying on experience buffers people of all ages against showing inconsistent preferences, but as the authors note, ignoring data when making a real-world medical decision could increase the risk of making an uninformed decision. Other research suggests that older adults are unwilling or even unable to ignore their experience (Horhota, Mienaltoski, & Blanchard-Fields, 2012). However, it has also been found that older adults switch from relying on experience to using a more analytical approach when information challenges their beliefs (Klaczynski & Robinson, 2000). These findings suggest that older adults' reliance on experiential versus deliberative skills may vary depending on motivation.

Summary. Our review illustrates how motivation may influence the deployment of deliberative, affective, and experiential skills that facilitate or undermine different facets of decision-making competence across the life span. Our review also draws attention to the importance of considering both individual characteristics and contextual demands when investigating decision-making competence. Clearly, further research is necessary to solidify the linkages outlined in our conceptual model. Hence, the final section of this chapter focuses on directions for future research.

CURRENT CHALLENGES AND DIRECTIONS FOR FUTURE RESEARCH

Linking Lab to Life. A central challenge for future research is to link performance on laboratory-based, behavioral decision-making tasks to real-world health and financial decisions (Fischhoff, 1996). Many important real-world decisions people face across the life span are tied to developmental tasks (Erikson, 1969) and life events (Norris & Murrell, 1984). In the United States, the transition to adulthood brings decisions about education, careers, long-term relationships, and starting a family. Midlife brings decisions about preventative health screening, health insurance, finances, caring for aging parents, and work–life balance. In later adulthood, medical decisions and putting one's affairs in order gain importance. Prior research on these decisions has focused more on demographic correlates (e.g., education, income) than on psychological processes.

Better performance on our A-DMC battery is associated with better life decision outcomes (e.g., not overdrawing bank accounts, not getting a DUI) as measured by our Decision Outcomes Inventory (DOI; Bruine de Bruin et al., 2007). However, decision outcomes relevant to later adulthood are not well-represented on the DOI. Research would benefit from a revised DOI, which could include outcomes corresponding to developmental tasks (e.g., making profitable financial investments, maintaining physical health, putting affairs in order) and other outcomes relevant to aging populations. For instance, in the United States, Medicare Part D requires older adults to choose a prescription plan, but their decisions often are irrational when judged in terms of their cost-effectiveness (Abaluck & Gruber, 2011). Hence, including decision outcomes corresponding to such domains could strengthen the validity of the DOI for understanding decision-making competence across the lifespan.

Another way to establish that performance on behavioral decision tasks is a valid indicator of decision-making competence is to link performance to decision-making outputs (i.e., the decisions themselves), such as financial planning, insurance purchases, and health-promotion behavior using criteria from normative theories to determine decision quality. Parker, Bruine de Bruin, Yoong, and Willis (2012) capitalized on an online panel of people of diverse ages, the American Life Panel (https://mmicdata.rand.org/alp/), to show that people with greater confidence in their knowledge were more likely to engage in retirement planning, even after controlling for actual knowledge (a measure related, but not identical, to the under/overconfidence measure in the A-DMC battery; Bruine de Bruin et al., 2007). Although useful, this approach is limited by the availability of data. Even though data on retirement and health decisions are available in large, publicly available datasets (e.g., American Life Panel; Health and Retirement Study), information about performance on behavioral decision tasks is not. Adding behavioral decision tasks to Sweden's longitudinal Betula study has facilitated understanding of how age-related memory declines affect decision-making competence (see Del Missier et al., this volume). Adding behavioral decision tasks to other national surveys could continue to address the gap in knowledge about how decision-making competence relates to real-world decisions. Data from national samples could then be used to establish norms for decision-making competence to guide judgments about decision-making capacity (see Moye, Marson, & Edelstein, 2013).

Linking performance on behavioral decision-making tasks to age-relevant, real-world decisions would also address concerns about the external validity of many phenomena identified by decision scientists in laboratory research, and the tasks used to measure those phenomena (e.g., Fischhoff, 1996). In other words, do heuristics, biases, and other decision-making phenomena observed in the laboratory translate into meaningful real-world consequences? Our initial work suggests that the answer to this question is "yes"; however, further research is necessary to solidify this conclusion.

Developing Effective Interventions. By identifying motivational, deliberative, affective, and experiential underpinnings of decision-making competencies, and linking these competencies to real-world outcomes, research can provide a basis for developing interventions to improve decisions about health and financial well-being across the life span. For example, since research shows that age-related memory declines are important for understanding age differences in some aspects of decision-making competence (e.g., Del Missier et al., 2013), reducing memory demands (e.g., by facilitating access to written information about options) and using memory training interventions (e.g., Rebok et al., 2014) could help older adults to make better use of the information provided to them. Moreover, if findings confirm that older adults pay more attention to affective information, decision aids and communication materials could aim to incorporate such information to benefit older adults' decisions (e.g., Peters et al., 2009).

Better understanding of the kinds of experiences people have had in particular decision-making contexts can inform interventions to improve decision making in those contexts (e.g., Bynum, Barre, Reed, & Passow, 2014). Ultimately, identifying individual differences in specific skills that predict different facets of decision-making competence will facilitate the development of behavioral skills training, and allow interventions to be tailored to a recipient's specific needs.

Measuring Other Elements of Decision-Making Competence. Another challenge to understanding aging and decision-making competence is the limited number of tasks that have been used to assess decision-making competence. Most studies focus on a single decision task, with few employing multiple tasks (cf. Bruine de Bruin et al., 2007; Finucane et al., 2002, 2005). The portfolio of tasks that comprise our A-DMC battery were chosen to correspond to key processes implicated by normative decision theory (Parker & Fischhoff, 2005). Well-documented age differences in affective processes and life experience (e.g., Charles & Carstensen, 2010) suggest the need to further study the skills that contribute to better decision-making competence. Because hypothetical tasks may not elicit strong emotions, it is important to study decision-making competence with real-world tasks.

Tasks developed by decision scientists studying college students in laboratories provide a starting point for identifying tasks that tap affective dimensions of decision-making competence. One candidate is a task that measures use of the affect heuristic. Risks and benefits are positively correlated in the real world, but *perceptions* of risks and benefits tend to be negatively correlated (Alhakami & Slovic, 1994). This correlation could be used as an affect-heuristic competence measure. Scores indicating higher negative correlations and greater differences in ratings of risks and benefits of technologies (e.g., nuclear power, chemotherapy) indicate greater use of the affect heuristic, signifying worse judgment (Alhakami & Slovic, 1994). Our recent work suggests that greater reliance on the affect heuristic is associated with less financial risk tolerance (Lemaster & Strough, 2014). To the extent that less financial risk tolerance predicts making less risky financial investments and therefore perhaps accruing less money, an affect heuristic task could be a useful addition to the A-DMC.

Another candidate is a task that measures the "if-only" error. Such a task involves judging the degree to which a negative outcome (e.g., a car accident) was caused by one's choices (e.g., to drive one's "typical" route versus a "new" route to enjoy the scenery; Epstein, Lipson, Holstein, & Huh, 1992). The "if-only" error occurs when less typical choices are perceived to have caused the negative outcome, which is inaccurate because the negative outcome would have been equally unpredictable. Irrational judgments are posited to stem from regret over not avoiding the seemingly more predictable negative outcome. Because older and younger adults use different coping strategies for dealing with negative events (e.g., Bruine de Bruin, Strough et al., 2014) and avoiding decision regret is important to older adults (Bjälkebring, Västjäfll, & Johannsson, 2013), their judgments may differ from those of younger adults (see Horhota et al., 2012).

Assessing preferences for temporal sequences of payment gains and losses (Loewenstein & Prelec, 1993) could tap other age-related shifts in decision competencies. When deciding about gains (e.g., salary, dividends) that increase or decrease over time, normative theories recommend choosing sequences in which larger payments are received sooner so as to optimize financial gain. Similarly, when deciding about losses (e.g., loan payments), it is recommended to make the larger payments later. However, many people choose the opposite, preferring to get losses over with and savor pending gains. Restricted life-span temporal horizons might facilitate normative decisions about temporal sequences of gains and losses. Indeed, older age has been associated with being less likely to devalue delayed monetary outcomes (e.g., Löckenhoff et al., 2011). However, such effects may depend on the larger cultural context, as well as individual differences in perceived health, among other factors (e.g., Chao, Szrek, Pereira, & Pauly, 2009).

Contextual Influences. More research is needed to understand how the immediate decision context and larger sociocultural historical context influence assessments of decision-making competence. For example, because many of the behavioral decision tasks used to assess decision-making competence were developed for use with younger adults, the content may not always motivate older adults to apply their deliberative skills. If so, standard tasks could underrepresent older adults' decision-making competence. Age-related declines in decision-making competence (e.g., Bruine de Bruin et al., 2012) could also reflect negative cultural stereotypes about aging that induce "stereotype threat," or concerns about confirming a negative stereotype. Such concerns influence older adults' memory performance (Barber & Mather, 2014) and could have similar negative consequences when assessing decision-making competence. Finally, another avenue ripe for research is to understand the social context in which individuals make important financial and health decisions. Even if a person has poor decision competence, they may not experience bad outcomes if they are able to compensate by relying on competent others. Hence, work that investigates decision making as a process that is shared (e.g., Dillard, Couper, & Zikmund-Fisher, 2010) or collaborative (see Queen, Berg, & Lowrance, this volume) may yield important insights. For example, work on everyday problem solving shows that older adults prefer to collaborate with others in domains where they perceive they have worse ability than same-age peers (Strough, Cheng, & Swenson, 2002). Preferences for collaborating with others to make decisions, for example, about health and finances, also may be domain-specific and depend upon personal views of one's ability relative to age peers.

Toward an Understanding of Decision-Making Competence Across the Life span. The generalizability of existing knowledge of aging and decision making is unclear because most studies use convenience samples to compare "extreme groups" of younger adults (often college students) to older adults. Middle-aged adults are rarely included. Yet, midlife is a distinct period of development (Lachman, 2004). Social reasoning (e.g., Hess, et al., 2005) and financial decision making (Agarwal, Driscoll, Gabaix, & Laibson, 2009) peak in midlife. Decisions made in midlife (e.g., engaging in preventative health screenings, saving for retirement) may determine outcomes experienced later in life, making it important to better understand decision-making competence during this age period. Research should also be directed toward understanding decision-making competence among those 60 and older. The "young old," "old old," and "oldest old" differ in important ways (Baltes & Smith, 2003), and decision-making competence may also vary among these groups (e.g., Finucane & Gullion, 2010).

Comparing college students to community-dwelling older adults introduces confounds that muddy the interpretation of age differences in decision-making competence. Because college students may come from different backgrounds (e.g., higher socioeconomic status) than community-dwelling adults, and people who reside in university towns may differ from adult populations more generally, such "town-gown" studies may lack external validity. Yet this approach is common in many studies, including our own (e.g., Strough et al., 2008). Using community volunteers of all ages instead of college students (e.g., Bruine de Bruin et al., 2007) or obtaining representative samples within a given city (e.g., Mikels et al., 2010) begins to address this issue. Using existing participant panels to investigate decision making is another way to address this issue. For example, the American Life Panel (described above) was designed to be nationally representative. In recent work, we leveraged this sample to examine knowledge, confidence in knowledge, and retirement planning decisions of a diverse group of adults aged 18–91 (Parker et al., 2012) and age-related improvement in decisions about sunk costs in adults aged 20–89 (Bruine de Bruin, Strough et al., 2014). Efforts to drag judgment and decision-making tasks out of psychology laboratories and introduce them to more diverse samples should continue.

As the research we have reviewed shows, the number of studies investigating age differences in decision making has increased substantially over the past 10 years. As this research area continues to grow, it will be important to begin to understand intra-individual changes in decision-making competence. To date, research can only speak to age differences, and the differences that have been identified may reflect cohort effects (e.g., Schaie, 1965), not developmental differences. Longitudinal-sequential studies are necessary to better understand developmental gains and losses in decision-making competence. Moreover, such efforts should focus on the entire life span, not just adulthood and aging (cf., Weller, Levin, Rose, & Bossard, 2012).

SUMMARY AND CONCLUSIONS

Efforts akin to Figure 2 are necessary to link judgment and decision-making research and life-span developmental theory. It is essential to obtain empirical evidence about the relative roles of motivational, experiential, and affective processes, considered as separate (although not unrelated) factors, in addition to deliberative processes. Future research should continue to investigate how performance on tasks that have been used in the judgment and decision-making literature to compare deliberative and affective/experiential decision making differ as a function of age, and how the links between decision-making competencies and life outcomes vary by age.

Existing research shows maintenance and even optimization of some aspects of decision-making competence with age, which is in accord with a key tenet of life-span theory: that development entails both losses and gains (Baltes et al., 2006). This work, however, is quite preliminary, and key pathways (e.g., the role of experience) are relatively poorly understood. Hence, future research should continue to investigate pathways that not only compensate for deliberative declines but also support maintenance and even improvement in judgment and decision making.

In closing, the challenges presented here provide fertile ground for improving the integration of judgment and decision-making research with life-span theory and research to understand the development of decision-making competence across the life span. Understanding how age-related maintenance and improvement in judgment and decision making are achieved despite age-related cognitive declines would significantly advance current understanding of aging and judgment and decision making. Ultimately, such research would inform the development of interventions for improving decisions in a variety of real-world domains and across the life span.

Acknowledgment

We gratefully acknowledge funding from the European Union Seventh Framework Program (Marie Curie Career Integration Grant 618522), the National Institute on Aging (P01AG026571), the National Institute on Drug Abuse (P50DA05605, R01DA033322), and the National Science Foundation (SES-0213782). We thank Nipat Pichayayothin, Philip Lemaster, and Rebecca Delaney for comments on a draft of this chapter and Rachel Stoiko for her assistance.

References

Abaluck, J., & Gruber, J. (2011). Heterogeneity in choice inconsistencies among the elderly: Evidence from prescription drug plan choice. *American Economic Review: Papers & Proceedings, 101*(3), 377–381.

Agarwal, S., Driscoll, J. C., Gabaix, X., & Laibson, D. (2009). The age of reason: Financial decisions over the lifecycle with implications for regulation. *Brookings Papers on Economic Activity, 2*, 51–117.

Alhakami, A. S., & Slovic, P. (1994). A psychological study of the inverse relationship between perceived risk and perceived benefit. *Risk Analysis, 14*, 1085–1096.

Arkes, H. R., & Blumer, C. (1985). The psychology of sunk cost. *Organizational Behavior and Human Decision Processes, 35*(1), 124–140.

Baltes, P. B., Lindenberger, U., & Staudinger, U. M. (2006). Life-span theory in developmental psychology. In R. M. Lerner, & W. Damon (Eds.), *Handbook of child psychology: Theoretical models of human development* (6th ed.) (Vol. 1, pp. 569–664). Hoboken, NJ: John Wiley & Sons.

Baltes, P. B., & Smith, J. (2003). New frontiers in the future of aging: from successful aging of the young old to the dilemmas of the fourth age. *Gerontology, 49*(2), 123–135.

Barber, S. J., & Mather, M. (2014). Stereotype threat in older adults: When and why does it occur, and who is most affected? In P. Verhaeghen, & C. Hertzog (Eds.), *The Oxford handbook of emotion, social cognition, and everyday problem solving during adulthood* (pp. 302–319). New York: Oxford University Press.

Bauer, A. S., Timpe, J. C., Edmonds, E. C., Bechara, A., Tranel, D., & Denburg, N. L. (2013). Myopia for the future or hypersensitivity to reward? Age-related changes in decision making on the Iowa gambling task. *Emotion, 13*(1), 19–24.

Berg, C. A., & Strough, J. (2011). Problem solving across the life span. In K. L. Fingerman, C. A. Berg, J. Smith, & T. C. Antonucci (Eds.), *Handbook of life-span development* (pp. 239–267). New York, NY: Springer Publishing Co.

Bernstein, D. M., Erdfelder, E., Meltzoff, A. N., Peria, W., & Loftus, G. R. (2011). Hindsight bias from 3 to 95 years of age. *Journal of Experimental Psychology: Learning, Memory, and Cognition, 37*(2), 378–391.

Bjälkebring, P., Västfjäll, D., & Johansson, B. (2013). Regulation of experienced and anticipated regret for daily decisions in younger and older adults in a Swedish one-week diary study. *Geropsych: The Journal of Gerontopsychology and Geriatric Psychiatry, 26*(4), 233–241.

Blanchard-Fields, F. (2007). Everyday problem solving and emotion: An adult developmental perspective. *Current Directions in Psychological Science, 16*(1), 26–31.

Bruine de Bruin, W., McNair, S. J., Taylor, A. L., Summers, B., & Strough, J. (July 2014). Thinking about numbers is not my idea of fun: Need for cognition mediates age differences in numeracy performance. *Medical Decision Making.* (Online in advance of print).

Bruine de Bruin, W., Parker, A. M., & Fischhoff, B. (2007). Individual differences in adult decision-making competence. *Journal of Personality & Social Psychology, 92*(5), 938–956.

Bruine de Bruin, W., Parker, A. M., & Fischhoff, B. (2012). Explaining adult age differences in decision-making competence. *Journal of Behavioral Decision Making, 25*, 352–360.

Bruine de Bruin, W., Parker, A. M., & Fischhoff, B. Individual differences in decision-making competence across the lifespan. In E. A. Wilhelms, & V. F. Reyna (Eds.), *Neuroeconomics, judgment, and decision making.* New York, NY: Psychology Press (in press).

Bruine de Bruin, W., Strough, J., & Parker, A. M. (2014). Getting older isn't all that bad: Better decisions and coping when facing sunk costs. *Psychology and Aging, 29*, 642–649.

Bynum, J. W., Barre, L., Reed, C., & Passow, H. (2014). Participation of very old adults in health care decisions. *Medical Decision Making, 34*(2), 216–230.

Carpenter, S. M., Peters, E., Västfjäll, D., & Isen, A. M. (2013). Positive feelings facilitate working memory and complex decision making among older adults. *Cognition and Emotion, 27*(1), 184–192.

Carstensen, L. L. (2006). The influence of a sense of time on human development. *Science, 312*(5782), 1913–1915.

Carstensen, L. L., Turan, B., Scheibe, S., Ram, N., Ersner-Hershfield, H., Samanez-Larkin, G. R., et al. (2011). Emotional experience improves with age: Evidence based on over 10 years of experience sampling. *Psychology and Aging, 26*(1), 21–33.

Chao, L. W., Szrek, H., Pereira, N. S., & Pauly, M. V. (2009). Time preference and its relationship with age, health, and survival probability. *Judgment and Decision Making, 4*, 1–19.

Charles, S., & Carstensen, L. (2010). Social and emotional aging. *Annual Review of Psychology, 61*, 383–409.

Crowe, E., & Higgins, E. (1997). Regulatory focus and strategic inclinations: Promotion and prevention in decision-making. *Organizational Behavior and Human Decision Processes, 69*(2), 117–132.

Damasio, A. R. (1994). *Descartes' error: Emotion, reason, and the human brain*. New York: Avon.

Del Missier, F., Mäntylä, T., Hansson, P., Bruine de Bruin, W., Parker, A. M., & Nilsson, L. (2013). The multifold relationship between memory and decision making: An individual-differences study. *Journal of Experimental Psychology: Learning, Memory, and Cognition, 39*(5), 1344–1364.

Depping, M. K., & Freund, A. M. (2013). When choice matters: Task-dependent memory effects in older adulthood. *Psychology and Aging, 28*(4), 923–936.

Diefendorff, J. M., Hall, R. J., Lord, R. G., & Strean, M. L. (2000). Action-state orientation: Construct validity of a revised measure and its relationship to work-related variables. *Journal of Applied Psychology, 85*(2), 250–263.

Dillard, A. J., Couper, M. P., & Zikmund-Fisher, B. J. (2010). Perceived risk of cancer and patient reports of participation in decisions about screening: The DECISIONS study. *Medical Decision Making, 30*(Suppl. 5), S96–S105.

Edwards, W. (1954). The theory of decision making. *Psychological Bulletin, 51*(4), 380–417.

Ennis, G. E., Hess, T. M., & Smith, B. T. (2013). The impact of age and motivation on cognitive effort: Implications for cognitive engagement in older adulthood. *Psychology and Aging, 28*(2), 495–504.

Epstein, S., Lipson, A., Holstein, C., & Huh, E. (1992). Irrational reactions to negative outcomes: Evidence for two conceptual systems. *Journal of Personality and Social Psychology, 62*(2), 328–339.

Erikson, E. H. (1969). *Identity: Youth and crisis*. New York, NY: Norton.

Evans, J. St. B. T. (2008). Dual-processing accounts of reasoning, judgment, and social cognition. *Annual Review of Psychology, 59*, 255–278.

Fennema, M. G., & Perkins, J. D. (2008). Mental budgeting versus marginal decision making: Training, experience, and justification effects on decisions involving sunk costs. *Journal of Behavioral Decision Making, 21*, 225–239.

Finucane, M. L., & Gullion, C. M. (2010). Developing a tool for measuring the decision-making competence of older adults. *Psychology and Aging, 25*(2), 271–288.

Finucane, M. L., Mertz, C. K., Slovic, P., & Schmidt, E. (2005). Task complexity and older adults' decision-making competence. *Psychology and Aging, 20*(1), 71–84.

Finucane, M. L., Slovic, P., Hibbard, J. H., Peters, E., Mertz, C. K., & MacGregor, D. G. (2002). Aging and decision-making competence: An analysis of comprehension and consistency skills in older versus younger adults considering health-plan options. *Journal of Behavioral Decision Making, 15*(2), 141–164.

Fischhoff, B. (1996). The real world: What good is it? *Organizational Behavior and Human Decision Processes, 65*(3), 232–248.

Gigerenzer, G. (2008). Why heuristics work. *Perspectives on Psychological Science, 3*(1), 20–29.

Hanoch, Y., Wood, S., & Rice, T. (2007). Bounded rationality, emotions and older adult decision making: Not so fast and yet so frugal. *Human Development, 50*(6), 333–358.

Henninger, D. E., Madden, D. J., & Huettel, S. A. (2010). Processing speed and memory mediate age-related differences in decision making. *Psychology and Aging*, *25*(2), 262–270.

Hess, T. M., Osowski, N. L., & Leclerc, C. M. (2005). Age and experience influences on the complexity of social inferences. *Psychology and Aging*, *20*(3), 447–459.

Hess, T. M., & Queen, T. L. (2014). Aging influences on judgment and decision processes: Interactions between ability and experience. In P. Verhaeghen, & C. Hertzog (Eds.), *Emotion, social cognition, and everyday problem solving during adulthood* (pp. 238–255). New York: Oxford University Press.

Hess, T. M., Queen, T. L., & Ennis, G. E. (2013). Age and self-relevance effects on information search during decision making. *Journals of Gerontology Series B: Psychological Sciences & Social Sciences*, *68*(5), 703–711.

Hess, T. M., Queen, T. L., & Patterson, T. R. (2012). To deliberate or not to deliberate: Interactions between age, task characteristics, and cognitive activity on decision making. *Journal of Behavioral Decision Making*, *25*(1), 29–40.

Horhota, M., Mienaltowski, A. M., & Blanchard-Fields, F. (2012). If only I had taken my usual route...age-related differences in counterfactual thinking. *Age, Neuropsychology and Cognition*, *19*(3), 339–361.

Isen, A. M., Nygren, T. E., & Ashby, F. G. (1988). Influence of positive affect on the subjective utility of gains and losses: It is just not worth the risk. *Journal of Personality and Social Psychology*, *55*, 710–717.

Jacobs, J. E., Greenwald, J. P., & Osgood, D. W. (1995). Developmental differences in baserate estimates of social behaviors and attitudes. *Social Development*, *4*, 165–181.

Johnson, E. J., & Tversky, A. (1983). Affect, generalization, and the perception of risk. *Journal of Personality and Social Psychology*, *45*, 20–31.

Kahneman, D. (2003). A perspective on judgment and choice: Mapping bounded rationality. *American Psychologist*, *58*(9), 697–720.

Kahneman, D., Slovic, P., & Tversky, A. (1982). *Judgment under uncertainty: Heuristics and biases*. Cambridge, England: Cambridge University Press.

Keren, G., & Bruine de Bruin, W. (2003). On the assessment of decision quality: Considerations regarding utility, conflict, and accountability. In D. Hardman, & L. Macchi (Eds.), *Thinking: Psychological perspectives on reasoning, judgment and decision making* (pp. 347–363). New York, NY: Wiley.

Kim, S., & Hasher, L. (2005). The attraction effect in decision making: Superior performance by older adults. *Quarterly Journal of Experimental Psychology*, *58A*(1), 120–133.

Klaczynski, P. A., & Robinson, B. (2000). Personal theories, intellectual ability, and epistemological beliefs: Adult age differences in everyday reasoning biases. *Psychology and Aging*, *15*(3), 400–416.

Kuhberger, A. (1998). The influence of framing on risky decisions: A meta-analysis. *Organizational Behavior and Human Decision Processes*, *75*, 23–55.

Lachman, M. E. (2004). Development in midlife. *Annual Review of Psychology*, *55*(1), 305–331.

Larrick, R. P., Morgan, J. N., & Nisbett, R. E. (1990). Teaching the use of cost-benefit reasoning in everyday life. *Psychological Science*, *1*(6), 362–370.

Lemaster, P., & Strough, J. (2014). Understanding age differences in financial risk tolerance: Temporal horizons and affect. In J. Strough, & C. Löckenhoff (Chairs), *Age differences in decision making: Balancing affect and reason in financial and healthcare settings. Symposium conducted at the meeting of Gerontological Society of America, Washington, D.C.*

Levin, I. P., & Gaeth, G. J. (1988a). How consumers are affected by the framing of attribute information before and after consuming the product. *Journal of Consumer Research*, *15*(3), 374–378.

Levin, I. P., & Gaeth, G. J. (1988b). Framing of attribute information before and after consuming the product. *Journal of Consumer Research*, *15*, 374–378.

Li, Y., Baldassi, M., Johnson, E. J., & Weber, E. U. (2013). Complementary cognitive capabilities, economic decision making, and aging. *Psychology and Aging*, *28*(3), 595–613.

Löckenhoff, C. E., & Carstensen, L. L. (2007). Aging, emotion, and health-related decision strategies: Motivational manipulations can reduce age differences. *Psychology and Aging, 22*(1), 134–146.

Löckenhoff, C. E., O'Donoghue, T., & Dunning, D. (2011). Age differences in temporal discounting: The role of dispositional affect and anticipated emotions. *Psychology and Aging, 26*(2), 274–284.

Loewenstein, G. W., & Prelec, D. (1993). Preferences for sequences of outcomes. *Psychological Review, 100*, 91–108.

Loewenstein, G. F., Weber, E. U., Hsee, C. K., & Welch, N. (2001). Risks as feelings. *Psychological Bulletin, 127*(2), 267–286.

Mata, R., Josef, A. K., Samanez-Larkin, G. R., & Hertwig, R. (2011). Age differences in risky choice: A meta-analysis. [Special issue]. *Annals of the New York Academy of Sciences, 1235*, 18–29.

Mata, R., Schooler, L. J., & Rieskamp, J. (2007). The aging decision maker: Cognitive aging and the adaptive selection of decision strategies. *Psychology and Aging, 22*, 796–810.

Mikels, J. A., Cheung, E., Cone, J., & Gilovich, T. (November 19, 2012). The dark side of intuition: Aging and increases in nonoptimal intuitive decisions. *Emotion, 13*(2), 189–195.

Mikels, J. A., Loeckenhoff, C. E., Maglio, S. J., Carstensen, L. L., Goldstein, M. K., & Garber, A. (2010). Following your heart or your head: Focusing on emotions versus information differentially influences the decisions of younger and older adults. *Journal of Experimental Psychology: Applied, 16*(1), 87–95.

Mikels, J. A., & Reed, A. E. (2009). Monetary losses do not loom large in later life: Age differences in the framing effect. *The Journals of Gerontology: Series B: Psychological Sciences and Social Sciences, 64B*(4), 457–460.

Molden, D., & Hui, C. (2011). Promoting de-escalation of commitment: A regulatory focus perspective on sunk costs. *Psychological Science, 22*(1), 8–12.

Moye, J., Marson, D. C., & Edelstein, B. (2013). Assessment of capacity in an aging society. *American Psychologist, 68*(3), 158–171.

Norris, F. H., & Murrell, S. A. (1984). Protective function of resources related to life events, global stress, and depression in older adults. *Journal of Health and Social Behavior, 25*, 424–437.

Osman, M. (2004). An evaluation of dual-process theories of reasoning. *Psychonomic Bulletin & Review, 11*(6), 988–1010.

Park, D. C., Lautenschlager, G., Hedden, T., Davidson, N. S., Smith, A. D., & Smith, P. K. (2002). Models of visuospatial and verbal memory across the adult life span. *Psychology and Aging, 17*(2), 299–320.

Parker, A. M., Bruine de Bruin, W., Yoong, J., & Willis, R. (2012). Inappropriate confidence and retirement planning: Four studies with a national sample. *Journal of Behavioral Decision Making, 25*, 382–389.

Parker, A. M., & Fischhoff, B. (2005). Decision-making competence: External validation through an individual-differences approach. *Journal of Behavioral Decision Making, 18*(1), 1–27.

Peters, E., & Bruine de Bruin, W. (2012). Aging and decision skills. In M. K. Dhami, A. Schlottmann, & M. Waldmann (Eds.), *Judgment and decision making as a skill: Learning, development, and evolution*. Cambridge University Press.

Peters, E., Dieckmann, N. F., Västfjäll, D., Mertz, C. K., Slovic, P., & Hibbard, J. H. (2009). Bringing meaning to numbers: The impact of evaluative categories on decisions. *Journal of Experimental Psychology: Applied, 15*(3), 213–227.

Peters, E., Dieckmann, N. E., & Weller, J. (2011). Age differences in complex decision making. In K. W. Schaie, & S. L. Willis (Eds.), *Handbook of the psychology of aging* (7th ed.) (pp. 133–151). San Diego, CA: Elsevier Academic Press.

Peters, E., Hess, T. M., Västfjäll, D., & Auman, C. (2007). Adult age differences in dual information processes: Implications for the role of affective and deliberative processes in older adults' decision making. *Perspectives on Psychological Sciences, 2*(1), 1–23.

Raiffa, H. (1968). *Decision analysis*. Reading, MA: Addison-Wesley.
Rebok, G., Ball, K., Guey, L. T., Jones, R. N., Kim, H., King, J., et al. (2014). Ten-year effects of the ACTIVE cognitive training trial on cognition and everyday functioning in older adults. *Journal of American Geriatrics Society, 62*, 16–24.
Reyna, V. F. (2004). How people make decisions that involve risk: A dual-process approach. *Current Directions in Psychological Science, 13*(2), 60–66.
Reyna, V. F., Chick, C. F., Corbin, J. C., & Hsia, A. N. (2014). Developmental reversals in risky decision making: Intelligence agents show larger decision biases than college students. *Psychological Science, 25*(1), 76–84.
Salthouse, T. A. (1996). The processing-speed theory of adult age differences in cognition. *Psychological Review, 103*(3), 403–428.
Salthouse, T. A. (2004). What and when of cognitive aging. *Current Directions in Psychological Science, 13*(4), 140–144.
Schaie, K. W. (1965). A general model for the study of developmental problems. *Psychological Bulletin, 64*(2), 92–107.
Shafir, E., & LeBoeuf, R. A. (2002). Rationality. *Annual Review of Psychology, 53*, 491–517.
Simon, H. A. (1956). Rational choice and the structure of the environment. *Psychological Review, 63*(2), 129–138.
Slovic, P., Finucane, M., Peters, E., & MacGregor, D. G. (2002). Rational actors or rational fools: Implications of the affect heuristic for behavioral economics. *The Journal of Socio-Economics, 31*(4), 329–342.
Strough, J., Cheng, S., & Swenson, S. (2002). Preferences for collaborative and individual everyday problem solving in later adulthood. *International Journal of Behavioral Development, 26*(1), 26–35.
Strough, J., Karns, T., & Schlosnagle, L. (2011). Decision-making heuristics and biases across the life span. [Special issue]. *Annals of the New York Academy of Sciences, 1235*, 57–74.
Strough, J., & Keener, E. J. (2014). Goals and strategies for solving interpersonal everyday problems across the life span. In P. Verhaeghen, & C. Hertzog (Eds.), *Emotion, social cognition and everyday problem solving during adulthood* (pp. 190–205). New York: Oxford University Press.
Strough, J., Mehta, C. M., McFall, J. P., & Schuller, K. L. (2008). Are older adults less subject to the sunk-cost fallacy than younger adults? *Psychological Science, 19*(7), 650–652.
Strough, J., Schlosnagle, L., & DiDonato, L. (2011). Understanding decisions about sunk costs from older and younger adults' perspectives. *The Journals of Gerontology Series B: Psychological Sciences and Social Sciences, 66B*(6), 681–686.
Strough, J., Schlosnagle, L., Karns, T., Lemaster, P., & Pichayayothin, N. (2014). No time to waste: Restricting life-span temporal horizons decreases the sunk-cost fallacy. *Journal of Behavioral Decision Making, 27*(1), 78–94.
Tentori, K., Osherson, D., Hasher, L., & May, C. (2001). Wisdom and aging: Irrational preferences in college students but not older adults. *Cognition, 81*(3), 87–96.
Thomas, A. K., & Millar, P. R. (2012). Reducing the framing effect in older and younger adults by encouraging analytic processing. *Journals of Gerontology Series B: Psychological Sciences & Social Sciences, 67B*(2), 139–149.
Tversky, A., & Kahneman, D. (1974). Judgment under uncertainty: Heuristics and biases. *Science, 185*(4157), 1124–1131.
Tversky, A., & Kahneman, D. (1981). The framing of decisions and the psychology of choice. *Science, 211*(4481), 453–458.
van Putten, M., Zeelenberg, M., & van Dijk, E. (2010). Who throws good money after bad? Action versus state orientation moderates the sunk cost fallacy. *Judgment and Decision Making, 5*(1), 33–36.
Weller, J. A., Levin, I. P., & Denburg, N. L. (2011). Trajectory of risky decision making for potential gains and losses from ages 5 to 85. *Journal of Behavioral Decision Making, 24*(4), 331–344.

Weller, J. A., Levin, I. P., Rose, J. P., & Bossard, E. (2012). Assessment of decision-making competence in preadolescence. *Journal of Behavioral Decision Making*, *25*(4), 414–426.

Wood, S., Busemeyer, J., Koling, A., Cox, C., & Davis, H. (2005). Older adults as adaptive decision makers: Evidence from the Iowa gambling task. *Psychology and Aging*, *20*, 220–225.

Wood, S., Hanoch, Y., Barnes, A., Liu, P., Cummings, J., Bhattacharya, C., et al. (2011). Numeracy and medicare Part D: The importance of choice and literacy for numbers in optimizing decision making for medicare's prescription drug program. *Psychology and Aging*, *26*(2), 295–307.

Woodhead, E. L., Lynch, E. B., & Edelstein, B. A. (2011). Decisional strategy determines whether frame influences treatment preferences for medical decisions. *Psychology and Aging*, *26*(2), 285–294.

Yates, J. F. (1990). *Judgment and decision making*. Englewood Cliffs, NJ: Prentice Hall.

Yates, J. F., & Patalano, A. L. (1999). Decision making and aging. In D. Park, R. Morrell, & K. Shifren (Eds.), *Processing of medical information in aging patients: Cognitive and human factors perspectives* (pp. 31–54). Mahwah, NJ: Erlbaum.

Zajonc, R. B. (1980). Feeling and thinking: Preferences need no inference. *American Psychologist*, *35*, 151–175.

SECTION 3

APPLIED PERSPECTIVES

CHAPTER

13

Decision Making and Health Literacy among Older Adults

Daniel Morrow, Jessie Chin

Department of Educational Psychology, University of Illinois at Urbana-Champaign, Champaign, IL, USA

INTRODUCTION

The health-care system is rapidly changing in ways that increase the importance of patient comprehension and decision making for managing health. Patient-centered care and shared decision-making paradigms, while intended to empower patients, also shift responsibility to them and contribute to the complexity of self-managing wellness and illness (McNutt, 2004). As a result, patients make many decisions when navigating the health-care system. They choose insurance plans that involve trade-offs of cost (premiums vs deductibles) and benefits (what is covered and at what level), especially with the implementation of the Affordable Care Act. They choose providers within the constraints imposed by insurance decisions. They make decisions about preventative care that involve balancing risks and benefits related to screening tests, diet, exercise, and other choices. They also decide when symptoms are worth a doctor visit, and may decide in collaboration with providers about diagnostic tests and treatment. Self-managing chronic illness requires decisions that may change lifestyle, such as developing and implementing self-care plans in the context of daily life (e.g., when and how to take medications, or whether a symptom is a side-effect of the medication or of the illness).

As these examples illustrate, health-related decisions made by patients are often *complex*. They require integration of dynamic and uncertain information from multiple sources (e.g., primary care physician, specialists, insurance companies, caregivers) in order to understand the problem or issue (Mitzner, Barg-Walkow, McBride, & Rogers, 2013). The decisions

http://dx.doi.org/10.1016/B978-0-12-417148-0.00013-3

are about emotional, value-laden issues (e.g., decisions about life-threatening illness and transitions of care). They may also interact (e.g., decisions about diet influence decisions about which medications to take and how). Whereas collaboration with providers can help patients understand and make health decisions, this collaboration can be inadequate because of limited coordination among multiple providers and caregivers that complicates information interpretation. Thus, patients' decisions can be compared to those made by experts in high-stakes domains (e.g., financial analysts, pilots), who make decisions under dynamic uncertain conditions that require understanding the problem situation. However, patients may lack the knowledge and experience that promote effective decision making under such conditions.

OLDER ADULTS AND HEALTH DECISIONS

Decision making is especially important to older adults' health. Older adults are the typical patient in our health-care system because they are more likely than younger adults to have chronic illness and therefore have to navigate the health-care system and make complex decisions (Centers for Disease Control and Prevention, 2011). In the present chapter, we consider decision making in the context of self-managing illness, which requires cognitive and affective processes. For example, understanding illness and working with providers to develop treatment plans (e.g., taking medications) require finding, understanding, and integrating relevant information in order to develop a plan of action, in part by evaluating options. These processes in turn require patient cognitive resources related to literacy and numeracy. They also depend on affective resources. For example, integrating and evaluating information about treatment options may turn on affective responses to illness and its impact on daily life. In this section we consider age-related changes in these resources in relation to health-care system support for decision making.

Health Literacy, Comprehension, and Decision Making

Health literacy (HL), or the ability to find, understand, communicate, and act on information needed to navigate the health-care system, is central to health decision making (Nielson-Bohlman, Panzer, & Kindig, 2004). It is often measured by simple tests such as the REALM (Rapid Estimate of Adult Literacy in Medicine), which involves pronouncing health-related words that vary in difficulty ("fat" vs "osteoporosis"; Davis et al., 1993), and the TOFHLA (Test of Functional Health Literacy in Adults), which involves reading and answering questions about health passages (Baker, 2006). Older adults with lower scores on such tests tend to use fewer preventative services, need more treatment services, receive less system support such as effective provider/patient communication, and are more likely to die at a younger age (Bostock & Steptoe, 2012).

It is generally agreed that HL is a multifaceted concept and there is a need to identify abilities that underlie relationships between HL measures and health behaviors and outcomes in order to develop interventions to support patients with diverse abilities (Berkman, Davis, & McCormack, 2010). Because HL requires reading and quantitative reasoning, abilities related to literacy and numeracy are central (Apter et al., 2008; DeWalt & Pignone, 2005). We have integrated the concept of HL with theories of cognitive aging and language comprehension to develop a process-knowledge framework that identifies HL-related cognitive abilities. In previous work, we focused on abilities that influence language comprehension (Chin et al., 2011). In the present chapter, we expand the framework to address HL-related abilities related to decision making. The expanded framework includes comprehension of numeric as well as linguistic information, and conceptualizes affect as well as cognition as patient resources relevant to HL. These additions are important for analyzing health-related decisions among older adults.

According to this framework, depicted in Figure 1, self-care behaviors require decisions that involve searching for and finding information, understanding the information and its implications for self-care, and developing a plan of action based on this understanding. These components in turn reflect complex abilities related to understanding linguistic information (literacy) and numeric information (numeracy). The latter ability requires understanding and using probabilistic and mathematical concepts (Apter et al., 2008). Literacy and numeracy in turn depend

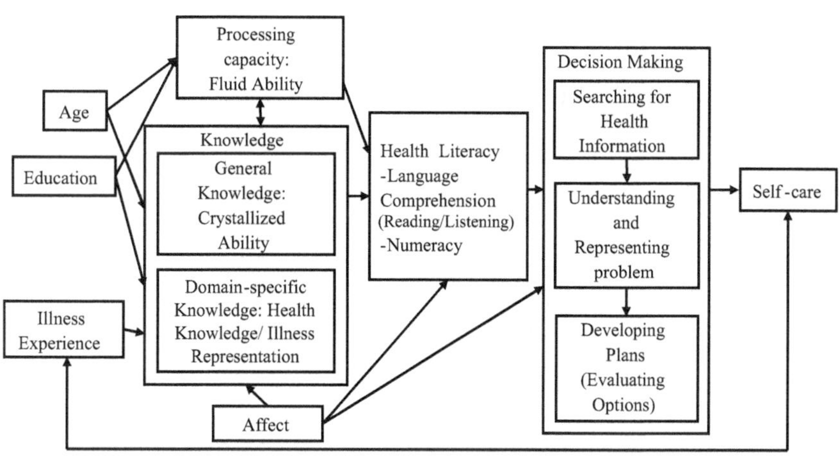

FIGURE 1 The process–knowledge model of health literacy. *Adapted from Chin et al. (2011).*

on broader cognitive abilities, or resources, related to processing capacity and knowledge. Because literacy and numeracy are influenced by affective processes, affect is conceptualized as another patient resource in the framework. An important implication of the framework is that HL reflects the interplay between age-related declines in some abilities or resources (e.g., processing capacity) and age-related gains in others (e.g., knowledge and affect; see Li, Baldassi, Johnson, & Weber, 2013 for a similar model applied to financial literacy and decision making).

In the rest of this section we focus on language comprehension as an example of how cognitive resources influence HL because of the large body of theoretical and empirical work on processes and representations involved in language comprehension. We then briefly consider comprehension of numeric information. In later sections of the chapter, we address decision making more directly, and return to comprehension as part of decision making.

The Role of Language Comprehension

Comprehension involves multiple levels: a verbatim representation of the message's linguistic form, a propositional representation of the meaning directly conveyed by the message (the textbase), and a situation model of the events described by the message (Kintsch, 1998). Whether viewed as concrete representations of perceptual-motor experience (Zwaan, 1999) or more abstract gist-based representations (Reyna, 2008), situation models created by patients help capture the "bottom line" of health information. They reflect high-level structure of the described situations, often organized around evaluative and affective categories (Is risk high or low? Is it increasing over time, and can it be reduced by treatment? Reyna, 2008). They are also more durable than text-based representations (Kintsch, 1998).

These representations are created by several processes. Word-level processes such as recognizing words and activating the associated concepts produce verbatim representations. Integrating these concepts into idea units or propositions and linking the propositions by coherence processes (e.g., identifying referents of anaphors) lead to the textbase. Elaborating the textbase with prior knowledge via inferences gives rise to the situation model (Kintsch, 1998). These processes in turn depend on several kinds of cognitive resources, as shown in Figure 1.

Processing Capacity

According to the process-knowledge framework, cognitive and sensory resources are central to explaining the impact of HL on health decisions, behaviors, and outcomes, especially through their impact on comprehension processes. Age declines in sensory function (e.g., visual acuity) and processing capacity (e.g., working memory) are associated with age differences in comprehension and learning, in part by reducing comprehension accuracy and thus the fidelity of representations. For example, age-related processing capacity declines undermine conceptual integration and impair the textbase, especially when comprehension is demanding (e.g., Stine-Morrow & Miller, 2009).

Not surprisingly then, processing capacity measures help explain performance on HL measures such as the REALM and STOFHLA (Chin et al., 2011). They account for a large amount of education- and age-related variance in performance on these measures (Chin et al., 2011; Levinthal et al., 2008; Wolf et al., 2012) and are more important than education for predicting health status (Gottfredson & Deary, 2004). This finding may reflect the fact that literacy and numeracy skills are both a product of education (Peters, Baker, Dieckmann, Leon, & Collins, 2010) and a prerequisite for educational advances (Ceci & Papierno, 2005).

Knowledge

While processing capacity tends to decline with age, general knowledge (linguistic/verbal knowledge, or crystallized ability) and domain-specific knowledge tend to remain unchanged or increase (Horn & Cattell, 1967). Knowledge gains reflect accumulating literacy experience that support word knowledge (Stanovich, West, & Harrison, 1995) and domain knowledge (Beier & Ackerman, 2005). Health knowledge can also increase with illness experience (Chin, D'Andrea, et al., 2009), perhaps reflecting illness-related literacy activities (Wister, Malloy-Weir, Rootman, & Desjardins, 2010) and accumulating general knowledge (Beier & Ackerman, 2005). Such knowledge is critical for helping older adults develop situation models that support health decisions and behaviors (Chin et al., 2014). Thus, inadequate health knowledge is a critical limitation on self-care among older adults with low HL.

Whereas age-related processing capacity limits can impair comprehension, knowledge gains streamline comprehension processes so that they depend less on processing capacity. Less common and longer words are accessed more quickly by high-verbal older adults, perhaps because word recognition processes are more likely automatized. Knowledge structures or schemas derived from literacy engagement facilitate conceptual integration (e.g., links between concepts mentioned in the text are readily available from long-term memory; Stine-Morrow & Miller, 2009), or support allocation of processing resources to integration (Chin et al., 2014) in order to create more accurate textbase and situation model representations. Similarly, illness experience can increase health knowledge, which facilitates word recognition and promotes resource allocation to conceptual integration, and in turn improves comprehension (Chin et al., 2014).

Consistent with these knowledge-related benefits for comprehension, knowledge also improves performance on tests of HL (Chin et al., 2011) and comprehension of health information (Chin et al., 2014; Miller, Stine-Morrow, Kirkorian, & Conroy, 2004), although little research has teased apart effects of general and health knowledge (but see Beier & Ackerman, 2005; Chin et al., 2014). Of course, these findings also suggest that patients with inadequate HL struggle to navigate the health system because they lack knowledge that supports effective comprehension and decision making.

Affect

Affect and emotion may be another age-related asset that is important for developing HL (Edwards, Wood, Davies, & Edwards, 2012) and for responding to health information (Fagerlin & Peters, 2011), in part because patients often face emotionally charged decisions and socioemotional goals may become more important in later life (Charles & Carstensen, 2010). Older adults often rely on affective information during comprehension, creating more affectively nuanced situation models with emotional information better remembered compared to younger adults (Charles & Carstensen, 2010). Affect influences learning of health information in part because of its impact on interest and motivation (Beier & Ackerman, 2005; Edwards et al., 2012). Affect and emotion influence decision making directly as well as through their influence on resource allocation to comprehension. According to dual-process models, older adults may rely more than younger adults do on intuitive, affect-based processes rather than on more deliberative processes such as evaluating options (Peters, Hess, Västfjäll, & Auman, 2007). This in turn may ease the strain on processing resources due to the low demands associated with processing affective content.

Illness Representation

The concept of illness representation integrates patient knowledge and affect in terms of self-care. According to patient-centered models of health care, patients make self-care decisions as part of making sense of their illness, which depends on illness representations (Meyer, Leventhal, & Gutmann, 1985) or explanatory models (Bokhour et al., 2012). These representations integrate illness knowledge (e.g., cause, time-course, consequences) with affective reactions to the impact of the illness on daily life, thus emphasizing that cognitive and affective resources relevant to HL interact to influence self-care through self-regulatory processes (Meyer et al., 1985). Patients with lower HL may have less adaptive illness representations that undermine self-care behaviors such as medication adherence. They are more likely to view their illness as acute rather than chronic and caused by temporary factors such as stress (Federman, Wisnivesky, Wolf, Leventhal, & Halm, 2010; also see Bokhour et al., 2012). These beliefs in turn may influence health decisions and behaviors (e.g., medication adherence).

Interplay of Processing Capacity, Knowledge, and Affect

The framework depicted in Figure 1, and the literature reviewed above, suggest that age-related knowledge gains, and perhaps an increasing role of affect, offset processing-capacity limits in order to support HL, decisions, behaviors, and outcomes. These resources may facilitate comprehension and reduce demands on processing capacity. Increasing reliance on knowledge and affect may also lead to more adaptive illness representations that promote allocation of processing capacity to support decision making.

Evidence for the prediction that knowledge offsets processing capacity comes from the finding that high levels of general or health knowledge are associated with better HL (Chin et al., 2011) and comprehension of self-care information (Chin et al., 2014) regardless of processing-capacity level; while among patients with less knowledge, processing capacity determines performance (see Li et al., 2013 for a similar interaction in predicting financial decision making). For example, older adults who know more about their hypertension tend to have more adaptive representations of their illness (better understanding, such as the fact that the illness is chronic; higher perceived control over the illness), which may support self-management (Chin, D'Andrea et al., 2009).

Numeracy

We briefly consider comprehension of numeric as well as linguistic information because of its importance to health decisions. For example, numeracy is often critical for understanding risk and other concepts important to evaluating options related to health (Brust-Renck, Royer, & Reyna, 2013). Like HL more generally, numeracy tends to be lower for older adults (Apter et al., 2008), perhaps because it is closely related to quantitative reasoning, which is associated with processing capacity (Carroll, 1993). Like words, numbers can be understood at a verbatim level (precise numeric values) and at a gist level. The latter reflects understanding numeric information in terms of goals and knowledge in order to act on the information to improve health. It often requires integrating cognitive meaning (e.g., How great is my risk of stroke given my family history?) and affective meaning (Do I feel reassured or threatened by this risk?) in terms of knowledge, including knowledge of numbers (Reyna, 2008).

Taken together, the studies reviewed in this section suggest that older adults integrate knowledge with affect to develop illness representations that support comprehension of linguistic and numeric information and decisions about their health, although we will see that this depends in part on the complexity of health decisions.

AGING, HEALTH LITERACY, AND HEALTH-RELATED DECISIONS

In the rest of the chapter, we review literature on aging and decision making in order to consider in more detail how relationships among HL-related resources influence older adults' health decisions. To do this, we integrate comprehension into a three-stage model of decision making related to self-managing chronic illness, as shown in Figure 1: (1) searching for and finding information, (2) understanding the information in order to represent the health problem or issue, and (3) developing an action plan, often involving choosing among options. We next briefly describe each stage, which will organize our review of studies about aging and decision making in self-care. While described sequentially, these stages often interact and overlap when people make health decisions.

Decision-Making Processes and Their Influence on Self-Care

Searching for Health Information

Patients often search for information on the Internet, which is increasingly the only source available for information needed to make health decisions (Bass, 2003). In the United States, 75–80% of Internet users look online for health information (American Life and Pew Internet Report, 2011). About 20% of adults over age 65 use the Internet and 80% search online for health information (American Life and Pew Internet Report, 2011). Furthermore, roughly one-third of older users claim their health-related decisions are influenced by online information (Flynn, Smith, & Freese, 2006). Among patients with chronic disease, 75% of those using the Internet report that their last health search affected a treatment decision.

In short, online health information has become an important second opinion for older patients making health-related decisions. However, finding this information is often challenging. Appropriate search terms must be generated in light of goals, search results must be evaluated, and search terms refined or the most relevant results chosen, requiring interpretation and selection of links. Knowledge may support search by streamlining processes (e.g., constraining search to the most relevant information; supporting integration of found information). These processes require processing capacity as well as general knowledge, health knowledge, and knowledge about the Internet (Sharit, Hernandez, Czaja, & Pirolli, 2008). Health technology has the potential to facilitate search for and interpretation of health information. For example, patient portals, a standard feature of many Electronic Health Record (EHR) systems, provide patients ready access to information about their conditions and treatments. However, portals currently function more as information repositories that are challenging to access and use than as tools that promote patient self-care (Morrow & Chin, 2012; Taha, Czaja, Sharit, & Morrow, 2013). Therefore, search for health information likely depends on the interplay between patients' processing capacity and knowledge, as well as characteristics of health tasks and technology.

Understanding Health Problems

Once found, patients interpret health information in terms of general knowledge and knowledge of their illness and treatment in order to create a situation model, or mental model of the problem situation ("situation awareness"; Durso, Rawson, & Girotto, 2007). These problem representations depend greatly on patients' illness representations, which can support self-care decisions and lead to better health outcomes (Leventhal, Safer, & Panagis, 1983; Petrie & Weinman, 2012). For example, older adults with more accurate illness representations (e.g., understanding their illness is chronic, which promotes sense of control over the illness) better adhere to medications (Ross, Walker, & MacLeod, 2004). Accurate illness representations can also reflect understanding of how self-care procedures, such as monitoring symptoms, influence illness progression (Lippa, Klein, & Shalin, 2008; Sun et al., 2013).

As outlined earlier, comprehension of health information is often challenging. Conceptually dense passages tax processing capacity and disadvantage older adults' comprehension (Stine-Morrow & Miller, 2009). Older adults also have difficulty understanding health-related passages that contain uncommon concepts and that are poorly organized (Morrow et al., 2005). Comprehension of numeric health information is particularly difficult for older adults (Gigerenzer, Gaissmaier, Kurz-Milcke, Schwartz, & Woloshin, 2008). Patients often must understand and reason about numeric information about benefits and risks of treatments or care plans as well. Health statistics are ubiquitous in the context of health decision making, such as the survival rate of a treatment plan, the morbidity rate of an illness, or the risk of medication side effects (e.g., Baker, 2006; Reyna, Nelson, Han, & Dieckmann, 2009). They are often presented in mathematically complex forms (e.g., conditional probabilities) that are difficult for many patients (and even physicians) to understand (Gigerenzer et al., 2008). For example, patients with hypertension need to interpret their systolic and diastolic blood pressure readings with respect to target values and to make appropriate decisions (e.g., contact their provider) if the readings change over time.

Domain knowledge helps older adults develop a situation model of the health problems despite cognitive declines. For example, in aviation, older and younger expert pilots are more likely than nonexperts to focus on the most relevant information when reading scenarios in which a flight problem occurs, and make better decisions about how to respond to the problem (Morrow et al., 2009). This advantage may reflect the ability to create gist representations of the problem situation (Reyna, 2011, pp. 111–120).

Developing an Action Plan and Choosing Options

After patients construct a representation of health-related problems, they must develop a plan for action, which often involves evaluating and choosing options. Patients are continually faced with choices in order to manage their health, and considering options is challenging. For example, about 70% of older adults judged the Medicare Modernization Act (i.e., Medicare Part D) to be complicated. Part of this complexity comes from the number of plans that patients need to consider, with most states having more than 50. Reed and colleagues found that older adults preferred half the number of options as younger adults across six domains about health care and everyday decisions (Reed, Mikels, & Simon, 2008). While older adults would prefer roughly four options each for drug plans, physicians, and hospitals (4.2, 4.8, and 3.6, respectively), current health-care policy offers 10 times that number. A similar issue may exist for older adults who are just entering the health insurance system in response to the Affordable Care Act requirements, especially considering that many of the newly eligible have limited education and HL. Evaluating options associated with self-care plans taxes processing-capacity resources, especially when options must be compared in terms of multiple attributes (e.g., comparing options requires working memory capacity), although knowledge about these options and attributes may reduce these demands.

This brief description of finding, interpreting, and acting on health information suggests that these phases often interact and overlap, so that it is difficult to investigate the phases in isolation. Comprehension and interpretation in particular are integral aspects of decision making. For this reason, in the following review we consider together studies that primarily investigate information search as it relates to comprehension and interpretation, and then consider studies that focus more on choice in relation to comprehension. The review will suggest that older adults' ability to find, understand, and make decisions about linguistic and numeric health information depends on the interplay between age-related resource limitations (processing capacity) and age-related gains (knowledge, affect).

Processing Capacity and Knowledge Trade-Offs in Health Decision Making

Searching For and Understanding Health Information

Theories of information search across the life span address possible trade-offs between processing capacity constraints and knowledge-related gains when patients search for and interpret information relevant to health decisions. Sinnott (1989) described younger and older information-processing styles in decision making. A "youthful style" for gathering and organizing information involves bottom-up processing, that is, search and integration processes that are driven by the input, or information itself. This style may be adopted by people with limited knowledge but adequate processing capacity. On the other hand, an "older style" relying on top-down or expectation-driven search processes that depends more on knowledge than the data or input may be adopted by people with relevant knowledge but limited processing capacity. According to this view, individual differences in search and decision-making styles depend on decision makers' processing capacity and knowledge.

Processing capacity and health knowledge shape patients' search for self-care information on the Internet (Chin, Fu, & Kannampallil, 2009; Chin & Fu, 2010, 2012). Compared to younger adults, older adults sometimes search for less information online but spend more time on a web page (Chin, Fu et al., 2009; Chin & Fu, 2010, 2012; Sharit et al., 2008), while those with more processing capacity search more quickly and broadly (Chin, Fu et al., 2009). Interestingly, older adults are also less likely than younger adults to follow the interface-based organization and more likely to browse links under the same category consecutively during search, suggesting an age-related shift to knowledge-based, top-down search strategies (Chin, Fu et al., 2009). In a follow-up study that manipulated how information was presented on the interface, older adults were more likely to use consistently the same strategies across different interface-based organizations, while younger adults' search behaviors were more influenced by changes in interface organization (Chin & Fu, 2010). Furthermore, older adults were likely to click on links that were organized to match their knowledge, while younger adults clicked on different links regardless of their knowledge structures (Chin & Fu, 2012). Thus, in line with Sinnott's "older style," older adults used more top-down knowledge-driven search strategies in online health information search tasks, viewing less information but spending more time integrating this information. Younger adults, on the other hand, used a "youthful style" involving more bottom-up interface-driven search strategies in which they gather more information from a greater number of pages.

Developing Plans by Evaluating Options

Like finding and interpreting health information, choosing a course of action when developing a plan more or less taxes processing capacity, depending on the number of options, the extent to which the options are evaluated, the amount of prior knowledge about the problem, and other factors.

Some studies of age differences in evaluation and choice processes tend to minimize the role of search by presenting pre-organized information about multiple options in a decision task (e.g., values of different cars or political candidates across the same set of attributes presented in a matrix). These studies may also limit the role of knowledge about the options because of the structured (and perhaps unfamiliar) presentation format. Payne (1982) distinguished compensatory and noncompensatory strategies for evaluating options, and argued that compensatory strategies require processing most of the presented information, such as comparing multiple options by summing all the attribute values for each option, which places heavy demands on processing capacity. Noncompensatory strategies, on the other hand, are less resource-demanding because they require less information to make a decision, such as comparing options in terms of one attribute. Some studies using similar techniques found age differences in the quality of decisions, reflecting age differences in processing capacity (Finucane, Mertz, Slovic, & Schmidt, 2005). Other studies have found few age differences in chosen options, although younger and older adults made these decisions through different processes (Johnson, 1990, 1993; Riggle & Johnson, 1996; Queen, Hess, Ennis, Dowd, & Gruhn, 2012). For example, older adults tended to look up less information about alternatives, but spent more time considering each piece of information compared to younger adults (Mata, Schooler, & Rieskamp, 2007).

Qualitative as well as quantitative differences related to age occur in decision-making strategies. Compared to younger adults, older adults are more likely to use an "attribute shift" strategy in which they compare alternatives in terms of one attribute, and are less likely to use an "alternative shift" strategy in which they compare alternatives in terms of multiple attributes (e.g., Johnson, 1990). Thus, in this situation, older adults tend to adopt strategies that require fewer processing resources—most likely because the alternative shift strategy is more resource-demanding (Russo & Dosher, 1983). Riggle and Johnson (1996) also suggested that older adults used more systematic and top-down strategies during decision making. In a simulated voting task, participants were given a list of candidates with their positions on a set of issues. Older adults were more likely than younger adults to view the information about a specific issue across candidates ("attribute-shift" strategy). Hence, older adults using the attribute-shift strategy and systematic search patterns viewed less information than younger adults, regardless of their final decisions. However, strategy selection differences could not be explained by differences in knowledge about the attributes and alternatives (Johnson, 1993), perhaps reflecting use of problems and formats that did not encourage knowledge use.

Other approaches have examined age differences in health decision-making in tasks in which experience and knowledge may play a larger role. Gigerenzer and colleagues have examined how decision-making heuristics reflect the "ecology" of cues in the physical and social world (Todd & Gigerenzer, 2007). These researchers emphasize that people who make decisions about familiar domains can use simple and frugal heuristics that rest on knowledge about cue relationships. With experience, people identify the structure of environments and adopt the corresponding simple heuristics from their "adaptive toolbox," or repertoire of heuristics, to make decisions with "good enough" outcomes (Gigerenzer, Todd & ABC group, 1999). In other words, decision makers first evaluate the statistical structure of the tasks, such as whether the attributes of options (e.g., physicians, insurance plans) are highly correlated, and then choose an appropriate heuristic. The problem space is compensatory when attributes are poorly correlated so that options cannot be effectively evaluated based on a single attribute. For example, a patient may choose one of several treatments whose attributes (e.g., survival rates and cost) are not associated. Thus, plans with higher survival rates may not be more expensive. In this case, the patient would do well to consider the different attributes to make a decision. However, a choice among options with highly correlated attributes allows noncompensatory strategies in which the choice is made based on a single property of the alternatives. For example, patients may need to choose a hospital from a set of alternatives with highly correlated attributes, such as hospitals with higher patient review scores also having higher quality of service. Now the patient could choose the hospital based only on patient reviews. Bröder (2003) suggested that adopting heuristics depends on processing capacity. People with less processing capacity have a smaller repertoire of heuristics, which in turn leads to suboptimal decisions. For example, they may use noncompensatory strategies in tasks that require compensatory strategies.

Older adults are able to use compensatory as well as noncompensatory strategies, depending on their processing capacity and experience in the problem domain (for a review, see Mata & Nunes, 2010). Mata and colleagues (Mata et al., 2007; Mata, von Helverson, & Rieskamp, 2010) examined age differences in strategy use. With the TALLY heuristic, people equally weigh the attributes of options in a choice task, then compare the sum of these values among the options, and pick the one with the highest value. People will use this information-intensive and cognitively demanding compensatory strategy for choices that involve options with uncorrelated attributes (Gigerenzer et al., 1999). On the other hand, the TTB (take the best) heuristic is more information-frugal and less resource-demanding, focusing on the single most important attribute to make a decision. If this attribute does not discriminate the alternatives, the decision maker moves to the next most important attribute. The TTB heuristic is used in tasks with highly redundant or correlated attributes. Older adults in one study were less likely to use the compensatory TALLY strategy and more likely to use noncompensatory strategies in multiattribute decision-making tasks (Mata et al., 2007). However, across multiple trials, older adults learned the attribute structure of the choice tasks and adopted compensatory heuristics in tasks with uncorrelated attributes. Even so, they still made more errors in the compensatory situation because of inadequate use of compensatory strategies, reflecting processing-capacity limitations (Mata et al., 2010).

As noted above, health information is increasingly provided through the Internet, requiring older adults to integrate information from multiple sources in order to evaluate options in health decisions. Older adults with lower HL often have trouble navigating health sites in order to find, interpret, and make decisions about health information. For example, they have difficulty choosing insurance plans offered through the Medicare Part D program (Czaja, Sharit, & Nair, 2008) and creating self-management plans based on information from their EHR portal (Taha et al., 2013). These challenges reflect limitations related to processing capacity, numeracy, and knowledge (Sharit et al., 2008; Taha et al., 2013). Limited knowledge may become even more of a barrier with the introduction of the Affordable Care Act, because more patients with limited experience with the health-care system will need to choose insurance plans and providers.

Health knowledge plays an important role in shaping strategies when patients make personally relevant decisions, such as evaluating choices related to treatment for their illnesses. Older and younger women make similar decisions about breast cancer treatment, although the older women often consider less treatment information and make the decision more quickly (Meyer, Russo, & Talbot, 1995). Meyer and colleagues suggested that treatment knowledge facilitates treatment decisions by supporting top-down strategies that focus on the most relevant information, similar to Sinnott's proposals about "older" information-processing styles in decision making. This difference may also reflect older adults' illness representations that increase motivation to act, as has been found for medication adherence (Park et al., 1999). Later findings by Meyer et al. (2007), however, suggested a more complex picture, with health knowledge interacting with processing capacity and interest. Older adults who had more knowledge but low interest in the topic tended to make immediate decisions with less intensive processing of the information, although they took more time when interested in the topic. Older adults with less knowledge and processing capacity made more rapid decisions, but took more time when supported by more processing capacity and interest in the topic. Therefore, the impact of knowledge-driven strategies on decision making depended on processing capacity and interest. Moreover, more processing capacity encouraged more information-intensive bottom-up strategies and delayed decisions, typical of Sinnott's "youthful style."

To sum up, older adults' use of strategies to make health-related choices reflects the interaction of processing-capacity constraints and gains in knowledge from experience in health domains. This literature also suggests that older adults rely on important affective and motivational resources to help support personally relevant health decisions. We next briefly review studies that more directly investigate the role of affect in making decisions about self-care, which may help offset declines in processing capacity.

The Role of Affect in Developing Plans and Evaluating Options

Affective-related resources as well as knowledge are important for guiding older adults' decisions about self-care. In general, affect plays a larger role in how people interpret, remember, and respond to information with increasing age (Charles & Carstensen, 2010). According to dual-process models as applied by Peters et al. (2007) to age-related decision making, decisions are influenced by both deliberative processes that are effortful, information-intensive, and analytic, and by affective processes that are more intuitive, implicit, and automatic. While the role of deliberative processes in decision making may decrease as processing capacity declines across the life span, affective processes become more prominent, perhaps reflecting increasing importance of socioemotional goals (also see Charles & Carstensen, 2010). Older adults sometimes make less effective health decisions because deliberative processes (e.g., evaluating options when choosing health plans) are impaired by processing-capacity declines (Finucane et al., 2005; Peters, Diefenbach, Hess, & Västfjäll, 2008). However, they may also make better decisions by relying on affective processes that offset decreased deliberative processes. Löckenhoff and Carstensen (2007) used a multiattribute decision-making task to examine information-gathering patterns of older adults in health contexts. Older adults showed a "positivity bias," recalling and reviewing more positive than negative information compared to younger adults, although when encouraged by instructions they tended to balance review and recall of both positive and negative health information related to their decisions. In addition, older adults can make better decisions when encouraged to evaluate options affectively rather than more analytically in health-related choice tasks (Mikels et al., 2010). Reliance on affective (especially positive) information can improve or impair health decisions, depending on how diagnostic of good options the information is in the task.

Affect also influences health decisions because it is integral to illness representations that support decisions despite processing-capacity limitations (Petrie & Weinman, 2012). It is critical to gist representations of risk, perhaps one reason why gist becomes more important with age (Reyna, 2011, pp. 111–120). Gist-based strategies may compromise decision making because they neglect precise information such as the reference class in risk probabilities. However, they can also improve decisions because they are organized around evaluative dimensions that capture critical features of the health situation and support top-down decision strategies that offset limited processing capacity (Brust-Renck et al., 2013). For example, gist representations developed from experience on a health task should highlight cues that discriminate options in health tasks and thus support use of heuristics. To sum up, affect, like general and health knowledge, can be an age-related asset that supports decisions about complex health issues such as choosing providers and treatments, or developing self-care plans.

CONCLUSIONS

The process-knowledge framework suggests older adults with lower HL tend to make less effective decisions that undermine health behaviors and outcomes in part because limited processing capacity and knowledge impair the ability to search for relevant information, to interpret found information to develop a representation of the health problem, or to develop an effective plan by evaluating options (see Figure 1). It also suggests that high levels of knowledge can offset processing-capacity limits to support health behaviors and outcomes. In this chapter, we expanded this framework to focus on how age-related declines in processing capacity impair the comprehension of numeric as well as linguistic information as possible constraints on health decision making, and on affect as well as knowledge as age-related strengths that can offset processing-capacity declines. Consistent with this framework, the reviewed research suggested that age-related differences in decision making are more likely to occur when limited processing capacity impairs comprehension and other components of decision making. For example, inadequate comprehension limits older adults' health-related decision making, especially for more complex decisions that tax processing capacity (e.g., Finucane et al., 2005; Hibbard, Slovic, Peters, Finucane, & Tusler, 2001; but see; Queen et al., 2012). Age differences in using numeric risk information to support decision making are more likely to occur for older adults with low numeracy skills (Peters et al., 2009). Older adults may fail to use compensatory strategies that would improve decisions when tasks impose heavy demands on processing capacity (Mata et al., 2010). Conversely, older adults with more processing capacity tend to consider more information relevant to evaluating treatment options, although there may not be differences in the quality of the resulting decisions (Meyer, Talbot, & Ranalli, 2007).

Older adults sometimes make as effective health decisions as do younger adults (Meyer et al., 2007; Stanley, Guido, Stanley, & Shortell, 1984; Tanius, Wood & Hanoch, 2009). The absence of age differences related to decisions in these studies may reflect the role of knowledge about illness and decision options (e.g., about treatments) that enable older adults to identify the most relevant information for understanding problems and for evaluating options to respond to them, especially when health situations can be represented by affect-based gist (Mikels et al., 2010; Reyna, 2011, pp. 111–120).

Implications. Our review suggests that older adults make better decisions about self-care when they can rely on resources that increase with age (e.g., knowledge) rather than on age-vulnerable resources (processing capacity). How can older adults who have limited knowledge, and therefore cannot rely on these resources to offset processing capacity limits, be helped to make better decisions about their health? One general approach is to reduce need for processing capacity by making decisions less complex. For example, reducing the number of options to be considered might be effective, because age differences in quality are less likely for decisions with fewer options (Tanius et al., 2009). In addition, numeracy-related constraints can be addressed by presenting numeric information in more "transparent" formats that are easier to interpret, such as using frequency instead of probability or conditional probability, absolute risks rather than relative risks, and mortality rates rather than survival rates (Gigerenzer et al., 2008). For example, instead of stating that "the treatment would reduce the risk of dying from the illness by about 40%," it would be more straightforward to state that "the treatment would reduce the risk of dying from the illness by about 2/1000, from about 5 in 1000 to about 3 in 1000." Using absolute risk with natural frequencies is likely to especially benefit older adults with more limited numeracy skills. Peters and colleagues have also found that older adults make better decisions when numeric information is conveyed by verbal evaluative labels and graphic support, regardless of numeracy level (Peters et al., 2009). More generally, well-designed graphics (e.g., bar charts) can present risk-related information in ways that highlight relevant features that promote understanding of risk by patients with limited numeracy (Brust-Renck et al., 2013). Both the transparent presentation of numerical information and use of verbal and graphic formats may improve comprehension and use of numerical information by supporting gist representations of risk.

A second general approach is to increase patients' reliance on general and health knowledge when making health decisions. Knowledge can be supported in several ways, such as organizing information to match patients' representations of the health task in order to improve comprehension (Morrow & Conner-Garcia, 2013). Diagrams, concept maps, or other graphics that highlight the organization of information in health-related documents can also improve memory for self-care information, although older adults with more health knowledge may benefit more than those with less knowledge (Morrow et al., 2012). Other approaches, such as using analogies that link unknown health concepts to well-known general concepts, might improve decision making by patients with little health knowledge, and may be effective education strategies that increase health knowledge. Finally, encouraging use of affective information relevant to health tasks may provide broad benefits for older adults who vary in HL (Mikels et al., 2010; see also Mikels, Shuster, & Thai, this volume).

Acknowledgments

Preparation of this chapter was supported by the National Institute of Aging (Grants R01 AG31718) and the National Institute of Nursing Research (Grant R01 NR011300). Any opinions, findings, and conclusions or recommendations expressed in this publication are those of the authors and do not necessarily reflect the views of the NIH.

References

American life & pew internet report. (2011). Health Topics. Retrieved from http://pewinternet.org/Reports/2011/HealthTopics.aspx.

Apter, A. J., Paasche-Orlow, M. K., Remillard, J. T., Bennett, I. M., Ben-Joseph, E. P., Batista, R. M., et al. (2008). Numeracy and communication with patients: They are counting on us. *Journal of General Internal Medicine, 23*, 2117–2124.

Baker, D. W. (2006). The meaning and the measure of health literacy. *Journal of General Internal Medicine, 21*, 878–883.

Bass, S. B. (2003). How will internet use affect the patient: A review of computer network and interactive technology studies and the implications in understanding how the use of the Internet affects patient populations. *Journal of Health Psychology, 8*, 25–38.

Beier, M. E., & Ackerman, P. L. (2005). Age, ability and the role of prior knowledge on the acquisition of new domain knowledge. *Psychology & Aging, 20*, 341–355.

Berkman, N. D., Davis, T. C., & McCormack, L. (2010). Health literacy: What is it? *Journal of Health Communication, 15*, 9–19.

Bokhour, B. G., Cohn, E. S., Cortes, D. E., et al. (2012). The role of patients' explanatory models and daily-lived experience in hypertension self-management. *Journal of General Internal Medicine, 27*, 1626–1634.

Bostock, S., & Steptoe, A. (2012). Association between low functional health literacy and mortality in older adults: Longitudinal cohort study. *British Medical Journal, 344*.

Bröder, A. (2003). Decision making with the "adaptive toolbox": Influence of environmental structure, intelligence, and working memory load. *Journal of Experimental Psychology: Learning, Memory, and Cognition, 29*, 611–625.

Brust-Renck, P. G., Royer, C. E., & Reyna, V. F. (2013). Communicating numerical risk: Human factors that aid understanding in health care. *Reviews of Human Factors and Ergonomics, 8*, 235–276.

Carroll, J. B. (1993). *Human cognitive abilities: A survey of factor-analytical studies*. New York: Cambridge University Press.

Ceci, S. J., & Papierno, P. B. (2005). The rhetoric and reality of gap closing: When the "have-nots" gain but the "haves" gain even more. *American Psychologist, 60*, 149–160.

Centers for Disease Control and Prevention (CDC). (2011). *National diabetes fact sheet: National estimates and general information on diabetes and prediabetes in the United States*. Atlanta, GA: U.S. Department of Health and Human Services, Centers for Disease Control and Prevention.

Charles, S. T., & Carstensen, L. L. (2010). Social and emotional aging. *Annual Review of Psychology, 61*, 383–409.

Chin, J., D'Andrea, L., Morrow, D. G., Stine-Morrow, E. A. L., Conner-Garcia, T., Murray, M. D., et al. (2009). Cognition and illness experience are associated with illness knowledge among older adults with hypertension. In *Proceedings of the 53rd annual meeting of the human factors and ergonomics society 2009* (pp. 116–120). San Antonio, TX: Human Factors and Ergonomics Society.

Chin, J., & Fu, W.-T. (2010). Interactive effects of age and interface differences on search strategies and performance. In *Proceedings of the 28th ACM conference on human factors in computing systems CHI'10* (pp. 403–412). Atlanta, GA: ACM Press.

Chin, J., & Fu, W.-T. (2012). Age differences in exploratory learning from a health information website. In *Proceedings of the 30th ACM conference on human factors in computing systems CHI'12* (pp. 3031–3040). Austin, TX: ACM Press.

Chin, J., Fu, W.-T., & Kannampallil, T. (2009). Adaptive information search: Age-dependent interactions between cognitive profiles and strategies. In *Proceedings of the 27th ACM conference on human factors in computing systems CHI'09* (pp. 1683–1692). Boston, MA: ACM Press.

Chin, J., Morrow, D., Stine-Morrow, E. A. L., Conner-Garcia, T., Graumlich, J. F., & Murray, M. D. (2011). The process-knowledge model of health literacy: Evidence from a componential analysis of two commonly used measures. *Journal of Health Communication, 16*, 222–241.

Chin, J., Payne, B., Gao, X., Conner-Garcia, T., Graumlich, J. F., Murray, M. D., Morrow, D. G., & Stine-Morrow, E. A. (2014). Memory and comprehension for health information among older adults: Distinguishing the effects of domain-general and domain-specific knowledge. *Memory, April, 30*, 1–13 epub ahead of print.

Czaja, S. J., Sharit, J., & Nair, S. N. (2008). Usability of the Medicare health web site. *JAMA, 300*(7), 790–792.

Davis, T. C., Long, S. W., Jackson, R. H., Mayeaux, E. J., George, R. B., Murphy, P. W., et al. (1993). Rapid estimate of adult literacy in medicine: A shortened screening instrument. *Family Medicine, 25*, 391.

DeWalt, D. A., & Pignone, M. P. (2005). Reading is fundamental: The relationship between literacy and health. *Archives of Internal Medicine, 165*, 1943–1944.

Durso, F. T., Rawson, K. A., & Girotto, S. (2007). Comprehension and situation awareness. In F. T. Durso, R. S. Nickerson, S. T. Dumais, S. Lewandowsky, & T. J. Perfect (Eds.), *Handbook of applied cognition* (pp. 163–194). Chichester, England: Wiley.

Edwards, M., Wood, F., Davies, M., & Edwards, A. (2012). The development of health literacy in patients with a long-term health condition: The health literacy pathway model. *BMC Public Health, 12*, 130.

Fagerlin, A., & Peters, E. (2011). Quantitative information. In B. Fischoff, N. Brewer, & J. Downs (Eds.), *Communicating risks and benefits: A users guide* (pp. 53–64). Washington DC: FDA.

Federman, A. D., Wisnivesky, J. P., Wolf, M. S., Leventhal, H., & Halm, E. A. (2010). Inadequate health literacy is associated with suboptimal health beliefs in older asthmatics. *Journal of Asthma, 47*, 620–626.

Finucane, M. L., Mertz, C. K., Slovic, P., & Schmidt, E. S. (2005). Task complexity and older adults' decision-making competence. *Psychology and Aging, 20*, 71–84.

Flynn, K. E., Smith, M. A., & Freese, J. (2006). When do older adults turn to the internet for health information? Findings from the Wisconsin longitudinal study. *Journal of General Internal Medicine, 21*, 1295–1301.

Gigerenzer, G., Gaissmaier, W., Kurz-Milcke, E., Schwartz, L. M., & Woloshin, S. (2008). Helping doctors and patients make sense of health statistics. *Psychological Science in the Public Interest, 8*, 53–96.

Gigerenzer, G., Todd, P. M., & the ABC Group. (1999). *Simple heuristics that make us smart*. New York: Oxford University Press.

Gottfredson, L. S., & Deary, I. J. (2004). Intelligence predicts health and longevity, but why? *Current Directions in Psychological Science, 13*, 1–10.

Hibbard, J. H., Slovic, P., Peters, E., Finucane, M. L., & Tusler, M. (2001). Is the informed-choice policy approach appropriate for medicare beneficiaries? *Health Affairs: The Policy Journal of the Health Sphere, 20*, 199–203.

Horn, J. L., & Cattell, R. B. (1967). Age differences in fluid and crystallized intelligence. *Acta Psychologica, 26*, 107–129.

Johnson, M. M. S. (1990). Age differences in decision making: A process methodology for examining strategic information processing. *Journal of Gerontology: Psychological Sciences, 45*, 75–78.

Johnson, M. M. S. (1993). Thinking about strategies during, before and after making a decision. *Psychology and Aging, 8*, 231–241.

Kintsch, W. (1998). *Comprehension: A paradigm for cognition*. New York, NY: Cambridge University Press.

Levinthal, B. R., Morrow, D. G., Tu, W., Wu, J., Young, J., Weiner, M., et al. (2008). Cognition and health literacy in patients with hypertension. *Journal of General Internal Medicine, 23*, 1172–1176.

Leventhal, H., Safer, M. A., & Panagis, D. M. (1983). The impact of communications on the self-regulation of health beliefs, decisions, and behavior. *Health Education & Behavior, 10*, 3–29.

Lippa, K. D., Klein, H. A., & Shalin, V. L. (2008). Everyday expertise: Cognitive demands in diabetes self-management. *Human Factors, 50*, 112–120.

Li, Y., Baldassi, M., Johnson, E. J., & Weber, E. U. (2013). Complementary cognitive capabilities, economic decision making, and aging. *Psychology and Aging, 28*, 595–613.

Löckenhoff, C. E., & Carstensen, L. L. (2007). Aging, emotion, and health-related decision strategies: Motivational manipulations can reduce age differences. *Psychology and Aging, 22*, 134–146.

Mata, R., & Nunes, L. (2010). When less is enough: Cognitive aging, information search, and decision quality in consumer choice. *Psychology and Aging, 25*, 289–298.

Mata, R., Schooler, L., & Rieskamp, J. (2007). The aging decision maker: Cognitive aging and the adaptive selection of decision strategies. *Psychology and Aging, 22*, 796–810.

Mata, R., von Helverson, B., & Rieskamp, J. (2010). Learning to choose: Cognitive aging and strategy selection learning in decision making. *Psychology and Aging, 25*, 299–309.

McNutt, R. A. (2004). Shared medical decision making: Problems, process, progress. *Journal of the American Medical Association, 292*, 2516–2518.

Meyer, B. J. F., Russo, C., & Talbot, A. (1995). Discourse comprehension and problem solving: Decisions about the treatment of breast cancer by women across the life span. *Psychology and Aging, 10*, 84–103.

Meyer, B. J. F., Talbot, A. P., & Ranalli, C. (2007). Why older adults make more immediate treatment decisions about cancer than younger adults. *Psychology and Aging, 22*, 505–524.

Meyer, D., Leventhal, H., & Gutmann, M. (1985). Common-sense models of illness: The example of hypertension. *Health Psychology, 4*, 115–135.

Mikels, J. A., Löckenhoff, C. E., Maglio, S. J., Carstensen, L. L., Goldstein, M. K., & Garber, A. (2010). Following your heart or your head: Focusing on emotions versus information differentially influences the decisions of younger and older adults. *Journal of Experimental Psychology: Applied, 16*, 87–95.

Miller, L. M. S., Stine-Morrow, E. A. L., Kirkorian, H. L., & Conroy, M. L. (2004). Adult age differences in knowledge-driven reading. *Journal of Educational Psychology, 96*, 811–821.

Mitzner, T. L., Barg-Walkow, H., McBride, S. E., & Rogers, W. (2013). Self-management of wellness and illness in an aging population. *Reviews of Human Factors and Ergonomics, 8*, 277–333.

Morrow, D. G., & Chin, J. (2012). Technological bridges between health care systems and older adults. In R. Hill, R. Zheng, & M. Gardner (Eds.), *Engaging older adults with modern technology: Internet use and information access needs* (pp. 59–79). Hershey, PA: IGI Publishing.

Morrow, D. G., & Conner-Garcia, T. (2013). Improving comprehension of medication information: Implications for nurse-patient communication. *Journal of Gerontological Nursing, 39*, 1–8.

Morrow, D. G., D'Andrea, L., Stine-Morrow, E. A. L., Shake, M., Bertel, S., Chin, J., Kopren, K., Gao, S., Conner-Garcia, T., Graumlich, J. F., & Murray, M. D. (2012). Comprehension of multimedia health information among older adults with chronic illness. *Visual Communication, 11*, 347–362.

Morrow, D. G., Miller, L. M. S., Ridolfo, H. E., Magnor, C., Fischer, U. M., Kokayeff, N. K., et al. (2009). Expertise and age differences in pilot decision making. *Aging, Neuropsychology, and Cognition, 16*, 33–55.

Morrow, D. G., Weiner, M., Young, J., Steinley, D., Deer, M., & Murray, M. D. (2005). Improving medication knowledge among older adults with heart failure: A patient-centered approach to instruction design. *The Gerontologist, 45*, 545–552.

Nielsen-Bohlman, L., Panzer, A. M., & Kindig, D. A. (2004). *Health literacy: A prescription to end confusion*. Washington, DC.: The National Academies Press.

Park, D. C., Hertzog, C., Leventhal, H., Morrell, R. W., Leventhal, E., Birchmore, D., et al. (1999). Medication adherence in rheumatoid arthritis patients: Older is wiser. *Journal of the American Geriatrics Society*, *47*, 172–183.

Payne, J. W. (1982). Contingent decision behavior. *Psychological Bulletin*, *92*, 382–402.

Peters, E. (2012). Beyond comprehension the role of numeracy in judgments and decisions. *Current Directions in Psychological Science*, *21*, 31–35.

Peters, E., Baker, D. P., Dieckmann, N. F., Leon, J., & Collins, J. (2010). Explaining the effect of education on health: A field study in Ghana. *Psychological Science*, *21*, 1369–1376.

Peters, E., Dieckmann, N. F., Västfjäll, D., Mertz, C. K., Slovic, P., & Hibbard, J. H. (2009). Bringing meaning to numbers: The impact of evaluative categories on decisions. *Journal of Experimental Psychology: Applied*, *15*, 213–227.

Peters, E., Diefenbach, M. A., Hess, T. M., & Västfjäll, D. (2008). Age differences in dual information-processing modes: Implications for cancer decision making. *Cancer*, *113*(12 Suppl.), 3556–3567.

Peters, E., Hess, T. M., Västfjäll, D., & Auman, C. (2007). Adult age differences in dual information processes and their influence on judgments and decisions: A review. *Perspectives on Psychological Science*, *2*, 1–23.

Petrie, K. J., & Weinman, J. (2012). Patients' perceptions of their illness: The dynamo of volition in health care. *Current Directions in Psychological Science*, *21*, 60–65.

Queen, T. L., Hess, T. M., Ennis, G. E., Dowd, K., & Gruhn, D. (2012). Information search and decision making: Effects of age and complexity on strategy use. *Psychology and Aging*, *27*, 817–824.

Reed, A. E., Mikels, J. A., & Simon, K. I. (2008). Older adults prefer less choice than young adults. *Psychology and Aging*, *23*, 671–675.

Reyna, V. F. (2008). A theory of medical decision making and health: Fuzzy-trace theory. *Medical Decision Making*, *28*, 850–865.

Reyna, V. F. (2011). *Across the life span. Communicating risks and benefits: An evidence-based user's guide*. Silver Springs, MD: Federal Drug Administration.

Reyna, V. F., Nelson, W. L., Han, P. K., & Dieckmann, N. F. (2009). How numeracy influences risk comprehension and medical decision making. *Psychological Bulletin*, *135*, 943–973.

Riggle, E. D. B., & Johnson, M. M. S. (1996). Age difference in political decision making: Strategies for evaluating political candidates. *Political Behavior*, *18*, 99–117.

Ross, S., Walker, A., & MacLeod, M. J. (2004). Patient compliance in hypertension: Role of illness perceptions and treatment beliefs. *Journal of Human Hypertension*, *18*, 607–613.

Russo, J. E., & Dosher, B. A. (1983). Strategies for multi-attribute binary choice. *Journal of Experimental Psychology: Learning, Memory and Cognition*, *9*, 676–696.

Sharit, J., Hernandez, M., Czaja, S., & Pirolli, P. (2008). Investigating the roles of knowledge and cognitive abilities in older adult information seeking on the web. *ACM Transactions on Computer- Human Interaction*, *15*, 11–25.

Sinnott, J. D. (1989). A model for solution of ill-structured problems: Implications for everyday and abstract problem solving. In J. D. Sinnott (Ed.), *Everyday problem solving: Theory and applications* (pp. 72–99). New York: Praeger.

Stanley, B., Guido, J., Stanley, M., & Shortell, D. (1984). The elderly patient and informed consent. *Journal of the American Medical Association*, *252*, 1302–1306.

Stanovich, K. E., West, R. F., & Harrison, M. R. (1995). Knowledge growth and maintenance across the life span: The role of print exposure. *Developmental Psychology*, *31*, 811–826.

Stine-Morrow, E. A., & Miller, L. (2009). Aging, self-regulation, and learning from text. *Psychology of Learning and Motivation*, *51*, 255–296.

Sun, X., Shi, Y., Zeng, Q., Wang, Y., Du, W., Wei, N., et al. (2013). Determinants of health literacy and health behavior regarding infectious respiratory diseases: A pathway model. *BMC Public Health*, *13*, 261.

Taha, J., Czaja, S. J., Sharit, J., & Morrow, D. G. (2013). Factors affecting usage of a personal health record (PHR) to manage health. *Psychology and Aging*, *28*, 1124–1139.

Tanius, B. E., Wood, S., Hanoch, Y., & Rice, T. (2009). Aging and choice: Applications to medicare part D. *Judgment and Decision Making*, *4*, 92–101.

Todd, P. M., & Gigerenzer, G. (2007). Environments that make us smart: Ecological rationality. *Current Directions in Psychological Science*, *16*(3), 167–171.

Wister, A. V., Malloy-Weir, L. J., Rootman, I., & Desjardins, R. (2010). Lifelong educational practices and resources in enabling health literacy among older adults. *Journal of Aging and Health*, *22*, 827–854.

Wolf, M. S., Curtis, L. M., Wilson, E. A. H., Revelle, W., Waite, K. R., Smith, S. G., Weintraub, S., & Baker, D. W. (2012). Literacy, cognitive function, and health: Results of the LitCog study. *Journal of General Internal Medicine*, *27*(10), 1300–1307.

Zwaan, R. A. (1999). Embodied cognition, perceptual symbols, and situation models. *Discourse Processes*, *28*, 81–88.

CHAPTER

14

Decisions and Actions for Life Patterns and Health Practices as We Age: A Bottom-up Approach

Howard Leventhal[1], *Jenna Herold*[2], *Elaine A. Leventhal*[3], *Edith Burns*[4], *Michael A. Diefenbach*[5]

[1]Institute for Health & Department of Psychology, Rutgers University, New Brunswick, NJ, USA; [2]Department of Psychology, Rutgers University, NJ, USA; [3]Department of Medicine, Robert Wood Johnson School of Medicine, Rutgers University, New Brunswick, NJ, USA; [4]Department of Medicine, Medical College of Wisconsin, Milwaukee, WI, USA; [5]Department of Medicine and Urology, North Shore-Long Island Jewish Health System, NY, USA

OVERVIEW

Our efforts to model the basic cognitive and affective mechanisms underlying health decisions suggest first, that decision making is most often automatic and nondeliberative, reflecting a process that is highly dependent upon perceptions and actions. Conscious comparison of two or more alternatives appear to be relatively rare in everyday health decisions in which "choices" reflect preferences that require little consideration of the attributes of alternative actions and outcomes. This perspective suggests that changes in physical health interacting with changes in executive function will play a major role in how threats to health are managed in the later years of life. Specifically, executive processes in these years face the problem of controlling and reorganizing schemas that were initially developed for managing acute conditions and may be inconsistent with managing the multiple chronic conditions common in later life. The

http://dx.doi.org/10.1016/B978-0-12-417148-0.00014-5

executive system may also face the need to overcome resistance to updating the self-system. Understanding how the history of responses to acute somatic crises affects management of multiple chronic and life-threatening conditions is a major focus of this chapter.

Our chapter is divided into two main sections. The first presents five themes underlying our conceptual approach to modeling health decisions, followed by a description of the content of the representations of health threats, the medical and life-style procedures for management, and the processes involved in their construction. The second section describes highly selected examples of empirical studies that played a major role in model development. The studies provide insights into the role of executive processes in three types of health decisions: (1) use of health care in response to minor illnesses of everyday life, (2) management of chronic asymptomatic (e.g., hypertension and diabetes) and episodic (e.g., asthma) conditions, and (3) preparation for treatment when terminally ill. The examples illuminate the developmental sequence involved in the generation of prototypes of illnesses that frame health decisions throughout life for the majority of individuals. The effects of age are commented upon throughout. A final, closing section summarizes what we now know and sets an agenda for future research and practice.

THEMES FOR MODELING HEALTH PREFERENCES AND DECISIONS

Our first theme is the assumption that a single complex system generates decisions and actions to manage health and illness in all contexts, from benign everyday ills through lifelong chronic conditions and terminal illness. The second posits that contextual variables are central factors in any model of health decisions. Context is usually conceptualized in terms of epidemiological variables such as socioeconomic status (SES), age, and gender. Though SES, age, and gender can identify the existence of populations with health problems, they typically fail to identify the specific variables and mechanisms underlying the preferences and decisions relevant to the problem. To understand the relationship of a specific marker such as age to decision making, it is essential to identify the specific factors nested within it. For example, advanced age involves both changes in executive function (e.g., short-term memory) and physical function, and either of these may be primarily responsible for its association with health decisions.

A third and related theme is that the physical and functional body anchors the self in a wider environment and plays a central role in the formation of concepts of space and time, and wellness and illness. As the body ages and is impacted by chronic diseases, somatic and functional changes set new targets and time-frames for action in addition to limiting the individual's ability to make decisions and act in managing health and illness.

Changes in the physical and functional body over the life span create mental models of illnesses that generate questions about causes, targets for actions, expected outcomes, and time-frames for preventing the onset or ameliorating the progress of illness (Leventhal et al., 2008; Leventhal, Idler, & Leventhal, 1999).

Fourth, prior decisions set the framework for current decisions. The utility of illnesses and procedures for management (e.g., medication, surgery); the perception of probabilities for prevention, cure, and control of disease progression; and the sense that one possesses the skills and resources to manage illness are key factors that shape decisions and actions at any given moment. Current preferences and decisions about treatment are affected by experience with similar past illnesses (e.g., was the prior illness cured and/or controlled by medication, an over-the-counter pill, or exercise and diet). A novel illness or an illness that recurs after being treated and "cured" can completely alter the decision process, as novelty and recurrence alter the utilities and probabilities associated with the condition and treatments. This is seen in the content and process of decisions to treat prostate cancer in the face of rising indicators of risk for a formerly treated and presumably cured disease (Johnson Shen et al., 2015).

Our fifth theme is the necessity of specifying the concrete referents of illnesses and treatments, and the concrete referents involved in planning as decisions and action are implemented in the physical world. A model of health decisions must examine the process from the bottom up as well as the top down.

MODELING THE PROCESSES UNDERLYING HEALTH DECISIONS AND ACTIONS

It is important to repeat that a model of the processes involved in health decisions must specify the referents for its theoretical concepts; that is, the physical and functional experiences and environmental cues that are referents for the self, an illness, and the illness causes and consequences (see Figure 2). This emphasis is important if we are to understand (1) how concepts emerge from experience and the mechanisms that connect experience to concepts; (2) how illness representations and treatment representations are linked to one another (i.e., when and how they form coherent packages); (3) how these packages become automatic bases for preferences and decisions; and (4) how executive processes form and implement action plans, evaluate outcomes, and then make and modify subsequent decisions and actions. As many illnesses in later life are chronic, executive processes will be critical for integrating behaviors into daily life for behavioral management of lifelong, chronic conditions. The Common-Sense Model (CSM) depicted in Figure 1 represents the cognitive and emotional mechanisms involved in decisions, planning, and action by people untrained in the medical professions.

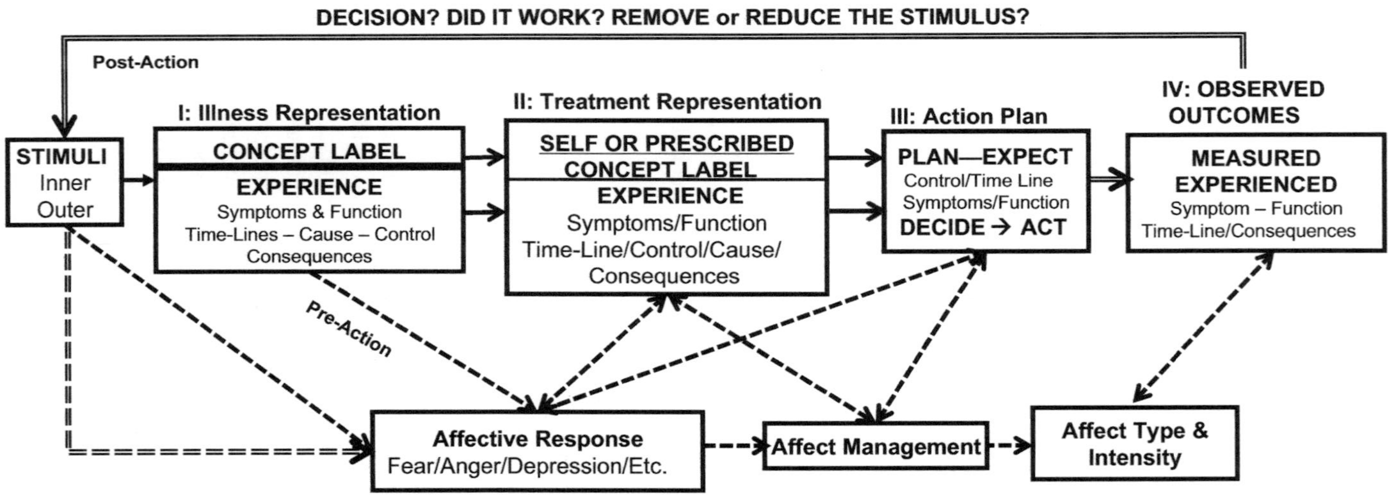

FIGURE 1 The Common-Sense Model (CSM) is a feedback model depicting the content and processes of the cognitive and affective system underlying responses to illness. Illness representations are generated by matching deviations from self to illness prototypes (see Figure 2); this can be automatic or involve active decisions. Illness representations activate treatment representations, which in turn lead to planning, and planning leads to decision to act and creates expectations for treatment outcomes: what is expected to change and how quickly. The processes involved in the construction of representations and those involved in planning and action can proceed independently; they are often related bidirectionally. Outcomes are evaluated either automatically or by conscious decisions. The conceptual and experiential levels can lead to different treatments, plans, and actions and different appraisals of outcomes; this is one of several sources of uncertainty in the cognitive behavioral system (others include failure of responses to meet expectations, uncertainty about the accuracy of each representation, etc.). The system is coherent when observed outcomes (IV) match expectations (III) generated by representations of illness (I) and treatment (II).

Representations in the Common-Sense Model

Illness representations frame the abstract and concrete targets, causal beliefs, and temporal expectations for evaluating and choosing one or another avenue for treatment. They are one of three important sets of variables that affect decisions and action.

Content of representations of illness. The factors defining specific diseases can be categorized into (1) identity, (2) time-lines, (3) cause, (4) control, and (5) consequences (Figure 1). *Identity* specifies the somatic sensations and functions (i.e., symptoms) and the associated concept and label. The connection of symptoms and functional changes to a disease label gives the concept depth. The concept provides breadth by uniting events occurring at different points in time and connects the package to a range of actions and outcomes allowing the decision maker to compare the relative utilities or efficacy of treatments. *Time-lines* set subjective and objective temporal expectations for the rates of onset, duration, and elimination and/or control. *Causal perceptions* can help to define a condition and suggest plausible approaches for control. *Control* defines expectations for eliminating symptoms, both in terms of control of cause and cure. Finally, *consequences* identify both immediate and longer disruptive impact of the disorder (Leventhal et al., 2011).

To understand how mental models of illnesses impact decisions and behavior requires addressing how both the concrete and abstract facets of the representation are generated and how these facets relate to representations of treatment and action plans. The effects of any single variable on a health decision will vary as a function of the other factors in the model, many of which are introduced by the social context. In addition, comparisons among alternatives are often biased by factors in addition to their immediate values. For example, gains in function from surgery to correct an arthritic joint may be discounted relative to living with current dysfunction, as the gains are "imagined" and the decision for surgery faces the immediate concerns of pain from the surgery as well as the elderly individual's fear of slow recovery. It is important, therefore, to understand the processes involved in creating and shaping representations to develop interventions that help patients make decisions consistent with their future biomedical experiences and outcomes.

Content of representations of treatments. Although the factors defining illness representations also apply to procedures for prevention and treatment (i.e., symptoms to be relieved by treatment and time-lines for benefits), they are not separately assessed in current studies. Instead of examining specific variables, Horne, Weinman, and Hankins (1999) developed two scales to assess general beliefs about medications—overuse (e.g., doctors use too many medicines) and harm (e.g., medicines do more harm than good); and two scales assessing patients' beliefs about their own medications—specific concerns (e.g., my medicines disrupt my life) and necessity (e.g., my health, at present, depends on medicine). Ratios of necessity over concerns of the patient obtained from these scales have been found to be moderate to strong predictors of medication adherence for an array of conditions (e.g., Horne et al., 2013). Such ratio scores do not, however, capture how each factor relates to adherence, and recent studies show that treating necessities and concerns as opposites and/or as a ratio ignores their specific contributions (Phillips, Diefenbach, Kronish, Negron, & Horowitz, 2014).

Studies such as those just cited illustrate our contention that predicting outcomes is not equivalent to identifying the specific factors that integrate the perceptions of treatment with the perceptions of an illness. For example, an intervention to encourage adherence to medication following surgical intervention for myocardial infarction (MI) may need to address specific components of the representations of both condition and surgical treatment, as the often severe and rapid onset of symptoms may encourage patients to represent MI as an acute condition. Representing MI as an acute event can lead a patient to expect a surgical cure, an expectation readily reinforced by an asymptomatic experience a few days post-surgery. This mental model may play a role in nonadherence to lifelong use of medications for preventing recurrence, perhaps helping to account for the fact that 52% of patients stop using ACE inhibitors and beta-blockers 2 years post-MI (Akincigil et al., 2007). An array of specific factors in addition to time-lines will be important in forming relationships between representations of illnesses and treatments that are coherent and form integrated packages or modules to sustain self-management over long periods of time.

As modeling common sense makes clear, the patient's targets (i.e., symptoms) and time-lines for observing treatment efficacy may not correspond to those set by a practitioner, and the patient may judge a treatment as a failure if it does not control or eliminate symptoms and dysfunctions as he or she expected. Coherence, or matching of attributes of illness to expectations for treatment at each step in CSM, is critical for adherence and both biomedical and quality-of-life outcomes. The difficulty in achieving coherence increases with advancing age given the age-associated increase in number of conditions and treatments that add to the complexity of management due both to the sheer number of treatments and the possibility of interactions among treatments. The increase in variability in later life with respect to factors such as medical literacy, cognitive functioning, and the organization of home environments adds to the challenges of forming coherent modules for effective self-management. As individual variability increases with age, uniform, age-related predictions are difficult.

Constructing Representations

A mental model of an illness or treatment must be constructed before it can provide a framework for guiding decisions, initiating actions, and evaluating outcomes. Construction involves the interaction of stimuli with the individual's knowledge base (i.e., prototypes of self, illnesses, and treatments). The details are important for developing and testing interventions to influence decisions and action.

Constructing illness representations: A computational process. Somatic sensations and physical and cognitive functions that deviate from the "normal" or usual self are likely the most common activators of illness representations. Whether the process becomes conscious and deliberative will depend upon the content of the initial match. For example, if a touch removes a barely noticed itch, the event will likely remain outside awareness; if it elicits an unexpected sensation, such as soreness, the process can become conscious. The content of the illness prototype involved in the initial match sets the stage for further decisions and action. Prototypes acquired through prior, direct experience and observations of illness in family members are highly available, particularly in the latter case when there is an element of similarity to self.

In the CSM, matching is computational as the weights assigned to the properties of an eliciting stimulus vary by the available prototypes or norms (Kahneman & Miller, 1986). Each prototype assigns weights to each property, including location, pattern, time-lines, consequences (e.g., disruption of specific motor and cognitive functions), and perceived causes, and the best match will result in an initial "self"-diagnosis. This process is depicted in Figure 2. For example, a deviation in structure and texture of a mole on the cheek that changes shape and color over time will match the prototype for melanoma for someone with a prior history of skin cancer or, alternatively, exposure to family members and friends with such histories. A similar mole with similar properties may not match the prototype for skin cancer if the skin is unexposed to sun but frequently abraded; location and perceived cause can shift the interpretation to an exacerbated, but otherwise benign irritation. Matching is often automatic when the eliciting stimulus and prototype are familiar and salient (e.g., a stress headache) and the features defining the pattern are quickly recognized (Bishop, 1991). As the number of chronic conditions increase over the life span, the number of available prototypes, both chronic and acute, can produce seemingly inconsistent outcomes, ranging from high levels of certainty to high levels of ambiguity. This can lead to social communication and "symptom sharing" often associated with older individuals (Stoller, Kart, & Portugal, 1997). The reasons for sharing may differ, however, depending on the situation. When deviations are unfamiliar and matching is uncertain, sharing will likely reflect a need for clarity. In contrast, if the stimulus appears to match a highly threatening prototype (e.g., colon cancer), decisions to share will likely reflect a need for reassurance. The variability in somatic stimuli adds a further level of uncertainty, reflecting changes in patterns and time-frames, resulting in an increase in the possible matches among the array of prototypes relevant to elderly individuals. CSM identifies processes that generate uncertainty, social communication, and decisional ambiguity.

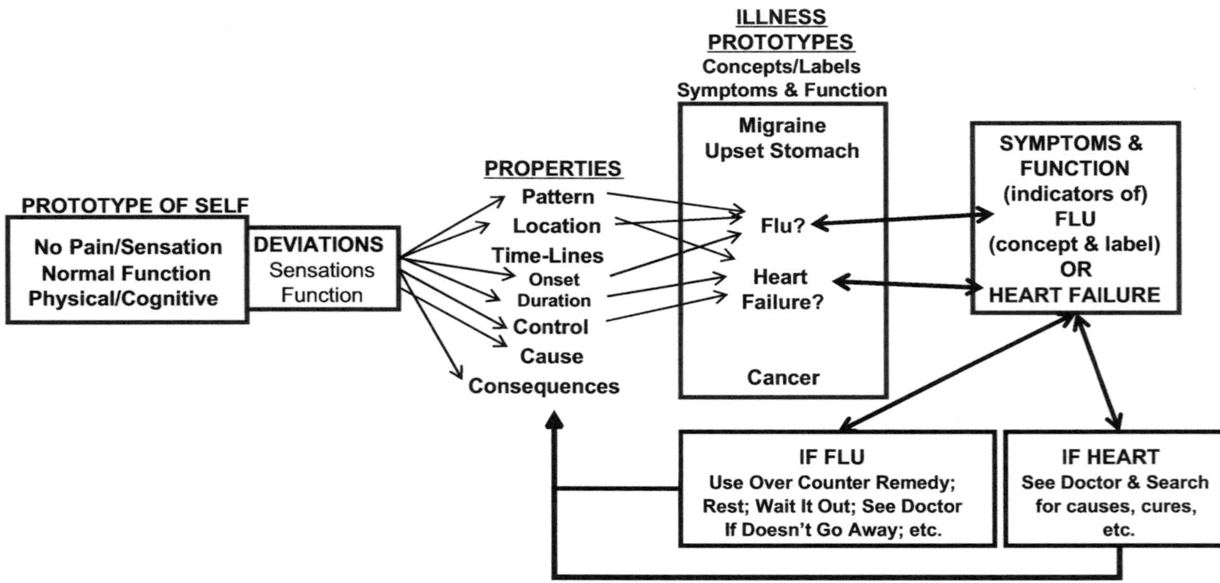

FIGURE 2 Matching deviations from self to illness prototypes. Prototypes are averages of a history of experiences with self and specific illnesses. The prototypes for flu and for heart failure share pattern and location of symptoms (obstructed breathing, fatigue), differ in time-lines (both can have episodic features though heart failure episodes constantly repeat), and they differ in control and outcomes. The process is computational, as each prototype assigns different weights to the deviations attributes. Repetition of attributes leads to the formation of modules (stomach problem, migraine, etc.) and higher-order, declarative structure, e.g., acute and chronic models. Uncertainty arises when properties fit two or more prototypes, and as the number of conditions increase with age there is increasing possibility of ambiguity in the construction of representations. Representations based on a lengthy history of repeated construction are activated rapidly and can interfere with the construction of new, biologically valid representations, a problem with the onset of many chronic, asymptomatic conditions in the later years of life.

The processes involved in self-diagnostic matching are similar in some respects to those involved in medical diagnoses; both are computational. Differences in level of expertise between and among patients and practitioners, however, can lead to dramatically different diagnostic outcomes and treatment recommendations, creating barriers for shared decisions. In addition to obvious differences in the number of prototypes available and their degree of details, patients and expert practitioners may differ in more subtle ways. For example, less experienced patients are more likely to reason backward from their common-sense diagnoses to observed stimuli (e.g., if I believe I have cancer, each symptom will fit this self-appraisal as everything is seen as "cancer"); whereas skilled practitioners reason forward, matching the observed events with more plausible and appropriate categories. Although differences of this type may seem minor, they can be involved in seemingly irreconcilable differences between patients and practitioners, with patients failing to perceive that their symptoms can be accounted for by a disease or nondisease process other than their most feared outcome. It is not uncommon for unskilled patients to make hasty decisions based on backward reasoning activated by highly threatening self-diagnoses inconsistent with biological realities and anathema for shared decision making.

Response evaluation: A feedback process. The utility of any treatment is influenced by directly experienced outcomes. Outcome expectations—that is, the targets and time-lines established by representations—are confirmed by reductions in symptoms and improved function. The effect of objective input from practitioners and family members will vary depending upon their consistency with the patient's representation. Duration of treatment, side effects, and economics add to the complexity of evaluation, especially for treatments lasting months or years, and inconsistencies between patient and practitioner perceptions are not always predictable and can be misunderstood when they arise. For example, investigators conducting randomized clinical trials often judge "side effects" as deficits or costs of treatment and assume patients assign side effects similar costs. Patients may, however, interpret side effects as signs that a medication is working—and they may be right (Cameron, Leventhal, Love, & Patrick-Miller, 2002; Leventhal, Nerenz, Love, Leventhal, & Bendena, 1991). When patients in clinical trials anticipate and then fail to experience side effects, they may assume they are in the placebo arm of the trial, drop out of the study, and seek out and volunteer for a different trial in the hope of assignment to the active arm. The perceived utility of a drug may also change if side effects are long lasting and severe. Far too little attention has been given to laypersons' common-sense computations of benefits and concerns in the presence of side effects, given the impact of their effects on adherence and the consequences of adherence on objective markers.

Coherence of representations of illness and treatment. As described earlier, coherence of a patient's mental model depends upon the match between treatment experience and prior expectations set by the representations of both illness and treatment. Efforts to assess coherence have faltered, however, as the coherence subscale of the Illness Perception Questionnaire (Weinman, Petrie, Moss-Morris, & Horne, 1996) measures distress caused by failure to understand the relationship of treatment to outcomes rather than perceptions of the match between factors (e.g., time-lines and symptoms) responsible for coherence (Tannenbaum, 2013). As coherence is critical for the formation of the habits needed to sustain treatment over the long term, improvement in its conceptualization and assessment is critical. Assessment is complex, however, as coherence is in the eye of the beholder, and will differ by disease, treatment, and patient. Insuring equivalence of assessment and findings across contexts will be further complicated by likely differences in the criteria (targets, time-frames, etc.) for evaluating feedback as a function of age-related changes in self-perception.

Age and the Knowledge Base: Prototypes of Self, Illnesses, and Treatments

Self: A prototype based on function. Physical and functional self-competencies are attributes of the self that create the framework for health decisions (Leventhal et al., 1999). These self-attributes set the norms or base rates for somatic sensations and physical and cognitive functions. As averages, they are highly available and easily recognized, even though never directly experienced. If self-assessments of health (SAH) are averages of prior experience, we can expect them to be a valid predictor of systems status, and SAH based on 5-point scales (1 = excellent, 5 = poor) have been found to be robust predictors of mortality over intervals as long as 20 years in 46 community samples (Benyamini & Idler, 1999; Idler & Benyamini, 1997). The predictive power of SAH holds after controlling for age, gender, ethnicity, chronic conditions, and other medical indicators. Studies with terminally ill patients find that SAH is often a stronger predictor of mortality than medical indicators (Shadbolt, Barresi, & Craft, 2002). Although daily physical and cognitive function, symptoms, and emotional states predict self-rated health in cross-sectional analyses, only self-reported physical and cognitive function predicts changes in SAH over time, and temporal declines in function add to the longitudinal decline in SAH (Mora, DiBonaventura, Idler, Leventhal, & Leventhal, 2008).

Deviations from the norm of the self generates the implicit and explicit processes involved in matching (Figure 2) and lead automatically or consciously through the steps and decisions depicted in Figure 1. As self-assessments are normative, we can expect them to change relatively little over the decades, even though few 70-year-olds will claim they feel as strong, robust, and energetic as they did 30 or 40 years earlier. How the self is sustained and updated over the life span is not well understood, though specific experiences such as outliving one's peers in the later decades of life (e.g., the 70s through 90s) provide an additional positive lift to self-assessment beyond the contribution of function and medical conditions (Idler, 1993). Predicting when a health event will lead to a dramatic decline in SAH is more complex than one might expect. We would expect the onset and treatment for breast or colon cancer to lead to downrating of health by a 65- or 70-year-old individual, if it is perceived to be caused by a deficit in the self (e.g., past history of heavy smoking, cancer in the family). If, however, the cancer is perceived to be precipitated by a transient external event, treatable and no different than any other treatable acute condition, the representation may protect against a negative impact on the self. Given the complexity of the self and its history, we have much to learn about how self-appraisals are made and whether the processes involved in self-appraisals by the elderly differ significantly from those affecting appraisals among young and middle-aged adults. As the self is an average of a lengthy history of somatic and functional experience, it can be a misleading target for post-illness and injury recovery; middle-aged and older adults are not as young as they believe, and expectations for rate and level of recovery can be unrealistic.

Illness and treatment prototypes. Many of the attributes involved in matching deviations with illness prototypes (e.g., location, pattern, time-lines) are built into our neurobiology; they are integral features of the self-system (Figure 2). These attributes and life experience construct the concepts or prototypes that define the utilities and expectations guiding decisions, actions, and the search for feedback (Figure 1; steps III and IV). Although one can identify symptom patterns that are related to higher-order concepts (e.g., coughs and headaches classified as acute colds), indicating that episodic experiences generate semantic memories or prototypes, and prototypes then modify episodic experiences (Nelson & Shiffrin, 2013), data on the developmental history of prototypes are limited. Conceptualizing and labeling conditions as cancers, cardiac conditions, stress headaches, and colds facilitates communication but can create a false sense of understanding as the experience-based features underlying these labels can vary widely across individuals. For example, prototypes for some persons may include but one or two attributes or some specific episodic event (e.g., cancer defined by the observation of a grandparent dying of lung cancer), whereas for others, they may be based on a rich history of personal experience (e.g., a migraine sufferer). These differences are important for examining how age affects health-care decisions as a history of experience with a specific illness can both increase certainty in an elder's appraisal of specific symptoms and introduce ambiguity if symptoms associated with a familiar acute condition now partially overlap with those of a late-life chronic condition.

Age and the transition from acute to chronic conditions. Although all but the most cognitively impaired elderly will "understand" the abstract meaning of chronic, the concrete experiences of a chronic illness can activate acute prototypes leading to interpretations of symptoms, decisions, actions, and outcome expectations inappropriate for the chronic malady. The shift from a lifetime of experience with the overlearned, highly structured acute prototype anchored in a history of concrete experiences and action, to addressing the demands of chronic conditions—a challenge at any age—may overwhelm the less-informed elderly who are not open to searching for information and restructuring everyday behaviors to manage chronic conditions (Leventhal & Crouch, 1997). A second factor adding to the complexity of this transition is the age-related increase in the number of chronic conditions. The typical 65- or 75-year-old adult may host four or more chronic conditions. An elder feeling a bit fatigued and distressed on a given day may be quite uncertain whether the distress is caused by the aging of the somatic system (e.g., sleep loss from joint pain) or from a flare of one or more chronic conditions caused by forgetting to take one or more of the eight or nine medications needed at multiple times during the day. The confusion may result in elders failing to treat chronic, stable, and mildly distressing symptoms that are wrongly attributed to age, while they remain vigilant and ready to seek care for symptoms that are unusual and threatening though of little medical significance (Prohaska, Leventhal, Leventhal, & Keller, 1985). The increased vigilance combined with willingness to tolerate and live with chronic but treatable conditions may also reflect an age-related perception of diminution of somatic resources. Awareness of the slowing of physical function, occasional gait instability, or other symptoms that increase feelings of vulnerability to unfamiliar symptoms may underlie what we have assessed as a motive to conserve resources by minimizing expenditure of energy (Leventhal, Leventhal, Schaefer, & Easterling, 1993). Conservation motivation can encourage rule-based decisions to minimize uncertainty and emotional distress. Park (1999) described scenarios for treatment decisions for two women diagnosed with Stage 2 breast cancer, one a 67-year-old widow with multiple chronic conditions, the other a 38-year-old investment banker. The widow minimized effort by leaving decisions to her oncologist and daughter, a rule-based approach, whereas the young, energetic banker sought second opinions and engaged in Internet searches, an analytic approach. The more limited life expectancy of the elderly widow lowered the value of expending time and resources searching for information and engaging in aggressive treatment to gain one or two years in her 70s or 80s. By contrast, the temporary investment of time and resource promises major lifetime gains for the younger banker. Classifying the widow's decision as rule-based and the banker's as analytic, however, ignores the many automatic and deliberative decisions prior to these final outcomes.

EXECUTIVE FUNCTION IN A COMMON-SENSE FRAMEWORK: SELECTIVE EVIDENCE

Executive Function: Action Plans and Planning

Consistent with other theoretical approaches, CSM assumes that planning, implementing, and evaluating the efficacy of specific actions involves the adaptive decision maker (i.e., executive function; Payne, Bettman, & Johnson, 1993). CSM represents executive processes as higher-order controls in a multilevel system (Carver & Scheier, 1981). CSM differs from earlier models of health decision making in two ways. First, it specifies the content and function of the lower level controls in the system: the representations of illnesses and treatments and the prototypes of self and illness. Second, the framework allows the generation of hypotheses respecting how executive processes implement and conduct action, set expectations, and evaluate outcomes. When actions fail, it is likely that these processes turn first to new actions, and if the new actions fail to meet expectations, the processes seem likely to revise the representation of the current condition and/or search for matches to an alternative illness prototype. In some cases executive processes face the challenge of revising the underlying knowledge base, that is, the prototypes of illness and the self. Describing how the executive interprets and organizes the concrete features of experience and action is essential for creating interventions to improve health outcomes. Understanding the effects of advancing age on these processes is important conceptually and practically, as the majority of chronic conditions that require complex decisions and drive health-care costs have their onset in later life.

As most data rely on after-the-fact verbal responses rather than online observations, our understanding of executive function is largely inferential. This is true for many dynamic models and true for most if not all predictions of decisions and action using linear regression. For example, self-efficacy is often a moderately strong predictor in decision and behavioral models, but assessments of self-efficacy do not tell us how it affects decisions or implementation of action, nor does the assessment of self-efficacy tell us how expectations, actions, and outcome appraisals led to the reports of response efficacy or self-efficacy. We will examine executive processes (e.g., attention, analysis, information seeking) in three areas: (1) decisions to prevent and manage everyday health threats, (2) managing chronic conditions, and (3) end-of-life planning. Empirical examples were selected to illustrate specific points, given that a comprehensive review of a substantial literature goes beyond the purpose and space limitations of our chapter.

Decisions to Prevent and Manage Everyday Health Threats

Early studies of the efficacy of fear messages for promoting preventive health behavior showed that both a threat and an action plan were required to move participants to action. For example, the threat component (e.g., a strong or mild description of the impact of tetanus) of a message generated attitudes and "motivation" favorable to be inoculated against tetanus, but action required the formation of a detailed plan (Leventhal, Singer, & Jones, 1965; Leventhal, 1970). The plan provided participants with a map of the campus—the environment in which action was to take place—and asked them to review their daily class changes and identify when a change brought them near the health service, at which point it recommended they step in to be inoculated. Little was left to the participants. In contrast, motivation in everyday life is activated by local events (e.g., somatic and functional changes observed in self or others), and the "executive self" must decide to create the plan for action and act. CSM provides a framework for understanding how this process unfolds.

Symptoms as triggers to decisions. A study of decisions to seek medical care by elderly adults (median age, 62 years; range, 45–80) supported the common-sense notion that care seeking is often triggered by somatic sensations (Cameron, Leventhal, & Leventhal, 1993). A group of 111 adults were interviewed while waiting to see their internist in a university-based practice, as were 111 non-care seekers who were matched in age, gender, and family size with the care seekers. The data were clear: 100% of the care seekers reported symptoms in comparison to 30% of the matched controls. The 70% difference between the two groups does not require a statistical test to conclude that symptoms played a critical role in decisions and action.

Stopping at that comparison, however, ignores a framework of prior decisions and social communications that led to the final decision to seek care. Specifically, in comparison to the symptoms reported by the 30% of control participants, symptoms reported by care seekers lasted longer (time-line), were more likely labeled (identity), were perceived as serious and disrupted daily life (consequences), and were less responsive to self-treatment (control); we can infer that a computational process matched the symptoms to an illness prototype. In addition, 92% of the care seekers reported talking to someone about their symptoms compared to 61% of the controls, and 50% of the care seekers versus 9% of the controls were advised to seek care. It is clear that symptoms alone were insufficient triggers for care seeking; decisions to seek care have a history involving a host of decisions prior to the final decision and action for care seeking (Prohaska et al., 1985). Decisions to seek care are seldom made de novo, and we can be certain that the "decision maker" acted both analytically and automatically, though we do not know precisely when either or a mix of the two were engaged, nor do we know if these decisions involved comparisons of ongoing experiences with a specific pre-illness baseline or with prototypes of possible alternative illnesses; the computational processes were not assessed.

In addition to the obvious role of symptoms, care-seeking decisions are affected by temporal factors in subtle though predictable ways. In a second study, Cameron, Leventhal, and Leventhal (1995) tested the hypothesis that people will be more likely to seek care for ambiguous symptoms when these symptoms are experienced in the context of a life stress of long as opposed to short duration. They first replicated prior findings showing that patients sought care when symptoms were severe, disruptive of daily function, and unresponsive to self-care; the symptoms were illness specific and not ambiguous or vague (e.g., fatigue). The percentage seeking care (~40%) was essentially the same for participants who were, and were not, experiencing life stress. As expected, care seeking was significantly lower for vague and ambiguous symptoms that are readily attributed to stress (e.g., malaise, irritability), and care seeking remained low if the symptoms were temporally coextensive with a life stress of recent onset (21%). Seeking care for ambiguous symptoms increased to 40%, however, for participants whose ambiguous symptoms occurred in the context of a life stress lasting 3 or more months. The increase in care seeking for ambiguous symptoms in combination with long-duration life stress appears rational when considered in relation to the finding of Cohen et al. (1998) that controlled exposure to rhinoviruses led to increased symptoms and objective indicators of upper respiratory illness for participants who reported exposure to life stresses of 3 months or longer; participants exposed to life stresses for shorter periods of time did not experience symptoms or signs of illness. We suggest, with due caution, that a causal time-line is built into the prototype for the acute schemata of the common cold.

Studies such as the above indicate that decisions and seeking medical care are based on a multicomponent process that includes (1) prototypes or base rates of specific illnesses generated from the individual's symptom history, (2) activation of illness representations by matching somatic experience and external conditions (e.g., duration of life stresses) to prototypes, (3) specific actions to reduce symptoms and alteration of action if initial actions fail to reduce symptoms and enhance function as expected, and (4) seeking advice from others who may or may not advise further action. Though some of these processes are automatic, others are conscious and analytic, and all are guided by prior expectancies. Updating mental representations is easy if it involves a shift from a familiar illness prototype (e.g., upper respiratory virus) to another familiar prototype (e.g., seasonal allergy), as is shifting from one treatment to another (e.g., antihistamine to antiviral). These transitions are facilitated if they share a higher-order concept (e.g., acute/infectious conditions), but more difficult if they require moving to a different concept (e.g., from acute to chronic illness). It also appears reasonable to conclude from these data that care-seeking decisions are "rational" given the actors' representations.

Confirmation of expectations affects response utility and coherence. Both automatic actions and explicit decisions for action reflect the perceived efficacy of the action, which is derived from a history of its coherence with the representations of illness. Specifically, did the action reduce or cure symptoms within the time-frames expected for a specific condition or for acute (or chronic) conditions in general? Treatments for minor colds and injuries are coherent across multiple features of both illness and treatment representations; for example, putting an antiseptic or antibiotic on a cut or taking an antacid for stomach upset address the location of the distress and are apt to alleviate the symptoms in the expected, relatively brief time-frame. There is often a "common-sense" overlap between the cause of a symptom and its treatment (e.g., what I ate caused the upset, and chewing an antacid tablet cleared the symptoms). Tannenbaum (2013) has shown that expectations—for example, taking X (aspirin) affects Y (headaches)—form schemata that are both coherent for specific conditions and generalized to classes of illnesses and treatments. Even when decisions and actions are biologically invalid, they can generate perceptions of response efficacy, and if frequent, they can enhance beliefs in one's ability to control health (Bandura, 1989).

Studies of the adoption of complementary and alternative medical treatments (CAM) provide a window into the development of perceived benefits and the emergence of self-efficacy for management of health. The review of Bishop, Yardley, and Lewith (2010) of CAM suggests that confidence in providers and treatments increase when users experience the concrete benefits suggested by providers. The finding for CAM users was supported in a study by Phillips, Leventhal, and Leventhal (2012) of patients in an internal medicine clinic. Specifically, if on the day post-visit they endorsed items stating that their doctor indicated what he or she was looking for, what they were supposed to do, and what they would observe when they did it, they reported good adherence, positive benefits, and fewer follow-up visits a month later. By contrast, patients who endorsed items that they felt they understood, and emotionally supported, but who did not report the details specific to action and experience, reported high levels of satisfaction but low levels of adherence and poor outcomes a month later. Thus, adherence and positive outcomes are more likely when physicians specify how to enact a treatment and create valid expectations regarding what and when change can be observed. These results are consistent with numerous studies of distress and adaptation during medical procedures such as endoscopy and childbirth (e.g., Johnson, 1975; Leventhal et al., 1989): action that validates the coherence of representations of condition and treatment leads to modules or scripts for initiation of effective self-management behavior.

Management of Chronic Illness

It is unusual for more than 40–60% of patients to adhere to treatment for chronic conditions such as hypertension, asthma, diabetes, and psychological disorders such as depression and schizophrenia. As stated by Cramer (2002), "Drugs don't work for patients who don't take them!" One among the many reasons for the deficit in adherence is that patients manage chronic conditions as acute, a practice that affects decision making and behavior in different ways for different conditions. Given the association between advanced age and the increased frequency of chronic conditions, one can expect that age will be positively associated with non-adherence and poor health outcomes. CSM also predicts that a sizable portion of non-adherence is due to the intrusion of the framework for management of acute conditions, as the acute prototype differs on multiple dimensions from the biology and treatment required for chronic conditions. Many chronic conditions are asymptomatic (e.g., diabetes and hypertension), some have episodic flares on a largely asymptomatic base (e.g., asthma), and others are asymptomatic during development (e.g., coronary conditions and cancers). These conditions and depression drive 80% or more of health-care costs (Anderson, 2010). Moreover, both prevention and control of chronic illnesses require adherence to life-styles and treatments that may generate little immediately perceptible benefit. Although patients can "understand" the differences between acute and chronic at an abstract level, their understanding may not override the perceptions that drive the actions and expectations at the concrete, experiential level.

Asymptomatic conditions: Hypertension, asthma, and diabetes. Patient management of hypertension, asthma, and diabetes illustrate predictable and surprising inconsistencies in executive processing. For example, an early study of patients in treatment for hypertension found that 80% of patients in ongoing treatment (i.e., had been adherent to appointments and treatment over multiple years) agreed with their doctors that "patients can't tell when their blood pressure is up." However, when asked, "Can you tell when your pressure is high," 92% said yes, and many of these patients were aware of the discrepancy between what they were told and what they believed, 64% stating spontaneously, "Don't tell my doctor what I told you" (Meyer, Leventhal, & Gutmann, 1985).

Among those who believed medication affected their symptoms, 70% were compliant and in better blood pressure control compared to 30% of the patients who did not report an effect of medication on their symptoms. For patients who were entering treatment for the first time, the effect was opposite; many more patients dropped out by the 9-month follow-up if they believed they could assess their pressure symptomatically in comparison to those who did not (60% vs 25%). New-to-treatment patients were confronting a discrepancy between their belief and the practitioner's for the first time, whereas the "executive decision maker" of continuing treatment patients was aware of and had navigated the discrepancy between experience and doctors' statements and succeeded in using an acute model to control a chronic condition by acting in accord with experience.

Multi-sided, seemingly contradictory statements were detected yet again in a study of adherence by asthmatic patients (median age, 49.9 years; range, 18–83), a condition common in many lower-income areas of U.S. cities (Halm, Mora, & Leventhal, 2006). Although the percentages can vary from one study to another, Halm and colleagues found that 80% of the adults in their sample agreed that they definitely or probably "will have asthma for the rest of their lives." However, 57% agreed that they definitely or probably only had "asthma when I have symptoms." The executive decision maker has little trouble agreeing with both statements, as the episodic flares are highly symptomatic and the underlying inflammatory process is asymptomatic (e.g., chronic, low levels of breathlessness). As expected, patients were efficient users of quick-relief medication to control attacks, but far fewer (45%) used medication to control the underlying inflammatory process if they believed they only had asthma when symptomatic; in contrast 70% of patients were adherent among those who said they have asthma when asymptomatic. The symptom-oriented group also failed to monitor their pulmonary function and were less likely to make routine visits to their provider when asymptomatic. Once again, decisions to medicate to relieve exacerbations and largely ignore the less dramatic underlying inflammatory process reflect prior history of management of acute conditions. In a review of nine studies of adherence to medication to control the inflammatory process underlying asthma, Kaptein, Klok, Moss-Morris, and Brand (2010) reinforce this conclusion, stating "Especially striking is the repeated finding that patients are liable to adopt an episodic or acute illness model of asthma (rather than more accurately considering asthma to be a chronic condition), which serves to discourage patients from properly adhering to anti-inflammatory medication, from long-term monitoring of pulmonary function, and from adequate self-management behavior." The decision process is consistent with stating that "I will have colds for the rest of my life" and "I only have colds when I have symptoms."

It is important to note, however, that mental models are not rigid; representations change over time. For example, whereas 70% of hypertensive patients new to treatment believed they could monitor pressure symptomatically; 92% believed this 9 months later (Meyer et al., 1985). Similarly, representations changed over time among asthmatic patients (Halm et al., 2006). The mental models actively shaping behavior at given time-points are responsive to feedback from behavior and information from others, though they gravitate toward one or more underlying models, such as the acute or chronic prototypes.

Misperceptions of symptoms: Acute coronary syndrome (ACS) and congestive heart failure (CHF). Decisions to seek care and adhere to treatment over the long term have proven to be a challenge not only for patients having ACS but for practitioners and the health-care system as well. Although it is recommended that patients be seen within 2h of symptom onset to avoid serious complications and death, few respond swiftly enough to meet this target. Women appear to delay because they misperceive symptoms or they are less severe than expected, and young adults, believing heart attacks are confined to elderly individuals, ignore symptoms and delay seeking care. Misattribution of symptoms to gastric distress also contributes to delay, whereas symptoms such as chest or arm pain, diaphoresis (sweating), and uncertainty contribute independently to swifter care seeking (Bunde & Martin, 2006). Randomized trials testing interventions to reduce the 1- to 12-h delay in seeking care post-symptom onset have addressed perception and interpretations of symptoms among patients with a prior history of myocardial infarct. Effective response to a MI requires, however, more than a valid representation of its presenting pattern. In addition to addressing the representation (Figure 1; step I), interventions need to address the output or response side of the system (Figure 1, step III). The CSM-based interventions addressing the representation of heart attacks (Dracup et al., 2009) produced significant improvements in patient's representations of their symptoms, but by overlooking action plans, the output side, failed to reduce delay to the recommended 2h or less post-symptom onset. Patients therefore, had not rehearsed calling the emergency medical service, what to say when calling, and had not visited their local emergency medical site and been reassured that it is important to call whether or not the episode proves to be a recurrence of MI. Decisions and action require a system that is coherent from the representations of illness and treatment, to plans for action in the individual's local environment; a module integrating all system components.

The intrusion of the acute module or script is only one of many factors capable of generating misperceptions of symptoms and delaying decisions and care seeking. Conceptual processes also can generate incorrect interpretations, decisions, and actions. For example, ACS and CHF share a common-sense label: both are "heart" diseases. They differ experientially, however, and require different decisions and actions. Unlike the fairly rapid onset of severe symptoms and need for prompt emergency care, the symptoms of CHF are chronic breathlessness, fatigue, and swelling of the legs. Management requires taking antidiuretic medication to control symptoms, and calling and visiting the practitioner when symptoms become severe. CHF patients, aware of the episodic pattern of heart attacks, do not recognize chronic experienced dyspnea, fatigue, and swollen feet as signs of heart disease and may not, therefore, perceive themselves as having heart disease. This is visible in the reports of patients who failed to seek care during serious episodes of CHF: "When you hear about having heart problems, you're supposed to feel maybe a pain in your left arm, maybe a pain in your chest, or pressure; it would have been more clear to me if I had chest pain then I would have said, okay, I'll call and say I'm having chest pain" (Horowitz, Rein, & Leventhal, 2004). The chronic and typically nondramatic symptoms of CHF do not match the heart prototype, and when interpreted as signs of aging they are symptoms to be tolerated rather than treated. There is little reason to treat such misinterpretations as relatively fixed, psychological traits; they are likely changeable with behavioral interventions that address the representations of both illness and treatment combined with action plans and valid outcome expectations to form coherent decision modules.

Life-Threatening Illnesses and End-of-Life Decisions

Efforts to empower and engage terminally ill patients in treatment decisions have led to requirements to complete advance directives when hospitalized. These documents ask patients to state their treatment preferences and designate someone to make critical decision in the event their lives are threatened and they are unable to make these decisions (Carr, 2011). Three aspects of end-of-life decisions of special interest psychologically are (1) the need to make decisions given limited or no direct experience with the events involved in a threatening and uncertain future, (2) the effect of prior patterns on current decisions, and (3) the importance of information sharing. How to address a basically unknowable, uncertain, and threatening future likely underlies data that fewer than 30% of adults have completed an advance directive, and many who have are unable to recall its content and/or where it is kept (Carr, 2011). Completion differs widely among ethnic groups. Both Hispanic and African Americans resist completing an advance directive, many believing that decisions as to when and how one dies are in God's hands (Carr, 2011). Studies of contextual moderators of the completion of advanced directives have not, however, examined the processes underlying how people project futures when making these decisions. We have begun

(Korovidov, 2009) to examine this processes by asking participants to briefly relate how they would prepare for specific events ranging from everyday happenings (e.g., visiting a new place; a 3- or 4-day bout of flu) to more serious issues (e.g., loss of income, becoming chronically ill, deciding for or against aggressive medical treatments if terminally ill). Using the methods for prospective memory (Addis, Wong, & Schachter, 2007), we replicated prior findings showing that younger participants generated more detailed narratives for everyday events than did their elders, but we found that difference decreased sharply as younger participants generated less detailed narratives when responding to health and end-of-life scenarios. The findings point to the importance of life experience and threat of the unknown for generating scene-specific details (Korovidov, 2009).

Recent studies suggest that decision making can shift from shared decisions to removing oneself from the process when the experience of a disease changes. Men previously diagnosed and treated for prostate cancer (median age, 69 years) report having been actively engaged in treatment decisions with their urological oncologist when first diagnosed (e.g., radiation vs surgery), but they leave decisions entirely in the hands of the oncologist given a subsequent rising prostate specific antigen (PSA) test (Johnson Shen et al., 2015). The changing PSA suggests that the initial decision and treatment did not cure the disease, implying that it is now a new and more virulent entity. Shifts in decision making of this type may vary across cancers, more likely for prostate cancers given the known, limited success of treatment following recurrence, but less so for breast cancer where treatment post-recurrence may stop progression. Treatment and screening decisions for cancer are clearly influenced by illness and treatment representations that are widely shared, and often based on the hope for cure intrinsic to the acute paradigm. The use of radical mastectomy in the 1940s and 1950s to fully extirpate and cure the disease suggest this outlook is at times shared by health professionals (Mukherjee, 2011). History highlights the role of political advocacy and publicly shared representations of illness and treatments on individual decisions.

SUMMARY AND THOUGHTS FOR THE FUTURE

Our description of the CSM and highly selective review of studies of decisions and actions for managing minor illnesses, chronic conditions, and terminal illness highlights themes applicable to decision making across the life span. First, specifying the referents for concepts is a critical step for decision theory. Second, decisions at any moment reflect both lifelong and episode-specific histories. Third, repeated experiences generate conceptual structures, modules, or scripts (Abelson, 1981) from features shared by multiple illnesses and treatments, and these scripts form higher-order abstractions that integrate properties common to these conditions and treatments (e.g., the acute and chronic models; Nelson & Shiffrin, 2013). These concepts, in turn, focus attention along with the acquisition and organization of information that affects decisions and action over the lifetime. Finally, contextual factors affect the salience, and therefore the content, of the variables active in health decisions. Many contextual factors are simply markers and do not specify the variables in the context that shape the content and action of the decision process.

The above themes have important implications for the study of health decisions and the role of executive processes in decision making. One concerns the assumption that reliable, multi-item scales to assess illness perceptions, self-efficacy, and conscientiousness, to predict adherence, quality of life, disease biomarkers, and other relevant factors will generate insights into the dynamics of decision making. Examining how executive processes maneuver the transition from acute to chronic conditions, or how they manage the seemingly less complex issue of developing a strategy for adhering to treatment for either an acute or chronic condition, will require a new approach using technologies for online assessments, aspects of which may present special challenges to those elderly patients unaccustomed to using computers and smart devices. Although valid scales are essential for assessing outcomes such as depression and quality of life in longitudinal studies and randomized, controlled trials, they are far less useful for identifying causal relationships in dynamic systems, and thus limited for guiding the development of interventions. Valid measures of self-efficacy or medical literacy may predict treatment adherence, but they do not tell us what these individuals did to adhere and how they acquired the skills to do so. As the association between such predictors and outcomes is far from perfect, it is likely that some individuals who are low in efficacy and literacy were adherent, and it is reasonable to ask whether they used the same or different strategies to adhere. For example, a subset of asthma patients adhere to anti-inflammatory medication by integrating its use into their daily routine (e.g., putting their inhaler in the bathroom, where it can be seen and used when washing and/or toileting), a practice little affected by education or literacy (Brooks et al., 2014). Identifying an effective strategy for adherence is not the same, however, as knowing how patients created this strategy. Did they focus attention and slowly review their daily routines to find a reliably repeatable routine and a place to put their inhaler so it would always be seen rather than focus on long-term goals such as avoiding severe attacks and hospitalization? Finding start points and engaging in a slow and careful review of context and behavioral sequences are strategies readily attributable to executive function and may be less frequently used by older than younger patients. It is also true that these strategies are not the same as knowing the most effective strategy for teaching patients how to discover and create adherence strategies in their home environments. Dynamic models are essential for understanding these processes and for modeling system changes over time.

Although modules such as the acute schema are stable, the mental representations or working models that shape interpretations and ongoing management can change rapidly, as can action plans, decision, and actions. The malleability of working mental representations may be related to the lack of visibility of underlying disease processes and initiating causes. Unlike injuries, the causal determinants of chronic and many acute conditions are remote from symptom onset and as shrouded in uncertainty as the internal disease processes themselves. The history of models for and treatments of cancer illustrates centuries—indeed millennia—of blindness to the processes underlying this disease (Mukherjee, 2011), and the same can be said for many medical and alternative practices.

Fear, depression, and other emotional reactions may focus attention on remote threats and interfere with the attention to start points and analysis of behavioral sequences. As emotions may be embedded in underlying prototypes, their activation will generate a mental model that includes the emotion, for example, fear of heart attack. Describing how emotions can affect executive processes such as attention to start points, monitoring behavioral sequences, and decisions to initiate actions, requires far more space than here available. By approaching health decisions and action within a framework designed to understand how the cognitive system works in real-world settings, CSM provides ample opportunity for discovering and modeling the details that operate in both the "cold" cognitive and "hot" affective domains. Studies motivated by CSM in both elderly and younger patients have alerted us to the computational processes underlying matching somatic changes to prototypes, generating and evaluating expectations, and have suggested a framework within which to examine how executive functions manage the transition from acute illnesses to the management of the uncertainties arising from an array of chronic conditions that arise primarily in the later years of life. Finally, CSM suggests new and combinations of existent approaches for helping patients discover how they can extract and understand the strategies and rules guiding everyday action and use these strategies in new ways and new places to better health and quality of life. Multiple challenges lie in waiting as we attempt to adapt this knowledge to the increasing levels of variability associated with a growing, aging population.

References

Abelson, R. P. (1981). Psychological status of the script concept. *American Psychologist, 36*, 715–729.

Addis, D. R., Wong, A. T., & Schacter, D. L. (2007). Remembering the past and imagining the future: Common and distinct neural substrates during event construction and elaboration. *Neuropsychologia, 45*, 1363–1377.

Akincigil, A., Bowblis, J. R., Levin, C., Jan, S., Patel, M., & Crystal, S. (2007). Long-term adherence to evidence based secondary prevention therapies after acute myocardial infarction. *Journal of General Internal Medicine, 23*, 115–121.

Anderson, G. (2010). *Chronic care: Making the case for ongoing care*. Retrieved from Robert Wood Johnson Foundation website: http://www.rwjf.org/content/dam/farm/reports/2010/rwjf54583.

Bandura, A. (1989). Human agency in social cognitive theory. *American Psychologist, 44*, 1175–1184.

Benyamini, Y., & Idler, E. L. (1999). Community studies reporting association between self-rated health and mortality additional studies, 1995 to 1998. *Research on Aging, 21*, 392–401.

Bishop, G. D. (1991). Understanding the understanding of illness: Lay disease representation. In J. A. Skelton, & R. T. Croyle (Eds.), *Mental representation in health and illness* (pp. 32–59). New York: Springer-Verlag.

Bishop, F. L., Yardley, L., & Lewith, G. T. (2010). Why consumers maintain complementary and alternative medicine use: A qualitative study. *Journal of Alternative and Complementary Medicine, 16*(2), 175–182.

Brooks, T. L., Leventhal, H., Wolf, M. S., O'Conor, R., Morillo, J., Martynenko, M., et al. (2014). Strategies used by older adults with asthma for adherence to inhaled corticosteroids. *Journal of General Internal Medicine, 29*(11), 1506–1512.

Bunde, J., & Martin, R. (2006). Depression and prehospital delay in the context of myocardial infarction. *Psychosomatic Medicine, 68*, 51–57.

Cameron, L., Leventhal, E. A., & Leventhal, H. (1993). Symptom representations and affect as determinants of care-seeking in a community dwelling adult sample population. *Health Psychology, 12*, 171–179.

Cameron, L., Leventhal, E. A., & Leventhal, H. (1995). Seeking medical care in response to symptoms and life stress. *Psychosomatic Medicine, 57*, 37–47.

Cameron, L. D., Leventhal, H., Love, R. R., & Patrick-Miller, L. J. (2002). Trait anxiety and tamoxifen effects on bone mineral density and sex hormone-binding globulin. *Psychosomatic Medicine, 64*, 612–620.

Carr, D. (2011). Racial differences in end-of-life planning: Why don't blacks and latinos prepare for the inevitable? *OMEGA–Journal of Death and Dying, 63*, 1–20.

Carver, C. S., & Scheier, M. F. (1981). *Attention and self-regulation*. New York: Springer-Verlag.

Cohen, S., Frank, E., Doyle, W. J., Skoner, D. P., Rabin, B. S., & Gwaltney, J. M. (1998). Types of stressors that increase susceptibility to the common cold in healthy adults. *Health Psychology, 17*, 214–223.

Cramer, J. A. (2002). Effect of partial compliance on cardiovascular medication effectiveness. *Heart, 88*, 203–206.

Dracup, K., McKinley, S., Riegel, B., Moser, D. K., Meischke, H., Doering, L. V., et al. (2009). A randomized clinical trial to reduce patient prehospital delay to treatment in acute coronary syndrome. *Circulation, Cardiovascular Quality Outcomes, 2*, 524–532.

Halm, E. A., Mora, P., & Leventhal, H. (2006). No symptoms, no asthma: The acute episodic disease belief is associated with poor self-management among inner-city adults with persistent asthma. *Chest, 129*, 573–580.

Horne, R., Chapman, S. C. E., Parham, R., Freemantle, N., Forbes, A., & Cooper, V. (2013). Understanding patients' adherence-related beliefs about medicines prescribed for long-term conditions: A meta-analytic review of the necessity-concerns framework. *PLoS ONE, 8*(12), e80633. http://dx.doi.org/10.1371/journal.pone.0080633.

Horne, R., Weinman, J., & Hankins, M. (1999). The beliefs about medicines questionnaire: The development and evaluation of a new method for assessing the cognitive representation of medication. *Psychology and Health, 14*, 1–24.

Horowitz, C. R., Rein, S. B., & Leventhal, H. (2004). A story of maladies, misconceptions and mishaps: Effective management of heart failure. *Social Science & Medicine, 58*, 631–643.

Idler, E. L. (1993). Age Differences in self-assessments of health: Age changes, cohort differences or survivorship? *Journal of Gerontology: Social Sciences, 48*(6), S289–S300.

Idler, E. L., & Benyamini, Y. (1997). Self-rated health and mortality: A review of twenty-seven community studies. *Journal of Health and Social Behavior, 38*, 21–37.

Johnson, J. E. (1975). Stress reduction through sensation information. In I. C. Sarason, & C. O. Speilberger (Eds.), *Stress and anxiety* (Vol. 2) (pp. 361–373). Washington: Hemisphere.

Johnson Shen, M., Nelson, C., Peters, E., Slovin, S., Hall, S., Hall, M., et al. (2015). Decision making processes among prostate cancer survivors with rising PSA levels: Results from a qualitative analysis. *Medical Decision Making* (in Press).

Kahneman, D., & Miller, D. T. (1986). Norm theory: Comparing reality to its alternatives. *Psychological Review, 93*, 136.

Kaptein, A. A., Klok, T., Moss-Morris, R., & Brand, P. L. (2010). Illness perceptions: Impact on self-management and control in asthma. *Current Opinion In Allergy and Clinical Immunology, 10*, 194–199.

Korovidov, D. (2009). Age related changes in episodic simulation of health events (Undergraduate Honors Thesis). Department of Psychology, Rutgers, University.

Leventhal, E. A., & Crouch, M. (1997). Are there differences in perceptions of illness across the life-span? In K. J. Petrie, & J. A. Wienman (Eds.), *Perceptions of health and illness: Current research and applications* (pp. 77–102). London: Harwood Academic Press.

Leventhal, E. A., Leventhal, H., Shacham, S., & Easterling, D. V. (1989). Active coping reduces reports of pain from childbirth. *Journal of Consulting and Clinical Psychology, 57*, 365–371.

Leventhal, H. (1970). Findings and theory in the study of fear communications. *Advances in Experimental Social Psychology, 5*, 119–186.

Leventhal, H., Idler, E. L., & Leventhal, E. A. (1999). The impact of chronic illness on the self-system. In R. J. Contrada, & R. D. Ashmore (Eds.), *Self, social identity, and physical health: Interdisciplinary explorations* (pp. 185–208). New York: Oxford University Press.

Leventhal, H., Leventhal, E. A., Cameron, L., Bodnar-Deren, S., Breland, J. Y., Hash-Converse, J., et al. (2011). Modeling health and illness behavior: The approach of the common sense model (CSM). In A. Baum, & T. A. Revenson (Eds.), *Handbook of health psychology* (2nd ed.).

Leventhal, H., Nerenz, D. R., Leventhal, E. A., Love, R. R., & Bendena, L. M. (1991). The behavioral dynamics of clinical trials. *Preventive Medicine, 20*, 132–146.

Leventhal, H., Singer, R., & Jones, S. (1965). Effects of fear and specificity of recommendation upon attitudes and behavior. *Journal of Personality and Social Psychology, 2*, 20.

Leventhal, H., Weinman, J., Leventhal, E. A., & Phillips, L. A. (2008). Health psychology: The search for pathways between behavior and health. *Annual Review of Psychology, 59*, 477–505.

Meyer, D., Leventhal, H., & Gutmann, M. (1985). Common-sense models of illness: The example of hypertension. *Health Psychology, 4*, 115.

Mora, P. A., DiBonaventura, M. D., Idler, E., Leventhal, E. A., & Leventhal, H. (2008). Psychological factors influencing self-assessments of health: Towards an understanding of the mechanisms underlying how people rate their own health. *Annals of Behavioral Medicine, 36*, 292–303.

Mukherjee, S. (2011). *The emperor of all maladies: A biography of cancer*. Simon and Schuster.

Nelson, A. B., & Shiffrin, R. M. (2013). The co-evolution of knowledge and event memory. *Psychological Review, 1230*(2), 356–394.

Park, D. (1999). Aging and the controlled and automatic processing of medical information and medical intentions. In D. C. Park, R. W. Morrell, & K. Shifren (Eds.), *Processing of medical information in aging patients: Cognitive and human factors perspectives* (pp. 3–22). Mahwah, NJ: Erlbaum.

Payne, J. W., Bettman, J. R., & Johnson, E. J. (1993). *The adaptive decision maker*. Cambridge: Cambridge University Press.

Phillips, L. A., Diefenbach, M. A., Kronish, I. M., Negron, R. M., & Horowitz, C. R. (2014). The necessity-concerns framework: A multidimensional theory benefits from multidimensional analysis. *Annals of Behavioral Medicine*, *48*(1), 7–16.

Phillips, L. A., Leventhal, H., & Leventhal, E. A. (2012). Physicians' communication of the common-sense self-regulation model results in greater reported adherence than physicians' use of interpersonal skills. *British Journal of Health Psychology*, *17*, 244–257.

Prohaska, T. R., Leventhal, E. A., Leventhal, H., & Keller, M. L. (1985). Health practices and illness cognition in young, middle aged, and elderly adults. *Journal of Gerontology*, *40*, 569–578.

Shadbolt, B., Barresi, J., & Craft, P. (2002). Self-rated health as a predictor of survival among patients with advanced cancer. *Journal of Clinical Oncology*, *20*, 2514–2519.

Stoller, E. P., Carry, S., & Portugal, S. S. (1997). Explaining pathways of care taken by elderly people: An analysis of responses to illness symptoms. *Sociological Focus*, *30*(2), 147–165.

Tanenbaum, M. L. (2013). *Learning what works: Illness coherence and self-monitoring of blood glucose in type2 diabetes management*. Yeshiva University: Ferkauf Graduate School of Psychology (Unpublished Dissertation).

Weinman, J., Petrie, K. J., Moss-Morris, R., & Horne, R. (1996). The illness perception questionnaire: A new method for assessing the cognitive representation of illness. *Psychology and Health*, *11*, 431–445.

CHAPTER

15

Choice and Aging: Less is More

Pi-Ju Liu[1], *Stacey Wood*[2], *Yaniv Hanoch*[3]

[1]Psychology Department, University of San Francisco, San Francisco, CA, USA; [2]Department of Psychology, Scripps College, Claremont, CA, USA; [3]School of Psychology, Plymouth University, Plymouth, Devon, UK

INTRODUCTION

The financial crisis that started in 2007–2008 has had a major impact on millions of people in the United States and across the globe. Unfortunately, as of 2014, its impact is still felt among older adults, as their capacity to compensate for losses is much more limited. Given older adults' unique position and challenges, it is no wonder that the popular press has been rife with stories on the financial difficulties older adults have encountered. A series of articles in the *New York Times*, for example, captured the diverse, and sometimes unexpected, ways the financial crisis has eroded older adults' financial standing. They discussed, among other topics, the need to return to work after retirement (Noor, 2009), the high rate of housing foreclosure among the elderly (Brown, 2012), how older adults became the family financial safety net (Daley, 2012), and the erosion of earning power among those near retirement (Rampell, 2013). Older adults are not only facing more financial challenges than ever before, but they have to do so in an increasingly complex and choice-rich environment.

Financial decision making involves analyzing related information, such as how much to save for retirement or which product to purchase. It is the process of selecting the right choice that has positive implications for a person's financial well-being. While the financial crisis has had a wide-ranging impact, one common thread among these articles is the link between economic hardship and health status. Interestingly, about a year prior to the emergence of the financial crisis, the Medicare Modernization Act (better known as Medicare Part D) had come into effect. Providing

Aging and Decision Making
http://dx.doi.org/10.1016/B978-0-12-417148-0.00015-7

prescription drug coverage for millions of beneficiaries, Medicare Part D has offered some financial reprieve for older adults. Yet a number of the program elements have been criticized, mainly due to the complex nature of the Medicare Part D decision environment. The criticism against the complexity of the program is in line with a growing body of evidence suggesting that the decision environment can enhance or impair individuals' decision making, with this perhaps being particularly true for older adults (McWilliams, Afendulis, Mcguire, & Landon, 2011). In this chapter, we use the Medicare Part D insurance choice as an example, for it can serve as a real-world decision environment to investigate older adults' decision-making capacity and preferences. We were particularly interested in the impact of choice set size on decision making in older adults for a couple of reasons. First, much of the work in decision making and aging is grounded theoretically in dual-process models. These models predict that increases in cognitive demands should disproportionally impact older adults. Second, in terms of policy, there is some debate regarding the optimal choice set size for consumers. On the one hand, consumers may benefit from a large degree of choice, because increased choice may increase the number of options and decrease cost. Alternatively, some have argued (e.g., Schwartz, 2004) that increasing choice decreases satisfaction with the decision, and hampers consumers' abilities to make decisions in their best interest. Medicare Part D provides something of a natural experiment to examine both of these issues. We review a number of key areas related to choice such as dual-process theories, cognitive ability, numeracy, and other related factors. We also provide results from one experiment that nicely captures many of the themes that develop in this chapter.

CHOICE PREFERENCE AND SIZE IN DECISION MAKING

In *The Paradox of Choice* (2004), Schwartz stated "More is less." Although having choices grants people a sense of autonomy, more options can become less advantageous when choices expand rapidly and become overwhelming. Decision quality, satisfaction, and preference can be impacted with a larger choice set size. Schwartz's idea corresponded to a body of literature that has found that as the number of choices increases, people have difficulties processing information and report overall lower levels of satisfaction with their choice (Botti & Iyengar, 2006; 2005; Schwartz et al., 2002; Wood et al., 2011). For example, in one study (Iyengar, Huberman, & Jiang, 2004), researchers assessed the retirement decision making of 80,000 U.S. workers. Overall, the study found that the more choices the employees had, the less likely they were to join any of the 401 (k) plans available to them.

As mentioned earlier, the U.S. government has created a decision environment for older adults where it is possible to study some of the relationships between cognitive resources and decision making. Medicare Part D was designed to foster market competition to allow older adults to purchase a drug plan that best fits their personal need. The program design, not surprisingly, has led to an abundance of insurance plans: Currently, more than 30 stand-alone plans exist in most states (Kaiser Family Foundation, 2013). Given the financial and health ramifications associated with choosing a Medicare prescription drug plan—as compared to other consumer products, such as jams—one might wonder whether older adults prefer to see many or fewer drug plan choices on the market.

Considerable empirical research explored the effect of choice size in relation to decision-making performance, and most indicated a negative impact of increasing options on performance (Botti & Iyengar, 2006; Iyengar & Lepper, 2000; Schwartz et al., 2002). In one of the first Medicare studies exploring the relationship between choice and decision making, Tanius, Wood, Hanoch, and Rice (2009) presented participants with either 6 or 24 different prescription drug plans and asked them to choose the best one (defined as the cheapest overall plan). Those presented with 24 options were less likely to pick the least expensive plan. Using a similar design, Barnes, Hanoch, Wood, Liu, and Rice (2012) found the same effect with 9 options versus 3 options. Moreover, in other studies examining Medicare Part D with different numbers of options (Besedes, Deck, Sarangi, & Shor, 2012; Hanoch, Rice, Cummings, & Wood, 2009; Hanoch, Wood, Barnes, Liu, & Rice, 2011; Szrek & Bundorf, 2013; Wood et al., 2011), both age and increased options decreased performance as well.

So far, only a limited number of studies have investigated age differences in the desired number of options (Cummings, Rice, & Hanoch, 2009; Reed, Mikels, & Löckenhoff, 2013; Reed, Mikels, & Simon, 2008). Reed et al. (2008) compared older and younger adults' desire for choice. Using a paper-and-pencil survey, they demonstrated that older adults (compared to younger ones) desired significantly less choice across six different choice domains (health care and everyday decisions, including cars, apartments, and jams). Furthermore, both age groups preferred less choice in the area of health care compared to daily decisions. Reed et al. (2013) further explored the relationship between age and choice preference across 12 different domains, and found an age-related decrease in desired number of options. Rice, Hanoch, and Cummings (2010) asked a representative panel of older adults whether they would prefer having dozens of plans for Medicare Part D or being offered a restricted number of plans. The majority (69%) of participants wanted to see Medicare take a more active role and restrict the number of plans. Findings from the above-mentioned studies exemplify a possible tension between what older adults report they want and the decision environment they currently face. In addition, what was crucially missing from this research is the investigation of the possible mechanisms underlying older adults' choice preferences. The following sections discuss potential explanations of choice preference and decision-making quality, including cognitive ability, numeracy, and other related factors.

DUAL-PROCESS MODELS AND IMPLICATIONS FOR DECISION MAKING IN OLDER ADULTS

Cognitive ability is one of the possible contributors to choice set-size performance as well as preference, and dual-process models have been postulated to characterize the role of cognitive ability in decision making. When making decisions, theorists proposed that information processing involves two types of procedures (e.g., Epstein, 1994; Kahneman, 2003): System 1, which refers to an affective/experiential system; and System 2, which refers to a more deliberative/analytical system. System 1 can be thought of as automatic, effortless, rigid, heuristic-based, affective, and implicit. It is the kind of decision that can be made almost unconsciously, such as stereotyping. In contrast, System 2 is described as effortful, conscious, analytical, slow, flexible, and more resource intensive. It requires attention and concentration, such as computing and comparing probabilities (Kahneman, 2011; Stanovich & West, 2000). The two systems can work simultaneously, and affective information can also influence deliberative thinking. However, System 2 can become depleted and less efficient with effort. Given the nature of health-related decision making, it is reasonable to assume that such decisions would involve both deliberate and affective components.

A number of researchers have capitalized on dual-process models to better understand life-span changes in decision-making abilities (Peters, Hess, Västfjäll, & Auman, 2007; Peters & Bruine de Bruin, 2012; see also Hess, in this volume). Overall, there is a general consensus by those studying aging and decision making that older adults will perform worse on tasks that are more heavily dependent on System 2 processes relative to those dependent on System 1, based on the findings that aging is associated with normative decline in specific cognitive abilities typically associated with System 2 (Peters & Bruine de Bruin, 2012). For example, changes in working memory and processing speed would more directly impact System 2 type deliberative processes than System 1 type processes (Evans, 2003).

Indeed, there are now ample data to argue that age effects on choice performance and strategies are most likely associated with System 2 type processes (e.g., Hanoch, Wood, & Rice, 2007), especially when the decision-making tasks are cognitively demanding or lack supportive environments for decisions (Finucane, Mertz, Slovic, & Schmidt, 2005; Yoon, Cole, & Lee, 2009). Declines in cognitive abilities make it more difficult for older adults to navigate a complex decision-making environment that requires concentration. For example, older adults are slower in terms of processing speed, which is associated with decreased performance on other cognitive tasks (Salthouse, 1996). Also, although it remains to be investigated in more depth, the tendency for older adults to seek less information in decision-making tasks might be related to decreased working memory capacity (for a review, see Mather, 2006). These findings from the cognitive aging literature imply that aging is associated with declines in fluid abilities, such as speed of processing, working memory, and executive functioning (Schaie & Willis, 2002), precisely the abilities that characterize System 2 processing and functioning. Whether older adults are cognizant of these changes and thus are more likely to actively prefer less demanding choice environments is an open empirical question. Regardless of preference, however, their performance in different choice environments may very well decline if these environments tax System 2 types of processes.

There is support for dual-process theories in the area of medical decision-making and aging. Because older adults tend to use more health-related services, more work was done in the health domain versus other areas of decision-making abilities. Hibbard, Slovic, Peters, Finucane, and Tusler (2001) have long been interested in older adults' abilities to understand health-related (e.g., insurance) information. In one study, they evaluated older and younger adults' comprehension of health and financial information about health insurance. Their results indicated that older adults are more likely to make mistakes compared to younger adults. Finucane et al. (2005), in a related investigation, focused on the association between age and decision quality by varying the complexity of tasks in a number of related domains: health, financial, and dietary. Their data showed that as the task became more complex, the number of errors increased as well, with older adults experiencing even greater difficulties than their younger participants. As such, one would predict that as the number of choices increases, older adults would be less likely to make optimal decisions compared with younger counterparts.

More evidence supports the relationship between cognitive resources and decision making in aging. Based on a series of studies, Johnson (1990, 1993) had amassed sufficient evidence to show that, when deciding about cars or apartments, older adults tend to evaluate less information, reexamine information more often, need longer time to review information, and use more simplified search strategies. Mata and colleagues (Mata, von Helversen, & Rieskamp, 2010; Mata, Schooler, & Rieskamp, 2007) have provided similar results, using somewhat different tasks. In their investigations, they were interested in the relationship between aging and the ability to utilize adaptive decision strategies in a number of different environmental structures. In line with Johnson's earlier work, Mata and colleagues found that older adults frequently use less information and require more time to evaluate it in their decision making. Furthermore, older adults often utilized simpler decision strategies due to, according to the authors, declines in cognitive abilities. A meta-analysis by Mata and Nunes (2010) provides further indication that older adults tend to use more heuristic-based decision strategies, as they often search and use less information in their decision-making process. However, other studies (Hess, Queen, & Ennis, 2013; Queen, Hess, Ennis, Dowd, & Grühn, 2013) found smaller differences in search strategies and highlight the importance of individual difference factors like education and search environment in strategy selection across the life span. Taken together, these findings appear to indicate that older adults are more likely than younger adults to adopt simpler strategies in their searches.

AN EMPIRICAL STUDY TESTING THE MEDIATING EFFECT OF COGNITIVE ABILITY ON CHOICE PREFERENCE

There is also evidence that most individuals will use different strategies based upon the task demands, and that age is only one factor to consider. Hanoch and Rice (2006) discussed the impact of Medicare Part D when it was newly introduced. They were concerned that many available options would be challenging for older adults in light of decline in cognitive ability across the life span. Their concern is consistent with findings on the decline of System 2 cognitive functioning with increasing age. Moreover, other researchers noted that as the number of options increases, the cognitive effort in evaluating those options also increases (Bundorf & Szrek, 2010; Keller & Staelin, 1987; Szrek & Bundorf, 2011). Consistent with that predication, older adults' Medicare Part D decision-making quality was found to be not as good as younger adults either, even though they were more confident in their choices (Hanoch et al., 2009). Based on the literature above, one straightforward prediction would be that older adults may express a preference for less choice when the complexity of decision-making increases (Finucane et al., 2002; Hanoch et al., 2011; Johnson, 1990; Mather, 2006; Meyer, Russo, & Talbot, 1995; Pinquart & Duberstein, 2004; Reed et al., 2013; Steginga & Occhipinti, 2002). To test this hypothesis, we conducted a study examining choice preferences and cognitive ability. It was predicted that performance in the cognitive domains relating to System 2 processes, including processing speed, working memory, and executive functioning, would mediate the relationship between age and preferred number of options.

Methods

A sample of 107 participants across the life-span (aged 18–91) were invited to our laboratory for a Medicare Part D decision-making study. Participants filled out a preference questionnaire from Reed et al. (2008) that contained questions related to choosing a Medicare prescription drug plan. Participants were asked to indicate their preferred number of options for Medicare plans (How many choices would you like to be available? How many choices, from 2 to 26, would make you most satisfied with your choice?). Following the suggestion of Reed et al., the mean was computed for analysis. Additionally, since personal importance could be another factor influencing participants' choice preference (detailed below), the degree to which a Medicare prescription drug plan was important to participants was assessed on a 5-point Likert scale (How important is a Medicare prescription drug plan to you?), ranging from "not important at all" to "very important." Cognitive measures included processing speed using digit comparison (Finucane et al., 2005), working memory using the two-back task (cognitivefun.net/test/4), and executive functioning using the Trail-Making Test A and B (Spreen & Strauss, 1998).

Results

Our analysis followed the Baron and Kenny (1986) framework by employing structural equation modeling (SEM) to analyze the mediated effects of cognitive ability on the relationship between age and preferences. The SEM model consisted of two observed variables (age and preferred number of options) and one latent variable (cognitive ability) that was measured by three indicators (processing speed, working memory, and executive functioning). As can be seen in Figure 1, a significant mediation effect for age to cognitive ability to preferred number of options was observed, meaning that age differences in choice preference can be statistically explained by cognition, such that individuals with lower cognitive ability overall preferred fewer choices. The finding provided support for the hypothesis such that performance in the cognitive domains mediated the relationship between age and preferred number of options (see Table 1 for path coefficient β, standard error, p-values, lower and upper bounds for bootstrap procedure).

Another decision-making study had a similar study design, but Henninger, Madden, and Huettel (2010) investigated decision-making performance rather than preference. They found that cognitive ability, including processing speed and working memory, plays a role in decision-making quality. As indicated in the study, age-related differences in participants' performance were mediated by age-related

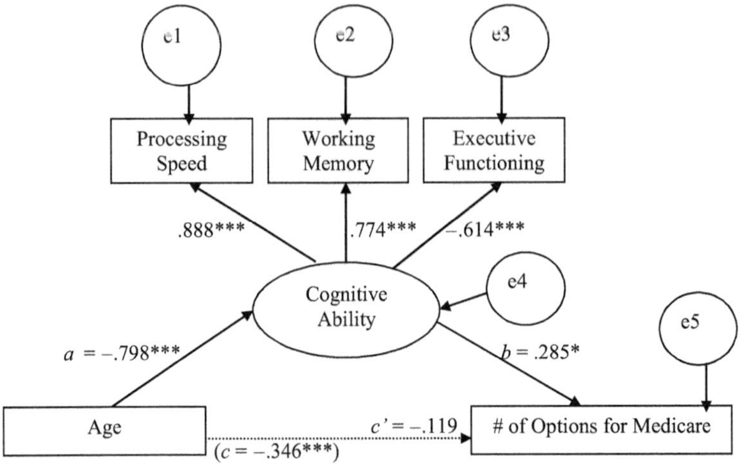

FIGURE 1 The model with cognitive ability as the mediator between age and preferred number of options for Medicare prescription drug plan. Path *c* showed an effect between age and the number of preferred options that could be mediated. Path *c*′ indicated the mediation effect after cognitive ability was included in the model. The values are standardized path coefficients. (***$p<0.001$, *$p<0.05$.)

TABLE 1 Bootstrap Mediation Methods on the Effect of Age on Preferred Number of Options Mediated Through Cognitive Ability

			Bootstrap 95% CI		
Effect	**Estimate**	**SE**	**Lower bounds**	**Upper bounds**	***p* (two-tailed)**
a	−0.798***	0.044	−0.873	−0.698	0.002
b	0.285*	0.201	−0.111	0.690	0.128
c	−0.346***	0.080	−0.512	−0.184	0.002
c′	−0.119	0.168	−0.446	0.217	0.454

***$p<0.001$, **$p<0.01$, *$p<0.05$.

change in cognitive capacities. One important caveat is that the data in both of these studies are cross-sectional by nature, and thus the mediation effects may simply represent spurious correlations as opposed to true functional relationships. We cannot infer casual relationships without conducting a longitudinal study (Lindenberger, von Oertzen, Ghisletta, & Hertzog, 2011). Overall though, the work from medical decision making supports the application of dual-process models to aging such that age differences mostly occurred in tasks that require System 2 processing.

NUMERACY AND CHOICE SET SIZE IN DECISION MAKING

In addition to cognitive ability, numeracy— or the ability to identify, understand, critically interpret and apply mathematical concepts, processes, and representations—is a second but related key factor important for financial decision making. An extensive line of research has shown that possessing financial literacy, including the ability to understand financial terms, be engaged in financial markets, or judge financial information, enables people to employ knowledge and skills to manage financial resources effectively for a lifetime of financial well-being (Lusardi & Mitchell, 2011). Numeracy appears to be independent of education and general intellectual abilities (IQ). Indeed, after reviewing earlier literature (e.g., Lipkus, Samsa, & Rimer, 2001) as well as their own findings, Brown et al. (2011) maintained that education level does not predict numeracy. In a series of studies, Peters et al. (2006) showed that high- and low-numeracy individuals process information differently. High-numeracy adults were at greater ease in transforming numbers from one unit of measurement to another, and more likely to utilize the correct numerical principles. Low-numeracy individuals, on the other hand, were "left with information that is less complete and less understood, lacking in the complexity and richness available to the more numerate" (2006, p. 412), suggesting that low-numeracy individuals processed information less efficiently.

There is ample evidence to show, for example, that higher numeracy and financial literacy are closely linked to the ability to understand a wide range of financial products, such as health insurance, stocks, saving, and borrowing. The pioneering work of Lusardi and colleagues provided some indication with regard to the poor nature of peoples' numeracy skills and ability to grapple and compute financial information. Lusardi and Mitchell (2011) included in the 2004 Health and Retirement Study (HRS) survey a number of financial questions, such as how much money a person will have after 5 years if they had $100 in a savings account and the interest rate was 2% per year. About one-third of the sample was unable to answer this question correctly, despite the fact that many have had extensive experience investing their money. The results of the U.S. Financial Capability Study (Lusardi & Mitchell, 2011), using the same questions, also exposed the low state of numeracy in the United States, as 13.5% of the participants indicated that they are not able to answer this question. What is even more alarming is the fact that participants in the aforementioned studies rarely had to make the computations themselves, which probably simplified the task.

Additionally, we know that the majority of the population is having difficulties with decision making that involves numbers based on data from the 2004 U.S. HRS survey, one of the largest surveys of individuals

50 and over in the United States (see http://hrsonline.isr.umich.edu/). For example, 50% of the participants could not answer correctly how much is 2million divided by 5. When it came to making a financial calculation, the rate of correct response dropped even further. Less than 20% of the participants were able to provide the correct answer to the following basic question: "*Let's say you have 200 dollars in a savings account. The account earns 10 percent interest* per *year. How much would you have in the account at the end of two years?*" (Lusardi & Mitchell, 2006, 2008). A study conducted in the United Kingdom among participants ranging in age from 18 to 79, with an additional two questions to the three used in the above study, also presented the dire level of numeracy among the general population. Only one out of 10 people was able to answer all five questions correctly. When the same five questions were presented to an American population the results remained the same (Atkinson, McKay, Kempson, & Collard, 2007). This fact further magnifies the extent to which numeracy is an issue.

The (in)ability to correctly answer these simple questions demonstrates the role of numeracy in financial decision making, which is vital for any discussion of older (as well as younger) adults' ability to understand health insurance information and make informed decisions. Indeed, a long line of research has precisely highlighted the key role numeracy plays in different medical decisions (Gigerenzer, Gaissmaier, Kurz-Milcke, Schwartz, & Woloshin, 2007). We know, for example, that low numeracy skills are related to poorer comprehension of screening information (Schwartz, Woloshin, Black, & Welch, 1997), lack of familiarity with the health-care structure (DeWalt, Berkman, Sheridan, Lohr, & Pignone, 2004), as well as worse health outcomes (Institute of Medicine, 2004). In our own studies (Wood et al., 2011), we have found that numeracy predicted performance on a medical insurance decision task. Furthermore, numeracy predicted success on this task, independent of other cognitive variables (processing speed, working memory, and executive functioning) or education. In other research looking at decision making within the Medicare Part D environment, Szrek and Bundorf (2011, 2013) reported similar findings, showing that numeracy plays a key, and unique, role in the decision-making process. Thus, our earlier studies (Hanoch et al., 2011; Wood et al., 2011) as well as others (Szrek & Bundorf, 2011, 2013) have demonstrated that higher numeracy levels are associated with better financial decision making, even after cognitive ability and education were taken into account. Other researchers (e.g., Brown et al., 2011) have reported similar trends related to the role of numeracy in making health decisions, including people's ability to interpret graphical breast cancer risk estimates. Reyna, Nelson, Han, and Diekman (2009) have argued that "on the basis of studies that have controlled for education, intelligence, literacy, and other factors, we can be reasonably sure that numeracy is a separate faculty" (p. 967) highlighting the importance of the complexity in understanding health decision making.

While to our knowledge only few studies examined numeracy skills across the life span, the existing literature suggests that, overall, older adults tend to possess lower numeracy abilities. One of the largest international surveys (OECD Skills Outlook, 2013) on literacy and numeracy has shown that older adults exhibit lower numeracy ability than younger counterparts. The findings by the OECD Skills Outlook mirror those reported in an earlier survey with a British population. The findings (Jenkins, Ackerman, Frumkin, Salter, & Vorhaus, 2011) revealed that the percentage of older adults who are classified as having low numeracy increases steadily from age 50 onward. In fact, while about 10% of those between 50 and 59 years of age were classified as low numeracy, among individuals 70 and over the rate increased to over 20% and to close to 30% among those over 80. As such, older adults are not only facing cognitive decline but also reduced numeracy ability to deal with complex and challenging decision environments, such as Medicare Part D. Nonetheless, the relatively new area of numeracy and choice preference is awaiting more extensive investigation. So far, only Reed et al. (2013) examined this question and found no bivariate relationship between numeracy and choice preference. Thus, whether lower levels of numeracy is also associated with preference for less choice is not clear, and may involve a more complex story.

ADDITIONAL FACTORS IN RELATION TO CHOICE SET SIZE AND PREFERENCE

Age differences in choice performance were the primary focus in the above studies, but the influence of individual variables (i.e., cost, brand names) in relation to the choice environment was not typically examined. Barnes et al. (2012) examined the effects of price frames, brand names, and choice set size using a mouse-laboratory style study (Bettman, Johnson, & Payne, 1990). Mouselab is a web-based decision environment which presents plan information in a grid. Participants must move over a square to reveal the information underneath. As such the program can trace the decision-making strategy of the participants, adding insight into how they are making their choice. As noted above, older adults are thought to rely more on System 1 type decision-making processes as a group, and may be more likely to rely on mental shortcuts such as heuristics in their decision processes. For example, brand names often serve as such a shortcut for all consumers (e.g., Ganther & Kreling, 2000). In the study of Barnes et al. (2012), they manipulated brand names and pricing information (real numerical dollar amounts vs a range indicated by dollar symbols $, $$, or $$$), in addition to number of plans. Overall, the study replicated the finding that choice set size matters, with older adults performing better overall with fewer choices. The authors also found that presenting price information as a symbol versus a number improved performance, perhaps because it lessened the burden of numeracy. It is also possible that the use of symbols evoked affective strategies similar to those reported in Hsee and Rottenstreich (2004); however, this was not explored in the original paper. In another Mouselab study, Hanoch et al. (2011) also indicated that the search strategy employed by older adults was less efficient than that used by younger adults in exploring the grid of information. In addition, although older adults tended to reveal more boxes for information, they also revisited the boxes they already looked at more frequently, perhaps reflecting poor memory for the already examined information.

Reviewing choice information more closely can also be related to personal relevance or significance (Hess et al., 2013; Reed et al., 2008). For example, individuals may desire more choices in domains that are highly relevant to them, and desire less in areas to which they are indifferent. Hess et al. (2013), also using Mouselab for choosing a prescription drug plan, found that personal relevance differentially affected extensiveness of search in older adults relative to younger adults. In another study, Zwahr, Park, and Shifren (1999) asked females to estimate the number of effective treatments for menopause. Older women perceived fewer options to be effective compared with younger women, consistent with a view that older adults prefer less choice. More interestingly, controlling for age, personal relevance of menopause was positively correlated with the number of treatments desired, indicating that for people of the same age, as relevance increased so did preference for choice options. In other words, higher importance ratings are related to preference for larger amounts of choice. Therefore, it is necessary to take both age and importance rating of individuals' into account. For instance, older adults who considered a decision to be less relevant may prefer fewer options, while older adults who considered the decision to be very relevant would prefer more options.

We examined the same dataset mentioned earlier in the chapter to test the hypothesis that personal relevance predicted choice preference above and beyond age (Liu & Wood, 2010). According to Reed et al. (2008), older adults preferred fewer options. According to Zwahr et al. (1999), health-related decisions should be important to some individuals affected by the decisions. Therefore, it was hypothesized that controlling for age, importance of the decision-making domain would predict preference for number of Medicare prescription drug plans, such that the higher the participants' importance rating, the more options they would prefer. The results indicated that Medicare prescription drug plans were rated as important in general, with older adults ($M=4.38$, $SD=1.00$) rating it, as expected, as more important than younger adults ($M=3.11$, $SD=1.34$, $p<0.01$). Regression results showed that overall, people preferred fewer options with increasing age; nonetheless, as predicted, for people of the same age, higher personal importance was associated with a preference

TABLE 2 Hierarchical Regression Predicting Preferred Number of Options

Step	Predictor	r	F	R^2 Added	Final B	SE (b)	β
1	Age	−0.33***	14.31***	0.12***	−0.10***	0.02	−0.44***
2	Medicare importance	−0.02	10.60***	0.05*	0.92*	0.47	0.21*
	Constant				10.73***	1.62	

***$p<0.001$, **$p<0.01$, *$p<0.05$. β values are from the second step, with age and importance in the model.

for more options (see Table 2 for results on hierarchal regression), indicating that personal relevance is another potential factor associated with choice preference.

In addition to the effects of cognitive ability and numeracy, a few other factors have been proposed to explain older adults' preference for fewer options. Older adults have been described as prioritizing emotional regulation, and it is possible that their desire to minimize unnecessary stress could result in a preference for less choice. A related factor, older adults' awareness of changes in their own cognitive ability, was also proposed as a mechanism underlying the preference for a smaller number of choices (Reed et al., 2008). However, although people prefer fewer options when a choice justification is asked for (Scheibehenne, Greifeneder, & Todd, 2009), it is not clear if older adults would provide managing stress or ability problems as reasons when a justification is requested. Reed et al. (2013) further examined whether personality traits, decision-making self-efficacy, maximizing (i.e., focus on selecting the optimal choice), and cognitive abilities (digit span, numeracy, and vocabulary) contributed in explaining choice preference after participant age was taken into account. Surprisingly, none of the factors did. In particular, the fact that ability was unrelated to performance is at odds with our own previously described study in the area. This may reflect differences in abilities sampled. The cognitive measures used by Reed et al. assessed short-term memory, numeracy, and verbal ability, whereas ours included processing speed, working memory, and executive functioning. Overall, these results are in line with other studies indicating that factors impacting choice performance and preference are complex, and that more research investigating mediation or moderation effects lies ahead for researchers to explore mechanisms that affect real-life decision making.

SUMMARY

Older adults are frequently faced with financial decisions that involve choices between an array of options. Current dual-process models predict that older adults will demonstrate relatively impaired decision making when effective performance relies on deliberative reasoning that taxes cognitive resources. Older adults are also, as a group, lower in numeracy, which can further hamper decisions that require reading tables or even making simple calculations. We found that cognitive ability, including processing speed, working memory, and executive functioning, is the factor that is most related to older adults' preference of Medicare prescription drug plans. An examination of older adults' insurance-purchasing decisions has allowed us to examine the above predictions in a real-world applied decision-making task.

When Medicare Part D was designed, policymakers presumed that a wide range of choices would benefit beneficiaries. Consequently, older adults have been required to choose from an array of well over 30 different Medicare prescription drug plans in some regions. Previous research has already demonstrated that the large numbers of prescription drug plans hindered older adults' decision-making abilities (Hanoch et al., 2009; Tanius et al., 2009; Wood et al., 2011). Nonetheless, little research had focused on older adults' desire for choice size, let alone the mechanisms underlying their preference (Reed et al., 2008, 2013).

The impact of numeracy on health-related decision making is profound. Low numeracy skills not only affected financial decision making in general but also increased errors in medical decisions. Although little has been done to investigate the relationships between aging, numeracy, and Medicare prescription drug plans (Szrek & Bundorf, 2013; Wood et al., 2011), the key role of numeracy in decision making can be inferred from the existing body of research (e.g., Peters et al., 2006). Since numeracy is independent of education and typically assessed cognitive abilities, strategies in constructing a user-friendly Medicare choice environment should limit reliance on numerical skills. Aiming to provide scaffolding would better assist older adults in making beneficial decisions. A study by Barnes et al. (2012) nicely demonstrated other viable approaches in mitigating the impact of low numeracy, such as transforming numerate amounts to dollar symbols.

Reed et al. (2008) proposed that the cognitive challenge of making Medicare plan decisions could help explain older adults' desire to want to choose between fewer options. Our study results presented in this chapter provided support for this hypothesis, demonstrating that cognitive ability serves as a mediator in the relationship between age and preferred number of options. Because the two age groups did not differ in their educational level, cognitive differences cannot be explained by education-related differences. Past research indicates that fluid cognition, including processing speed, working memory, and executive functioning, decline with age (e.g., Mather, 2006; Salthouse, 1985). As the mediation model indicates, cognitive abilities could help explain older adults' preference for fewer options. In other words, older adults' preference for fewer options may be the result of greater difficulties in processing information about many alternatives. Our data thus fit nicely with the results reported by previous studies (Cummings et al., 2009; Reed et al., 2008).

One of the other factors influencing choice preference that was tested using the empirical data was personal relevance (Hess et al., 2013; Reed et al., 2008). Both younger and older adults rated Medicare prescription drug plans to be a personally relevant domain of decision making, though older adults rated Medicare as more relevant to themselves than younger adults. Research has demonstrated a relationship between importance ratings and choice preference above and beyond age. When choosing a Medicare prescription drug plan, higher ratings on personal importance were related to preference for more options within groups of same-aged individuals. It is interesting to note that age differences on importance ratings exist, with older adults rating Medicare prescription drug plans as being more important than younger adults. In spite of greater importance ratings, however, older adults still preferred fewer options compared to younger adults, supporting a general shift to a preference for less choice in later life.

Overall, older adults prefer fewer options, and cognitive ability appears to be one of the underlying mechanisms explaining this desire (though longitudinal data are urgently needed to support this claim). The current design of Medicare Part D thus might place older adults in a disadvantageous choice environment. In our studies, older adults faced about 20 Medicare prescription drug plans at most, which is far less than the actual number of choices they must face in the real world (Kliff, 2011). Considering the fact that cognition declines with age, older adults might be the targeted age group that would benefit from having fewer well-designed (rather than more) choices (Wood et al., 2011).

The Medicare Part D program has aided millions of older adults in reducing their health-care bills while improving access to health care. This is, of course, a welcome reprieve for many older adults whose financial situation has worsened since the financial crisis. Indeed, with a much more limited time horizon to recuperate from losses, increasing health-care needs, and reduced access to the job market, financial issues are of top concerns to many older adults. Improving their ability to manage their financial position is, therefore, of key importance. Actively using math concepts or numeracy skills in daily life may help sharpen one's financial decision making, for example, by making one more cognizant of how much or what percentage of money is spent on transportation or groceries every week. While the focus in this chapter was on the Medicare Part D program, our study results and our review of existing literature have implications for other possible domains. First, as with earlier studies, the importance of numeracy is highlighted in making sound and erudite financial decisions, whether in the financial or the medical domain.

As such, improving adults' numeracy skills could serve to help them make better financial and medical related decisions. Second, designing decision environments that are more ecologically sensitive to their abilities (e.g., with fewer choices) will better match older adults' wishes and improve their decision outcome. In line with presenting fewer options, introducing a few default options that satisfy the needs of an older adult's age and background may decrease the stress in search for the best plan. Considering ways to best present or convey information would also help. For example, changing the presentation of price from numbers to symbols, or disseminating easy-to-read comparative brochures that assist the decision-making process, could help support older adults' decision-making. How to design better decision environments for older adults is a major challenge, but one that has received relatively little attention from researchers. We hope that this chapter (and book) will stimulate discussion on this issue and generate novel and exciting possibilities.

References

Atkinson, A., McKay, S., Kempson, E., & Collard, S. (2007). Levels of financial capability in the UK: Results of a baseline survey. *Public Money & Management, 27*, 29–36.

Barnes, A. J., Hanoch, Y., Wood, S., Liu, P., & Rice, T. (2012). One fish, two fish, red fish, blue fish: Effects of price frames, brand names, and choice set size in medicare Part D insurance plan decisions. *Medical Care Research and Review, 69*(4), 460–473.

Baron, R. M., & Kenny, D. A. (1986). The moderator-mediator distinction in social psychological research: Conceptual, strategic, and statistical considerations. *Journal of Personality and Social Psychology, 51*, 1173–1182.

Besedes, T., Deck, C., Sarangi, S., & Shor, M. (2012). Age effects and heuristics in decision-making. *Review of Economics and Statistics, 94*, 580–595.

Bettman, J. R., Johnson, E. J., & Payne, J. W. (1990). A componential analysis of cognitive effort in choice. *Organizational Behavior and Human Decision Processes, 45*, 111–139.

Botti, S., & Iyengar, S. S. (2006). The dark side of choice: When choice impairs social welfare. *Journal of Public Policy & Marketing, 25*, 24–38.

Brown, R. (July 19, 2012). *Facing foreclosure after 50*. The New York Times. Retrieved from http://www.nytimes.com/2012/07/19/us/foreclosure-rates-surge-for-older-americans-aarp-says.html.

Brown, S. M., Culver, J. O., Osann, K. E., MacDonald, D. J., Sand, S., Thornton, A. A., et al. (2011). Health literacy, numeracy, and interpretation of graphical breast cancer risk estimates. *Patient Education and Counseling, 83*, 92–98.

Bundorf, M. K., & Szrek, H. (2010). Choice set size and decision-making: The case of medicare Part D prescription drug plans. *Medical Decision-Making, 30*, 582–593.

Cummings, J., Rice, T., & Hanoch, Y. (2009). Who thinks that Part D is too complicated? Survey results on the medicare prescription drug benefit. *Medical Care Research and Review, 66*, 97–115.

Daley, S. (July 28, 2012). *Spain's jobless rely on family, a frail crutch.* The New York Times. http://www.nytimes.com/2012/07/29/world/europe/spains-elders-bearing-burden-of-recession.html?pagewanted=1.

DeWalt, D. A., Berkman, N. D., Sheridan, S., Lohr, K. N., & Pignone, M. P. (2004). Literacy and health outcomes: A systematic review of the literature. *Journal of General Internal Medicine, 19*, 1228–1239.

Epstein, S. (1994). Integration of the cognitive and the psychodynamic unconscious. *American Psychologist, 49*, 709–724.

Evans, J. S. B.T. (2003). In two minds: Dual-processing accounts of reasoning. *TRENDS in Cognitive Sciences, 7*, 454–459.

Finucane, M. L., Mertz, C. K., Slovic, P., & Schmidt, E. (2005). Task complexity and older adults' decision-making competence. *Psychology and Aging, 20*, 71–84.

Finucane, M. L., Slovic, P., Hibbard, J. H., Peters, E., Mertz, C. K., & MacGregor, D. G. (2002). Aging and decision-making competence: An analysis of comprehension and consistency skills in older versus younger adults considering health-plan options. *Journal of Behavioral Decision-Making, 15*, 441–464.

Ganther, J. M., & Kreling, D. H. (2000). Consumer perceptions of risk and required cost savings for generic prescription drugs. *Journal of the American Pharmaceutical Association, 40*, 378–383.

Gigerenzer, G., Gaissmaier, W., Kurz-Milcke, E., Schwartz, L. M., & Woloshin, S. (2007). Helping doctors and patients make sense of health statistics. *Psychological Science in the Public Interest, 8*, 53–96.

Hanoch, Y., & Rice, T. (2006). Can limiting choice increase social welfare? The elderly and health insurance. *Milibank Quarterly, 84*(1), 37–73.

Hanoch, Y., Rice, T., Cummings, J., & Wood, S. (2009). How much choice is too much? The case of the medicare prescription drug benefit. *Health Services Research, 44*, 1157–1168.

Hanoch, Y., Wood, S., Barnes, A., Liu, P., & Rice, T. (2011). Choosing the right medicare prescription drug plan: The effect of age, strategy selection, and choice set size. *Health Psychology, 30*, 719–727.

Hanoch, Y., Wood, S., & Rice, T. (2007). Bounded rationality, emotions and older adult decision-making: Not so fast and yet so frugal. *Human Development, 50*, 333–358.

Henninger, D. E., Madden, D. J., & Huettel, S. A. (2010). Processing speed and memory mediate age-related differences in decision-making. *Psychology and Aging, 25*, 262–270.

Hess, T. M., Queen, T. L., & Ennis, G. E. (2013). Age and self-relevance effects on information search during decision-making. *Journals of Gerontology Series B: Psychological Sciences and Social Sciences, 68*, 703–711.

Hibbard, J. H., Slovic, P., Peters, E., Finucane, M. L., & Tusler, M. (2001). Is the informed-choice policy approach appropriate for medicare beneficiaries? *Health Affairs, 20*, 199–203.

Hsee, C. K., & Rottenstreich, Y. (2004). Music, pandas, and muggers: On the affective psychology of value. *Journal of Experimental Psychology: General, 133*, 23–30.

Institute of Medicine. (2004). *Health literacy: a prescription to end confusion*. https://hospitals.unm.edu/health_literacy/pdfs/HealthLiteracyExecutiveSummary.pdf.

Iyengar, S., Huberman, G., & Jiang, W. (2004). How much choice is too much? Contributions to 401(k) retirement plans. In O. S. Mitchell, & S. Utkus (Eds.), *Pension design and structure: New lessons from behavioral finance* (pp. 83–95). Oxford: Oxford University Press.

Iyengar, S. S., & Lepper, M. R. (2000). When choice is demotivating: Can one desire too much of a good thing? *Journal of Personality and Social Psychology, 79*, 995–1006.

Jenkins, A., Ackerman, R., Frumkin, L., Salter, E., & Vorhaus, J. (2011). *Literacy, numeracy and disadvantage among older adults in England*. National Research and Development Centre (NRDC).

Johnson, M. M. (1990). Age differences in decision-making: A process methodology for examining strategic information processing. *Journal of Gerontology, 45*, 75–78.

Johnson, M. M. (1993). Thinking about strategies during, before, and after making a decision. *Psychology and Aging, 8*, 231–241.

Kahneman, D. (2003). A perspective on judgment and choice: Mapping bounded rationality. *American Psychologist, 58*, 697–720.

Kahneman, D. (2011). *Thinking, fast and slow*. New York, NY: Farrar, Straus & Giroux.

Kaiser Family Foundation. (2013). *The medicare prescription drug benefit fact sheet*. The Henry J. Kaiser Family Foundation Headquarters, Washington, DC. Available at http://kff.org/medicare/fact-sheet/the-medicare-prescription-drug-benefit-fact-sheet/.

Keller, K. L., & Staelin, R. (1987). Effects of quality and quantity of information on decision effectiveness. *Journal of Consumer Research, 14*, 200–213.

Kliff, S. (August 2011). Too many choices decrease medicare enrollment. *The Washington Post*. Available at http://www.washingtonpost.com/blogs/ezra-klein/post/too-many-choices-decrease-medicare-enrollment/2011/08/22/gIQADxsXWJ_blog.html.

Lindenberger, U., von Oertzen, T., Ghisletta, P., & Hertzog, C. (2011). Cross-sectional age variance extraction: What's change got to do with it? *Psychology and Aging, 26*(1), 34–47.

Lipkus, I. M., Samsa, G., & Rimer, B. K. (2001). General performance on a numeracy scale among highly educated samples. *Medical Decision-Making, 21*, 37–44.

Liu, P., & Wood, S. (April 2010). Do older adults prefer less choice? The influence of choice set size and relevance of importance on preferred number of options. In *Poster session presented at Cognitive Aging Conference, Atlanta, GA*.

Lusardi, A., & Mitchell, O. S. (2006). *Financial literacy and planning: implications for retirement wellbeing*. Working Paper. Pension Research Council, Wharton School, University of Pennsylvania.

Lusardi, A., & Mitchell, O. S. (2008). Financial literacy and retirement preparedness: Evidence and implications for financial education. *Business Economics, 54*, 35–44.

Lusardi, A., & Mitchell, O. S. (2011). Financial literacy and retirement planning in the United States. *Journal of Pension Economics and Finance, 10*, 509–525.

Mata, R., & Nunes, L. (2010). When less is enough: Cognitive aging, information search, and decision quality in consumer choice. *Psychology and Aging, 25*, 289–298.

Mata, R., Schooler, L. J., & Rieskamp, J. (2007). The aging decision maker: Cognitive aging and the adaptive selection of decision strategies. *Psychology and Aging, 22*, 796–810.

Mata, R., von Helversen, B., & Rieskamp, J. (2010). Learning to choose: Cognitive aging and strategy selection learning in decision-making. *Psychology and Aging, 25*, 299–309.

Mather, M. (2006). A review of decision-making processes: Weighing the risks and benefits of aging. In L. L. Carstensen, & C. R. Hartel (Eds.), *When I'm 64: Committee on aging frontiers in social psychology personality, and adult developmental psychology* (pp. 145–173). Washington, DC: The National Academies Press.

McWilliams, J. M., Afendulis, C. C., Mcguire, T. G., & Landon, B. E. (2011). Complex medicare advantage choices may overwhelm seniors—especially those with impaired decision-making. *Health Affairs, 30*, 1786–1794.

Meyer, B. J. E., Russo, C., & Talbot, A. (1995). Discourse comprehension and problem solving: Decisions about the treatment of breast cancer by women across the life span. *Psychology and Aging, 10*, 84–103.

Noor, M. (February 6, 2009). *Losing the glint of the golden years*. The New York Times. Retrieved from http://www.nytimes.com/2009/02/08/nyregion/long-island/08Rseniors.html?_r=0.

OECD. (2013). *OECD skills outlook 2013: first results from the survey of adult skills*. OECD Publishing.

Peters, E. M., & Bruine de Bruin, W. (2012). Aging and decision skills. In M. K. Dhami, A. Schlottmann, & M. Waldmann (Eds.), *Judgment and decision-making as a skill: Learning, development, and evolution*. New York, NY: Cambridge University Press.

Peters, E., Hess, T. M., Västfjäll, D., & Auman, C. (2007). Adult age differences in dual information processing: Implications for the role of affective and deliberate processes in older adults' decision-making. *Perspectives on Psychological Science, 2*, 1–23.

Peters, E., Västfjäll, D., Slovic, P., Mertz, C. K., Mazzocco, K., & Dickert, S. (2006). Numeracy and decision-making. *Psychological Science, 17*, 407–413.

Pinquart, M., & Duberstein, P. R. (2004). Information needs and decision-making process in older cancer patients. *Critical Reviews in Oncology/Hematology, 51*, 69–80.

Queen, T. L., Hess, T. M., Ennis, G. E., Dowd, K., & Grühn, D. (2013). Information search and decision-making: The effects of age and complexity on strategy use. *Psychology and Aging, 27*(4), 817–824.

Rampell, C. (February 2, 2013). *In hard economy for all ages, older isn't better...it is brutal.* The New York Times. http://www.nytimes.com/2013/02/03/business/americans-closest-to-retirement-were-hardest-hit-by-recession.html?_r=0.
Reed, A. E., Mikels, J. A., & Löckenhoff, C. E. (2013). Preferences for choice across adulthood: Age trajectories and potential mechanisms. *Psychology and Aging, 28*, 625–632.
Reed, A. E., Mikels, J. A., & Simon, K. I. (2008). Older adults prefer less choice than young adults. *Psychology and Aging, 23*, 671–675.
Reyna, V., Nelson, W. L., Han, P. K., & Diekman, N. F. (2009). How numeracy influences risk comprehension and medical decision-making. *Psychological Bulletin, 135*, 943–973.
Rice, T., Hanoch, Y., & Cummings, J. (2010). What factors influence seniors' desire for choice among health insurance options? Survey results on the medicare prescription drug benefit. *Health Economics, Policy and Law, 5*, 437–457.
Salthouse, T. A. (1985). *A theory of cognitive aging*. Amsterdam: North-Holland.
Salthouse, T. A. (1996). The processing-speed theory of adult age differences in cognition. *Psychological Review, 103*, 403–428.
Schaie, K. W., & Willis, S. L. (2002). *Adult development and aging* (5th ed.). Upper Saddle River, NJ: Prentice-Hall.
Scheibehenne, B., Greifeneder, R., & Todd, P. M. (2009). What moderates the too-much-choice effect? *Psychology & Marketing, 26*, 229–253.
Schwartz, B. (2004). *The paradox of choice: Why more is less*. New York, NY: HarperCollins Publishers.
Schwartz, B., Ward, A., Monterosso, J., Lyubomirsky, S., White, K., & Lehman, D. R. (2002). Maximizing versus satisficing: Happiness is a matter of choice. *Journal of Personality and Social Psychology, 83*, 1178–1197.
Schwartz, L. M., Woloshin, S., Black, W. C., & Welch, H. G. (1997). The role of numeracy in understanding the benefit of screening mammography. *Annals of Internal Medicine, 127*, 966–972.
Spreen, O., & Strauss, E. (1998). *A compendium of neuropsychological tests: Administration, norms and commentary* (2nd ed.). New York, NY: Oxford University Press.
Stanovich, K. E., & West, R. F. (2000). Individual differences in reasoning: Implications for the rationality debate? *Behavioral and Brain Sciences, 23*, 645–726.
Steginga, S. K., & Occhipinti, S. (2002). Decision-making about treatment of hypothetical prostate cancer: Is deferring a decision an expert-opinion heuristic? *Journal of Psychological Oncology, 20*, 69–84.
Szrek, H., & Bundorf, M. (2011). Age and the purchase of prescription drug insurance by older adults. *Psychology and Aging, 26*, 308–320.
Szrek, H., & Bundorf, M. (2013). Enrollment in prescription drug insurance: The interaction of numeracy and choice set size. *Health Psychology, 33*(4), 340–348.
Tanius, B., Wood, S., Hanoch, Y., & Rice, T. (2009). Aging and choice: Application to medicare Part D. *Judgment and Decision-Making, 4*, 92–101.
Wood, S., Hanoch, Y., Barnes, A., Liu, P., Cummings, J., Bhattacharya, C., et al. (2011). Numeracy and medicare Part D: The importance of choice & literacy for numbers in optimizing decision-making for medicare's prescription drug program. *Psychology and Aging, 26*(2), 295–307.
Yoon, C., Cole, C. A., & Lee, M. P. (2009). Consumer decision-making and aging: Current knowledge and future directions. *Journal of Consumer Psychology, 19*, 2–16.
Zwahr, M. D., Park, D. C., & Shifren, K. (1999). Judgments about estrogen replacement therapy: The role of age, cognitive abilities and beliefs. *Psychology and Aging, 14*, 179–191.

CHAPTER

16

Financial Decision Making across the Adult Life Span: Dynamic Cognitive Capacities and Real-World Competence

Douglas A. Hershey[1], *James T. Austin*[2], *Helen C. Gutierrez*[3]

[1]Department of Psychology, Oklahoma State University, Stillwater, OK, USA; [2]College of Education and Human Ecology, Ohio State University, Columbus, OH, USA; [3]Department of Psychology, Oklahoma State University, Stillwater, OK, USA

There is perhaps no decision-making domain that has greater real-world significance than decisions involving personal finance. Most of us, over the course of our lives, will be called upon to make thousands of decisions of an economic or financial nature. Moreover, in light of recent increases in the variety of financial products and services that have become available on the market, during the course of the next few decades we should expect to see an increase in the range and complexity of personal financial decisions individuals are expected to make (Weierich et al., 2011), and perhaps, in the requirements that enable one to make those decisions. Yet despite the ubiquitous nature of financial decision making, this remains a domain in which individuals receive little in the way of formal training. We can readily bring to mind some people we consider to be particularly skilled and adept at managing their finances, and we can just as readily think of others who seem prone to making shortsighted financial decisions. This chapter focuses on two broad, related questions of theoretical and applied significance. The first is, what are the cognitive and intellectual capacities that underlie competence when it comes to real-world personal financial decision making (e.g., balancing a checkbook, saving and investing,

Aging and Decision Making
http://dx.doi.org/10.1016/B978-0-12-417148-0.00016-9

purchasing a house), and how do those competencies change over the life span? The second is, to what extent can individuals at different ages be trained to make better personal financial decisions?

A variety of cognitive resources go into decline with advancing age, but the attenuation of these basic abilities is to some extent offset by the development of one's general knowledge about the world, and specifically, age-related increases in knowledge of and experience with personal financial matters. In light of the large body of literature that shows fluid intellectual abilities undergo significant declines around the third decade of life (Baltes, 1987; Horn, 1988; Salthouse & Davis, 2006), it is interesting to consider why, as a society, we tend to seek out older individuals to manage many of our most important and sensitive decisions. In the public finance arena, the average age of appointment among chairs of the Federal Reserve Bank is 55 years, yet they are subject to mandatory retirement upon reaching the age of 65 (Federal Reserve Bank, 2014). In industry, chief financial officers tend to be in their 50s and 60s (Bower, 2007). Even the American president, who is responsible for shaping national budgetary priorities, is required by the United States Constitution to be *at least* 35 years of age. The competence of older decision makers also extends to the area of personal finance. Individuals over the age of 65, who make up only 13% of the American population, hold 34% of the nation's wealth (Laibson, 2011). From a theoretical perspective, it is interesting to understand how older adults maintain high-level cognitive competence in the face of declines in basic processing resources. Also key is understanding the unique circumstances under which competence may be compromised, which suggest boundary conditions under which respect for elders' abilities may be misplaced.

It is important to recognize at the outset of this chapter that there exist trade-offs between basic cognitive abilities, the pragmatics of intelligence, and domain-specific financial expertise (Li, Baldassi, Johnson, & Weber, 2013; Walsh & Hershey, 1993). That being the case, in the following section we seek to characterize the dynamic forces that underlie differing levels of financial competence at different points in the adult life span.

FLUID ABILITIES, CRYSTALLIZED ABILITIES, AND FINANCIAL KNOWLEDGE

The theory of fluid and crystallized intelligence (Horn & Cattell, 1966; Horn, 1988) posits the existence of two distinct types of intellectual abilities. Fluid reasoning abilities encompass the set of basic cognitive processing abilities necessary to assimilate and integrate critical information about a problem or decision. Crystallized abilities, in contrast, involve an understanding of culturally-based values and knowledge about the world. Additional details about this theory as they apply to aging and decision making can be found in two other chapters in this volume. There exists a large and growing body of research to suggest that as we pass through adolescence into adulthood and old age, these dual intellectual capacities undergo change (Baltes, 1987; Li et al., 2004). Crystallized abilities (world knowledge) increase throughout young adulthood and middle-age, and then plateau, showing little or no growth into old age (Li et al., 2004). Financial knowledge can be thought of as one of many different subtypes of crystallized abilities. Fluid abilities, in contrast, show a pattern of increasing development throughout young adulthood, but then a slow pattern of decline beginning in middle-adulthood which continues throughout old age (Li et al., 2004).

Based on the assumption that both fluid and crystallized abilities jointly contribute to our ability to make complex financial decisions (Li et al., 2013), it is plausible that younger and older adults demonstrate differing degrees of financial competence at their respective points in the life span for different reasons. That is, when making everyday financial decisions, older adults facing declines in fluid abilities would be expected to rely more heavily on crystallized knowledge gained through personal experience. Younger adults, on the other hand, would be expected to rely more heavily on fluid reasoning abilities when confronted with a novel financial problem, given their (relative) lack of domain-specific knowledge. Consistent with this notion of trade-offs between fluid and crystallized abilities, Agarwal, Driscoll, Gabaix, and Laibson (2009) concluded that financial mistakes surrounding a variety of different credit behaviors is minimized around the age of 53, which is when crystallized knowledge has nearly peaked and fluid abilities have yet to substantially decline. One implication of this finding is that we could expect to see increases in within-person variability in the quality of individuals' financial decisions as we stray from the 50s (Laibson, 2011), with poorer performance (i.e., increased decision error) down the age range into the 40s and 30s (due to limited experiential knowledge), and up the age range into the 60s and 70s (due to declining fluid resources).

Another factor believed to influence financial decision making—domain-specific financial knowledge—has been found to be one of the more powerful determinants of financial decision-making performance. One's experiential knowledge of a financial task (i.e., expertise), in the form of habits, computational strategies, or decision-making scripts (Hershey, Jacobs-Lawson, & Walsh, 2003), is in most circumstances likely to outweigh the relative value of more general crystallized knowledge and fluid abilities.

Domain-specific knowledge increases in a cumulative fashion over the course of adulthood, as individuals encounter different types of financial tasks and have repeated experiences with many of the same types of decisions. The slope of this knowledge-acquisition function is presumably steeper for some and flatter for others depending on the nature of their exposure to, interest in, and involvement with different types of personal financial decisions. Moreover, domain-specific knowledge slopes for some individuals may be linear, but that need not be the case. Life circumstances may lead some individuals to have broad exposure to financial issues (or formal educational training) early in life, resulting in a negatively accelerated growth function. Alternatively, the growth function for "slow starters" may demonstrate a pattern of exponential development that accelerates late in life. Individuals' domain-specific knowledge may even show a downturn late in life, in cases in which individuals are reticent to embrace new financial technologies, unwilling to explore new decision domains, and losing competence at financial tasks they had previously mastered. In light of these decision dynamics, we now turn our attention to a discussion of the essential nature of various types of financial decisions.

THE NATURE OF FINANCIAL DECISION-MAKING TASKS

Financial decision making is in certain ways unique relative to other real-world decision domains. One reason for this is because certain tasks are linked to a particular age or life stage. Take, for instance, day-to-day money management tasks such as paying bills, budgeting, and balancing a checkbook. These are important tasks that individuals typically first experience early in adulthood, and they remain relevant over the remainder of one's life. Other financial tasks are often linked to a later age or life stage. Examples include selecting the right investment vehicle to save for a child's college education, selecting the most appropriate home mortgage, deciding how assets should be disbursed as part of the estate-planning process, and deciding whether one can afford to retire. Each of these tasks typically emerges in middle age or late life, and often, surrounding specific circumstances (e.g., turning 65 years of age). That being the case, one could expect that individual differences in exposure to different types of financial tasks over the course of adulthood would result in different levels of financial knowledge and expertise.

The diagram of a trapezoid shown in Figure 1 identifies a sample of commonly experienced financial decision-making tasks. The tasks shown are not intended to be comprehensive, but rather, representative of a limited range of financial decisions one might face over one's lifetime. As seen in the figure, one's developmental trajectory (i.e., indexed by age) is graphically represented along the right side of the hierarchy. This dimension suggests that different financial tasks become relevant at different points in the adult life span, or at different life stages. A number of the

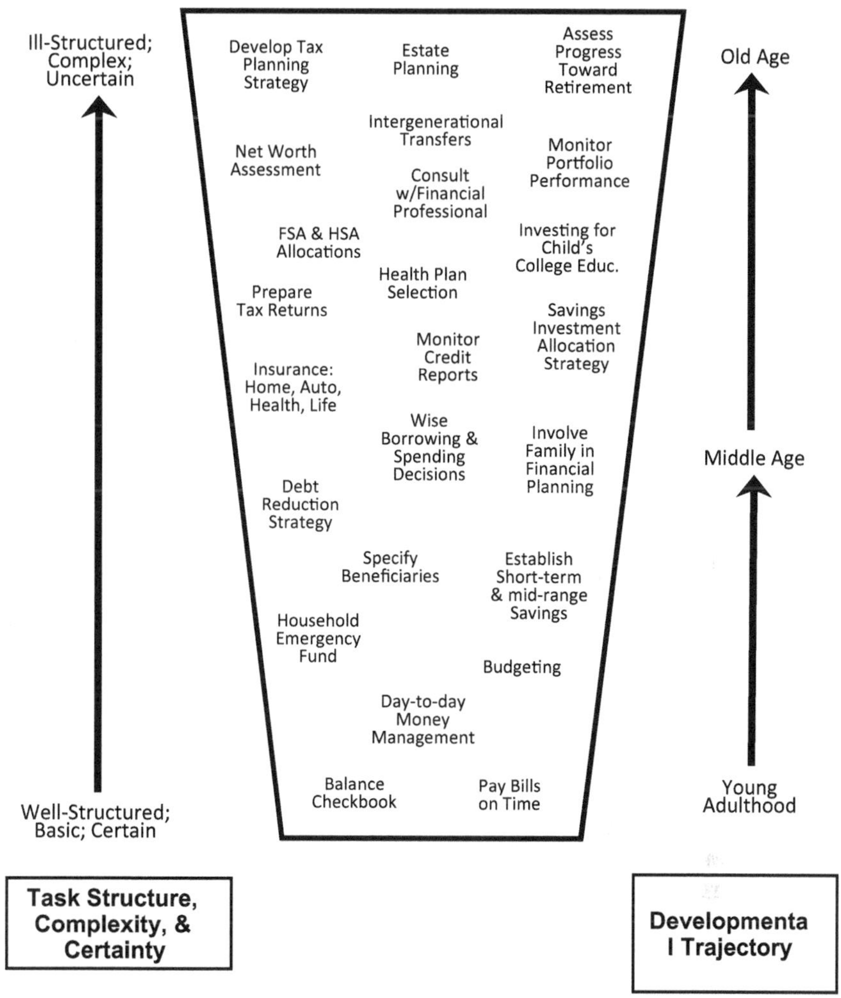

FIGURE 1 Developmentally-based hierarchical arrangement of household financial tasks. Tasks arranged from the bottom of the trapezoid to the top become increasingly ill-structured, complex, and uncertain, and their resolution requires an increasingly complex set of cognitive skills.

tasks adults in their 20s face are fairly basic in nature, and many of them accompany independence from one's parents (e.g., creating a budget, maintaining a checkbook, payment of bills). But as one grows into middle-age, the odds of starting a family, purchasing a house, and landing a job with health and retirement benefit options all become increasingly likely, and the financial decisions one faces at this stage of life become increasingly complex (i.e., tasks that involve more information to consider in formulating a decision strategy). The complexity and uncertainty of financial decisions once again increases as one enters older adulthood, with many tasks at this stage of life requiring the development of a coherent and internally consistent strategic plan. The age-linked progression of tasks described above is not immutable; that is, a 20-year-old could purchase a house, develop a tax-planning strategy, or develop an estate plan for her elderly parents. But the notion that age is normatively associated with increases in task complexity (in terms of the cognitive processes involved) is well founded, and for most individuals advancing age is accompanied by an increase in the range of financial tasks in which one is likely to engage (Carpenter & Yoon, 2011). This is why the walls of the trapezoid flare out from bottom to top. It is also worth noting that normative developmental trajectories in relation to financial decisions may be moderated by factors such as socioeconomic status, ethnicity, social forces, and other cultural influences.

As seen on the left side of the diagram, it is possible to think of household financial tasks as varying in terms of their structure (i.e., whether they are well-structured or ill-structured; Laxman, 2010; Simon, 1973); complexity (Probst & Bassi, 2014); and degree of uncertainty (i.e., extent to which the dynamics of a particular decision allow the decision maker to know, with a degree of certainty, the quality of his or her decision) (Demange & Laroque, 2006). Certain tasks, such as balancing a checkbook, are well structured and lacking in complexity. Moreover, in the case of reconciling a checking account, there is little in the way of uncertainty and ambiguity. That said, however, even "basic" financial tasks—such as creating a household budget—may be marked by uncertainty, such as not knowing whether one has set aside sufficient short-term savings for the coming month. Other tasks, such as day-to-day money management, require moderately high levels of fluid abilities, but relatively little in the way of advanced analysis, synthesis of information, and strategic planning.

Tasks closer to the top of the hierarchy, in contrast, are inherently complex, ill-structured, and marked by a high degree of uncertainty. Take, for instance, assessing one's progress toward saving for retirement, which is a task more likely to be engaged in by middle-aged and older adults. This task is complex, ill-structured, and marked by multiple uncertainties such as knowing how long one is likely to live, whether one will experience costly health problems in old age, and how potentially volatile financial markets will affect one's retirement nest egg over time. When one considers the variability inherent in the essential nature of these different types of tasks, it becomes clear that the nature of the tasks (i.e., structure, complexity, and uncertainty) is likely to interact with age-related changes in various cognitive and intellectual abilities.

Relative to tasks near the bottom of the hierarchy, those near the top tend to be associated with a higher degree of risk, which generally stem from uncertain parameters (e.g., the chance that *all* of one's children will attend college; whether the size of one's estate will be appreciable upon passing).

As financial decisions become increasingly risky and complex (as in the case of entrepreneurial endeavors, estate planning, and certain tax planning scenarios), individuals become increasingly likely to seek out external assistance or professional help before they can be confident the strategy adopted will lead to success. However, outsourcing aspects of personal financial decisions to an adviser is something many individuals are hesitant to do (Gerrans & Hershey, 2013; Gutierrez, Hershey, & Gerrans, 2011), based on concerns about disclosing personal information or being negatively evaluated by the adviser for poor prior decisions. Nevertheless, the likelihood of engaging a financial professional increases as a function of age during adulthood, as "mature consumers" face new decision challenges that are linked to important life transitions such as changing employers, paying off a house, or transitioning into retirement (Milner & Rosenstreich, 2013).

Tacitly represented in the trapezoid are a range of cognitive skills required to carry out the various financial tasks. Basic tasks, such as those near the bottom of the trapezoid, involve little more than recognition of the fact that a decision needs to be made (i.e., problem identification), fundamental numeracy abilities, and a degree of computational competence. However, just because a decision is a basic one does not mean individuals will choose wisely, as evidenced by the appreciable percentage of individuals who overspend and struggle with day-to-day money management and the balancing of accounts.

Mid-level tasks are more complex, requiring relevant data to be sought out, analyzed, and synthesized. Tasks at this level also involve lower-level abilities such as numeracy and computational competence, but the hallmark of mid-level tasks is that the individual is called upon to compare and contrast different dimensions of the decision in a rational and analytic fashion. Relative to the most basic tasks, there is more room for error when one is engaged in mid-level tasks, as all relevant information may not be available to the decision maker, or the information needed may not be complete or aggregated inappropriately.

For most individuals, tasks near the top of the trapezoid are those that are relevant late in life, and they require extensive strategic planning. Furthermore, for high-level financial tasks there may be no one right decision, but rather, a range of alternative solutions that lead to different outcomes bearing differing utilities. After analysis of a high-level financial decision has been carried out and a strategic plan is adopted, the decision needs to be implemented. In assessing savings progress toward retirement, for example, one must first assess the balance between anticipated future resource streams, current investments, and anticipated postemployment expenditures, before determining whether one's savings are on track. Conclusions reached during this process require the decision maker to either stay the course or adjust his or her investment strategy. Any indicated change in one's investment strategy then needs to be implemented. Unlike tasks near the bottom of the trapezoid in which outcomes are rather certain, for high-level tasks the quality of one's decision may not be known for years. In some instances the quality of the decision outcome may never be known, which is why in such cases individuals are wise to focus on the use of normative strategies (i.e., a course of action that maximizes the probability of a beneficial outcome) and the efficient processing of task information in the hopes that doing so will result in a positive outcome. The various cognitive skills required for tasks at different levels of the hierarchy correspond well to existing decision taxonomies (e.g., Scherpereel, 2006).

We would be remiss if we failed to mention that there exists a segment of the population who live on the margins of society, whose experience with finances fails to be captured by the tasks represented in the trapezoidal hierarchy. These American adults are effectively "financially disenfranchised" from mainstream financial institutions. Many live with physical, cognitive, or emotional disabilities; others are migratory workers and day laborers; and still others adopt this lifestyle as a matter of choice. These individuals may or may not be homeless; they would likely lack steady employment, a health insurance plan, or even a bank account. Members of these cohorts are often targeted by individuals and merchants for necessary financial transactions (Gallmeyer & Roberts, 2009; Johnson, 2010). Living on a day-to-day or week-to-week basis, these individuals live their lives engaging in financial tasks that would conceptually be located *outside* the confines of the trapezoid. It is difficult to estimate the size of this segment of the population, but suffice it to say that it is substantial and their experience of everyday finance is qualitatively different than what most of the population experiences (Houser, D'Andrea, & Daniels, 1992).

REASONS WHY INDIVIDUALS MAKE POOR FINANCIAL DECISIONS

There exist a variety of reasons why individuals make sub-optimal decisions in the financial arena. Poor decisions may result from a lack of familiarity with the task and low levels of financial literacy, insufficient levels of basic cognitive abilities, decision biases that skew one's performance, and situational and contextual influences that hinder sound reasoning. Importantly, for various reasons these factors may exert different degrees of influence at different points in the adult life span. Each of these factors is examined separately, next.

Task Familiarity and Financial Literacy

One of the chief determinants of financial decision-making competence (i.e., the ability to make decisions successfully or efficiently) is arguably one's level of financial knowledge and financial literacy (Croy, Gerrans, &

Speelman, 2010; Lusardi & Mitchell, 2013). According to the United Nations Educational, Scientific, and Cultural Organization, financial literacy involves the ability to identify, interpret, understand, and use written materials to function effectively in the financial arena (UNESCO, 2004). Indeed, a growing body of literature from the fields of psychology, finance, and economics suggests that on the whole, American consumers lack familiarity with a wide range of real-world financial products, and this limited experience results in limited levels of domain-specific knowledge. Without an appropriate knowledge base, individuals are hampered in their ability to effectively evaluate different decision options and implement a rational financial plan. From stock market participation, to debt reduction, to retirement planning, to mortgage defaults, low levels of financial literacy and numeracy have been identified as the root cause of poor saving and investment decisions (Gerardi, Goette, & Meier, 2013), ultimately leading to significant out-of-pocket expenses and low levels of financial satisfaction (Xiao, Chen, & Chen, 2013).

Data from the U.S. National Financial Capability Study (Lusardi & Mitchell, 2011a) reveal that literacy levels are particularly low among less-educated individuals and women. Furthermore, African-Americans and Hispanics in that study scored lowest, on average, on a set of key financial literacy concepts. Paradoxically, all participants in the study viewed themselves as financially competent, which reveals a halo effect operating (Thorndike, 1920) when it comes to self-perceptions in the financial realm. Low levels of financial literacy are not just a problem in the United States, however. As Lusardi and Mitchell (2011b) point out, insufficient financial knowledge is a problem in numerous other countries around the world in which financial markets are well developed, such as Germany, the Netherlands, Sweden, Japan, and Italy. Future solutions to the problem of suboptimal financial decision making will necessarily involve interventions that seek to raise financial awareness.

Boyle et al. (2013) suggest that financial literacy is particularly a problem among adults over the age of 65, despite the fact that members of this age group would be assumed to have relatively high levels of financial knowledge. Thus, after decades of improvement in financial literacy, it appears that in later adulthood there is a downturn in the acquisition and use of financial knowledge. According to Boyle et al., literacy deficits among older individuals stem from low levels of formal education, insufficient word knowledge associated with new and different types of financial and investment products, and ultimately, declines in basic cognitive abilities such as episodic memory capacity and executive functioning. At the other end of the age spectrum, a cross-sectional study on the financial literacy among over 3000 Australian adults (ANZ, 2011) revealed that individuals under the age of 25 exhibited particularly low levels of financial literacy, presumably due to a limited involvement with various financial products. Otherwise, the survey revealed age to be positively related to behavioral indicators of financial literacy (saving on a regular basis; maintaining a household budget) among those 25 years of age and older. Lusardi, Mitchell, and Curto (2010) also reported that young adults have troubling low levels of financial literacy, which they argued would make them less likely to participate in the stock market, choose mutual funds with lower fees, accumulate and manage wealth effectively, and plan for retirement.

Insufficient Basic Cognitive Abilities and Resources

In light of the fact that many financial decision-making tasks are associated with information-rich domains, it is no surprise that in studies of adult development and aging, basic cognitive resources, abilities, predispositions, and strategies have been implicated in the quality of individuals' decision-making efforts. Age-linked attentional and working memory constraints are likely to lead to diminished executive functioning when the information load and computational demands of a task are high (McDowd & Hoffman, 2008; Naveh-Benjamin, Cowan, Kilb, & Chen, 2007). The capacity to plan effectively has also been singled out as a vulnerable ability, with one recent study showing that older adults (age 65–76) failed to plan ahead as effectively as adults under 65 years of age when engaged in a laboratory planning task (Köstering, Stahl, Leonhart, Weiller, & Kaller, 2014). Moreover, in the decision-making domain, Tymulaa, Belmakerb, Rudermanb, Glimcherc, and Levy (2013) found that older adults not only demonstrated a cognitive bias toward being more risk averse when making financial decisions, but they were also strikingly inconsistent in their choices compared to younger adults. This led the researchers to call into question the rationality of older adults in decision-making contexts. Consistent with this finding, researchers (Besede, Deck, Sarangi, and Shor, 2012; Walsh & Hershey, 1993) have reported that relative to younger counterparts, older individuals are more likely to use suboptimal heuristics (approaches) and occasionally make random selections when solving financial problems, which lead to objectively worse choices with age. Some have speculated that age-related differences, such as those cited above, are due to changes that occur during late adulthood at the level of the neural substrate (Kuhnen & Knutson, 2005; Samanez-Larkin, Wagner, & Knutson, 2011).

Decision Biases That Compromise Performance

There exists a growing body of literature that examines age-related differences in decision biases (Strough, Karns, & Schlosnagle, 2011). Biases do not simply cause individuals to err when faced with a reasoning or decision-making task; rather, they predispose individuals to make *systematic errors* (Shleifer, 2000). Unfortunately, all too often those errors are of a self-serving nature, resulting more times than not in decision performance that leaves individuals in a deficit position. Why is it that individuals routinely purchase with great confidence "more house" than they can reasonably afford (Scatinga, 2009), or why do individuals typically misestimate their longevity when planning for retirement (Post & Hanewald, 2013), yet they feel their estimates are reasonable and robust? The answer is that we are all prone to different types of cognitive biases that limit our general financial competence.

Nofsinger (2001) identifies more than a dozen cognitive biases that predispose individuals to make poor personal economic decisions. From the topic of overconfidence to sunk-cost effects, he describes the reasons why individuals make the mistakes they do, and points out ways those financial mistakes can be avoided. Similarly, in a chapter on effective financial planning for retirement, Hershey, Jacobs-Lawson, and Austin (2012) identified some 40 different cognitive biases that stand to compromise one's personal economic decisions. Examples of just three of these biases when it comes to investing include the familiarity bias, in which individuals buy the stock of companies they are familiar with; the overconfidence bias, in which investors believe the stocks they have chosen will perform above average in the future; and the status quo bias, in which due to inertia the investor fails to take action (i.e., maintain the status quo) when action is indicated. All three biases can work to the detriment of investors.

Another cognitive bias—resistance to sunk costs (which is often implicated in investment decisions)—has been related to late life changes in semantic memory (Del Missier et al., 2013). According to Del Missier et al., resistance to this bias is positively linked to age due to older adults' increased awareness of sunk cost traps. Resistance to framing, which has been linked to late life changes in working memory, also improves with age when individual differences in working memory capacity are statistically controlled. Yet another bias, consistency in the application of decision rules (which is also related to working memory), however, demonstrates a negative relationship with advancing age (Del Missier et al., 2013). This latter finding is in agreement with the findings of Tymulaa et al. (2013) cited in the preceding section, which suggests older adults are often inconsistent when making choices. The impact of these latter two biases (resistance to framing and application of decision rules) would not be uncommon to find operating in situations in which individuals have to make insurance purchases or select a workplace health plan.

The insidious aspect of cognitive biases is that the distorted perceptions they create are often invisible to the decision maker, which makes them difficult to identify and circumvent, and therefore, resistant to intervention. Interestingly, individuals are quick to spot biases in reasoning except in cases when those biases are their own (Pronin, 2007). This suggests an important role for objective third-party advisors (such as certified financial planners) who are equipped to identify situations in which our financial-reasoning processes might fail.

Situational and Contextual Influences

Financial decisions are always made in a situational context and sometimes, for better or worse, that context will determine one's decision. Take, for instance, the range of possible contexts and individual difference dimensions surrounding "one-off" life events such as choosing to retire, receiving an inheritance, receiving a large pension payout, or being forced to retire by one's employer. Each of these situations has been found to be related to the decision to seek professional financial advice among Australian adults 40–69 years of age (Milner & Rosenstreich, 2013), which suggests that the complexity inherent in the decision is in part driven by perceptions of the context in which that decision is embedded. Other studies have found that a contextual factor as innocuous as an asset's name can affect investor behavior (Rau, Patel, Osobov, Khorana, & Cooper, 2002). When person–context–task fit is high, older adults have been shown to use their experiential knowledge to overcome age-related declines in cognitive abilities. But when person–context–task fit is low (such as when a novel task is attempted), older adults face the need to adapt existing strategies to fit the demands of the situation (Yoon, Cole, & Lee, 2009).

Perhaps an even more surprising contextual finding is that investors are more willing to purchase risky assets on days in which there is good weather (Hirshleifer & Shumway, 2003). Kliger and Levy (2003) explain this seemingly odd finding in terms of a priming effect, in which cloudy weather conditions prime investors to be in a bad mood, thereby leading them to prefer low-risk options. Gilad and Kliger (2008) demonstrated that even investment professionals are not impervious to "cloudy weather" priming effects. These authors found that CPAs and investment advisors for commercial banks were *more* susceptible to weather condition-priming influences than a comparison group of undergraduate students, which led the investigators to conclude that the financial professionals' decisions were based largely on intuition. In a different priming investigation (Kliger & Gilad, 2012), asset valuations were examined as a function of whether details about the asset were printed on red or green paper. In this study, respondents estimated a value for the asset and assessed the probability of the asset's future gain or loss. Based on preexisting positive and negative associations with the colors green and red, respondents considered an asset description printed on green paper to be of greater value and more likely to result in investment gains than the very same description printed on red paper. Whether these seemingly ephemeral contextual cues from the priming literature covary with age has yet to be determined. However, Hess,

Waters, and Bolstad (2000) identified age differences in affective priming, with older adults being more susceptible to such effects. All financial decisions are made in a specific context or in the face of certain life events, and our susceptibility to biases stemming from those contexts and events likely has a very real impact on the nature of the decisions we make.

Consistent with the Life Course Perspective principle of linked lives (Elder, 1994; Mortimer & Shanahan, 2003), it is critical to recognize that *all* financial and economic decisions take place in a social context. Decisions regarding consumption, spending, credit use, debt management, savings, and fiscal responsibility are all influenced by the messages we receive from others, and our perceptions of what constitutes socially normative behavior. Evidence for this is found in studies that have shown parental financial values shape the financial values and investment orientations of their adult children (Hira, Sabri, & Loibl, 2013; Koposko & Hershey, in press). Other research has demonstrated that the opinions of one's spouse, friends, and colleagues color our attitudes toward investing in new business ventures, saving for retirement, and general financial planning practices (Hershey, Henkens, & Van Dalen, 2010; Loibl & Hira, 2006; Werbel & Danes, 2010; Yang & DeVaney, 2012). Still other investigations reveal that credit-based spending decisions and patterns of charitable giving are shaped by individuals' perceptions of descriptive societal norms (Sotiropoulos & d'Astous, 2013). When well-informed social support is high, we are prone to make better financial decisions. But the opposite also holds true as well. When social support is low and normative social reference information is either incorrectly perceived or absent, then the quality of one's personal financial decisions is likely to suffer.

In much the same way that low levels of social support can affect us when making financial decisions, low levels of environmental support can also compromise the choices individuals make. Environmental support could be considered high in cases in which task-relevant information is readily available and presented in an easily interpretable fashion. However, in the world of personal finance, this is often not the case. For instance, it is not uncommon for credit offers to present information regarding exorbitant finance charges in small print, or to encounter debt-reduction services that charge nearly as much in fees as the debt they are likely to dismiss. Many have struggled with complicated mortgage financing offers that contain hidden fees, and others have encountered "too good to be true" used car offers. When confronted with risky product offerings, older adults need high levels of environmental support in order to function at an optimal level (Craik & Anderson, 1999), in part, because they sometimes lack the basic processing resources and literacy levels required to evaluate complex offers. That said, everyone—not just older adults—could benefit from tighter regulatory controls on financial offers in the marketplace.

INTERVENTIONS DESIGNED TO IMPROVE FINANCIAL DECISION MAKING

Interventions, in any area, harness research to design, deploy, and evaluate training programs and other support systems. The objective for interventions in financial decision making as we view it in this chapter is to improve awareness, literacy (Lusardi & Mitchell, 2013), domain-specific knowledge (Walsh & Hershey, 1993), and ultimately to ameliorate maladaptive decision strategies (Nofsinger, 2001; Su, 2013). However, given the dynamic nature of financial decision competence and the different trajectories associated with performance we have portrayed above, no single universal intervention platform is likely to remediate performance on all financial tasks. Our review located financial interventions informed by work in program evaluation (Morell, 2010) and implemented across disciplines that include neuroscience (Samanez-Larkin et al., 2011) and consumer psychology (Moschis, Mosteller, & Fatt, 2011; Yoon et al., 2009).

Although not a focus of this chapter, it is worthwhile to review the use of content and performance standards (for children or adults) to ensure individuals receive sufficient training to perform at or above a baseline level of competence. An example is the Equipped for the Future standards developed by the National Institute for Literacy. These approaches rely on specification of life tasks or similar concepts, ordered along a developmental continuum sufficiently common across individuals to support research and practice. Elder's (1994) concept of the life course is representative (cf. Mortimer & Shanahan, 2003). It is instructive to consider the forms of training, intervention, and socialization practices that would be appropriate for children and adolescents as they mature, acquire crystallized knowledge, then enter the workforce. Important roles are played by parents/caregivers, educators, employers, and community members.

A theme across research reviewed in this chapter is the potential of various nudges and supports. Youth development accounts (Shobe & Sturm, 2007), for example, help to initiate saving and a pattern of life-long financial responsibility. We found a similar strategy for low- and moderate-income families in the SaveUSA project, initiated in 2011 and supported by a private–public Social Innovation Fund partnership. The basis for this intervention encouraged interested tax filers in four cities ($N=1554$) to save part of their tax return up to $1000 for a period of 1 year in order to receive a 50% match. The logic of this intervention is that even small savings can assist individuals or families in emergency situations to avoid risky, less effective choices (payday loans). An interim evaluation of this intervention, using randomized assignment, reported statistically significant results (Azurdia, Freedman, Hamilton, & Schultz, 2014). It is noteworthy that follow-ups are planned to study maintenance of effects. We noted attempts to intervene with elderly adults in the workforce through educational seminars, tax counseling, financial independence training, and employer assistance (Council on Adult and Experiential Learning, 2012; Houser et al., 1992).

A neuroscience framework of financial risk-taking developed by Kuhnen and Knutson (2005) was used in a study that suggests features of future interventions. Samanez-Larkin et al. (2011) investigated, in two studies, financial risk-taking across multiple ages. A first study used functional neuroimaging with an investment task; a second manipulated expected value information, discrete and integrated, in two age groups over blocked trials of the investment task. Findings were suggestive but not conclusive about mesolimbic involvement in addition to declarative knowledge.

Another feature of intervention in financial decision making that may covary with age is nature of the delivery system. More active forms of intervention provided earlier in life are followed by passive interventions that continue through adulthood. We found interventions summarized in various reports that range from active (i.e., in school, direct intervention through teachers and aides using content standards) through passive (websites, financial calculators).

What conclusions can be drawn from intervention practice? Current approaches to intervention, whether active or passive, seem to be unintegrated. This suggests the need for coordination of services along the entire life span and prescription of a range of potential interventions from a portfolio. Implementation of a comprehensive skills training approach that ensures a minimal level of financial competence for all adults remains a goal rather than reality. Specific predictable deficits lead to suboptimal decisions (for example, trying to balance content suggests that work on assets may not be required for those in poverty, whereas managing liabilities such as debt is very important).

The work of Lusardi (2012) and others shows a mismatch between financial capabilities, assessed through small sets of questions in large-scale surveys, and confidence in financial capabilities, which tends to be high. The idea of "nudges" (Thaler & Sunstein, 2008)—that is, choice architectures that alter individuals' financial behaviors in a positive way—may be relevant, but their ultimate success will require a solid understanding of decision dynamics prior to their deployment within intervention strategies. The SMarT retirement savings program advanced by Thaler and Benartzi (2012) is an example of one such choice architecture. The program results in high levels of saving compliance by asking individuals to allocate to retirement savings moneys linked to future workplace pay increases. We mentioned above the SaveUSA project, which similarly incentivizes savings through matches to tax returns saved for one year.

It is worth mentioning one other topic—financial elder abuse—prior to concluding this section on intervention. Common forms of financial abuse include fraud, theft, illegal property transfers, and misuse of powers of attorney (Rabiner, Brown, & O'Keefe, 2004), which are carried out by family members, predatory individuals (some named as guardians), and unscrupulous professionals (National Committee for the Prevention of Elder Abuse, 2008). Of course, any older individual is a potential target of financial elder abuse, but those who are experiencing some degree of cognitive decline are particularly vulnerable due, in part, to lapses in critical judgment, unwarranted levels of trust in others, or the tendency to acquiesce when providing informed consent in the face of insufficient information (Griffiths & Harmon, 2011).

We agree with Agarwal et al. (2009) that it will be difficult to stem the rising tide of abuse unless tighter regulatory controls are put in place through, among other things, "disclosures, nudges, financial driving licenses, advanced directives, fiduciaries, [and] asset safe harbors" (p. 1). Also needed are more effective clinical means of financial competency testing for older adults, using either structural interviews or behavioral indices of performance. Competency testing could potentially be beneficial for individuals not only at the late end of the age spectrum, but also early in adulthood as a way to ensure young adults have the basic skills necessary to make decisions of reasonable quality. Also of value would be improved methods for training social workers to detect cases of financial elder abuse (Davies et al., 2011) and forensic approaches that would help to prosecute those who seek to victimize elders (Navarro, Gassoumis, & Wilber, 2013).

SUMMARY AND CONCLUSION

This chapter makes a compelling case for the notion that human adults are less than perfect decision makers when it comes to matters of personal finance. The reasons for our errors, however, differ at different points in the adult life span. Suboptimal financial decisions are most likely to be exhibited by young adults and very old adults, but for different reasons. Young adults are likely to suffer from a lack of world knowledge and insufficient prior experience at making financial decisions. Older adults possess real-world financial decision-making expertise and knowledge, but they are at an age at which they are likely to be experiencing declines in basic cognitive abilities that stand to hinder executive functioning. Based on the three determinants of financial competence outlined in this chapter—fluid abilities, crystallized abilities, and domain-specific knowledge—it is concluded that those between the ages of 40 and 60 are the most likely to execute high-quality personal financial decisions, a conclusion consistent with the findings of Agarwal et al. (2009).

One unique contribution of this chapter to the extant literature on financial decision making is a hierarchical taxonomy of household financial tasks. This taxonomy ranges in intellectual complexity from simple and mundane decisions at one end of the spectrum to complex and nuanced decisions at the other. Tasks within the taxonomy also differ as a function of their structure, degree of uncertainty, and the types of requisite cognitive skills required to reach closure. The tasks in the hierarchy also routinely occur in predictable situational contexts, sometimes predisposing the individual to certain biases and other times not. It is hoped this taxonomy will be useful to practitioners who seek to work effectively with clients needing different levels of professional support to accomplish their decision-making objectives.

We concluded the chapter by describing various types of developmentally-appropriate interventions that follow from the issues raised in the chapter. At this point in time, a comprehensive, forward-thinking wrap-around approach to life span intervention and financial services is needed. The goal of this approach is to anticipate and remediate weaknesses in decision performance prior to a point at which those weaknesses manifest themselves. Toward that end, early identification and risk factors should be carefully monitored on an ongoing basis.

Clearly, we have our work cut out for us. It has yet to be determined whether the tools and ideas we have at our disposal will prove sufficient to foment positive change. Ultimately, the metric of our success in the decades to come will be assessed through increases in individual levels of financial satisfaction and an overall improvement in societal quality of life.

Acknowledgment

This chapter was prepared while the first author was a guest researcher at the Netherlands Interdisciplinary Demographic Institute in The Hague. He is sincerely indebted to the Institute for their support of this work.

References

Agarwal, S., Driscoll, J. C., Gabaix, X., & Laibson, D. (2009). *The age of reason: Financial decisions over the life-cycle with implications for regulation*. Social Science Research Network. Working paper #973790.

ANZ. (2011). *Adult financial literacy in Australia (full report)*. Melbourne, Australia: Social Research Centre.

Azurdia, G., Freedman, S., Hamilton, G., & Schultz, C. (April 2014). *Encouraging low- and moderate income tax filers to save: Implementation and interim impact findings from the SaveUSA evaluation*. New York: MDRC.

Baltes, P. B. (1987). Theoretical propositions of life-span developmental psychology: On the dynamics between growth and decline. *Developmental Psychology*, *23*, 611–626.

Besede, T., Deck, C., Sarangic, S., & Shore, M. (2012). Decision-making strategies and performance among seniors. *Journal of Economic Behavior and Organization*, *81*, 524–533.

Bower, J. L. (2007). *The CEO within: Why inside outsiders are the key to succession*. Boston: Harvard Business Review Press.

Boyle, P. A., Yu, L., Wilson, R. S., Segawa, E., Buchman, A. S., & Bennett, D. A. (2013). Cognitive decline impairs financial and health literacy among community-based older persons without dementia. *Psychology and Aging*, *28*, 614–624.

Carpenter, S. M., & Yoon, C. (2011). Aging and consumer decision making. *Annals of the New York Academy of Sciences*, *1235*, E1–E12.

Council on Adult and Experiential Learning. (2012). *Financial literacy and retirement decisions: The choices facing older workers*. New York: Author.

Craik, F. M., & Anderson, N. D. (1999). Applying cognitive research to problems of aging. In D. Gopher, & A. Koriat (Eds.), *Attention and performance XVII: Cognitive regulation of performance: Interaction of theory and application* (pp. 583–615). Cambridge, MA: The MIT Press.

Croy, G., Gerrans, P., & Speelman, C. (2010). The role and relevance of domain knowledge, perceptions of planning importance, and risk tolerance in predicting savings intentions. *Journal of Economic Psychology*, *31*, 860–871.

Davies, M., Harries, P., Cairns, D., Stanley, D., Gilhooly, M., Gilhooly, K., et al. (2011). Factors used in the detection of elder financial abuse: A judgment and decision-making study of social workers and their managers. *International Social Work*, *54*, 404–420.

Del Missier, F., Mäntylä, T., Hansson, P., Bruine de Bruin, W., Parker, A. M., & Nilsson, L. (2013). The multifold relationship between memory and decision making: An individual-differences study. *Journal of Experimental Psychology: Learning, Memory, and Cognition*, *39*(5), 1344–1364.

Demange, G., & Laroque, G. (2006). *Finance and the economics of uncertainty*. Hoboken, NJ: Wiley-Blackwell.

Elder, G. H. (1994). Time, human agency, and social change: Perspectives on the life course. *Social Psychology Quarterly*, *57*, 4–15.

Federal Reserve Bank. (2014). *Federal Reserve bank presidents*. Federal Reserve Bank of St. Louis. Retrieved from http://www.federalreserve.gov/aboutthefed/bios/banks/default.htm.

Gallmeyer, A., & Roberts, W. T. (2009). Payday lenders and economically distressed communities: A spatial analysis of financial predation. *The Social Science Journal*, *46*, 521–538.

Gerardi, K., Goette, L., & Meier, S. (2013). Numerical ability predicts mortgage default. *Proceedings of the National Academy of Sciences*, *110*, 11267–11271.

Gerrans, P., & Hershey, D. A. (2013). *The role of financial literacy and financial adviser anxiety in older Australians' advice seeking*. Canberra: Technical Report Published by the National Seniors Australia Productive Ageing Centre. National Seniors Productive Ageing Centre, ISBN: 978-0-9874598-2-4.

Gilad, D., & Kliger, D. (2008). Priming the risk attitudes of professionals in financial decision making. *Review of Finance*, *12*, 567–586.

Griffiths, M. A., & Harmon, T. R. (2011). Aging consumer vulnerabilities influencing factors of acquiescence to informed consent. *Journal of Consumer Affairs*, *45*, 445–466.

Gutierrez, H. C., Hershey, D. A., & Gerrans, P. (2011). What to do when clients are afraid to share. *CSA: Certified Senior Advisor*, *49*, 39–44.

Hershey, D. A., Henkens, K., & Van Dalen, H. P. (2010). Aging and financial planning for retirement: Interdisciplinary influences viewed through a cross-cultural lens. *The International Journal of Aging and Human Development*, *70*, 1–38.

Hershey, D. A., Jacobs-Lawson, J. M., & Austin, J. T. (2012). Effective financial planning for retirement. In M. Wang (Ed.), *Oxford handbook of retirement* (pp. 402–430). New York: Oxford University Press.

Hershey, D. A., Jacobs-Lawson, J. M., & Walsh, D. A. (2003). Influences of age and training on script development. *Aging, Neuropsychology, and Cognition*, *10*, 1–19.

Hess, T. M., Waters, S. J., & Bolstad, C. A. (2000). Motivational and cognitive influences on affective priming in adulthood. *Journal of Gerontology: Psychological Sciences*, *55B*, 193–204.

Hira, T. K., Sabri, M., & Loibl, C. (2013). Financial socialization's impact on investment orientation and household net worth. *International Journal of Consumer Studies, 37*, 29–35.

Hirshleifer, D., & Shumway, T. (2003). Good day sunshine: Stock returns and the weather. *Journal of Finance, 58*, 1009–1032.

Horn, J. (1988). Thinking about human abilities. In J. R. Nesselroade, & R. B. Cattell (Eds.), *Handbook of multivariate experimental psychology* (2nd ed.) (pp. 645–685). New York, NY: Plenum Press.

Horn, J. L., & Cattell, R. B. (1966). Refinement and test of the theory of fluid and crystallized general intelligences. *Journal of Educational Psychology, 57*, 253–270.

Houser, R., D'Andrea, M., & Daniels, J. (1992). Fostering financial independence self-efficacy in AFDC recipients participating in a vocational training program. *Journal of Employment Counseling, 29*, 117–127.

Johnson, C. (2010). The magic of group identity: How predatory lenders use minorities to target communities of color. *Georgetown Journal on Poverty Law & Policy, 17*, 165–172.

Kliger, D., & Gilad, D. (2012). Red light, green light: Color priming in financial decisions. *The Journal of Socio-Economics, 41*, 738–745.

Kliger, D., & Levy, O. (2003). Mood-induced variation in risk preferences. *Journal of Economic Behavior & Organization, 52*, 573–584.

Koposko J.L. & Hershey D.A. Parental and early influences on expectations of financial planning for retirement. *Journal of Personal Finance* (in press).

Köstering, L., Stahl, C., Leonhart, R., Weiller, C., & Kaller, C. P. (2014). Development of planning abilities in normal aging: Differential effects of specific cognitive demands. *Developmental Psychology, 50*, 293–303.

Kuhnen, C. M., & Knutson, B. (2005). The neural basis of financial risk taking. *Neuron, 47*, 763–770.

Laibson, D. (June 2011). Age of reason. In *Closing keynote presentation at the 23rd annual Morningstar Investment conference, Chicago, IL*. Retrieved from http://www.academia.edu/2667799/The_Age_of_Reason.

Laxman, K. (2010). A conceptual framework mapping the application of information search strategies to well and ill-structured problem solving. *Computers & Education, 55*, 513–526.

Li, Y., Baldassi, M., Johnson, E. J., & Weber, E. U. (2013). Complementary cognitive capabilities, economic decision making, and aging. *Psychology and Aging, 28*, 595–613.

Li, S., Lindenberger, U., Hommel, B., Aschersleben, G., Prinz, W., & Baltes, P. B. (2004). Transformations in the couplings among intellectual abilities and constituent cognitive processes across the lifespan. *Psychological Science, 15*, 155–163.

Loibl, C., & Hira, T. K. (2006). A workplace and gender-related perspective on financial planning information sources and knowledge outcomes. *Financial Services Review, 15*, 21–42.

Lusardi, A. (2012, Summer). Financial literacy and financial decision-making in older adults. *Generations, 36*, 25–31.

Lusardi, A., & Mitchell, O. S. (2011a). Financial literacy and retirement planning in the United States. *Journal of Pension Economics and Finance, 10*, 509–525.

Lusardi, A., & Mitchell, O. S. (2011b). Financial literacy around the world. *An Overview Journal of Pension Economics and Finance, 10*, 497–508.

Lusardi, A., & Mitchell, O. S. (2013). *The economic importance of financial literacy: Theory and evidence* (Working paper #18952). Retrieved from the National Bureau of Economic Research website http://www.nber.org/papers/w18952.

Lusardi, A., Mitchell, O. S., & Curto, V. (2010). *Financial literacy among the young: Evidence and implications for consumer policy* (Working paper #2010/09). Retrieved from the Center for Financial Studies website http://nbn-resolving.de/urn:nbn:de:hebis:30-78626.

McDowd, J. M., & Hoffman, L. (2008). Challenges in attention: Measures, methods, and applications. In S. M. Hofer, & D. F. Alwin (Eds.), *Handbook of cognitive aging: interdisciplinary perspectives* (pp. 122–133). Thousand Oaks, CA: Sage Publications, Inc.

Milner, T., & Rosenstreich, D. (2013). Insights into mature consumers of financial services. *Journal of Consumer Marketing, 30*, 248–257.

Morell, J. A. (2010). *Evaluation in the face of uncertainty: Anticipating surprise and responding.* New York: Guilford Press.

Mortimer, J. T., & Shanahan, M. J. (2003). *Handbook of the life course.* New York: Plenum.

Moschis, G. P., Mosteller, J., & Fatt, C. K. (2011). Research frontiers on older consumers' vulnerability. *Journal of Consumer Affairs, 45*, 467–491.

National Committee on the Prevention of Elder Abuse. (2008). *Fact sheet on financial elder abuse.* Retrieved from the NCPEA website http://www.preventelderabuse.org/elderabuse/fin_abuse.html.

Navarro, A. E., Gassoumis, Z. D., & Wilber, K. H. (2013). Holding abusers accountable: An elder abuse forensic center increases criminal prosecution of financial exploitation. *The Gerontologist, 53*, 303–312.

Naveh-Benjamin, M., Cowan, N., Kilb, A., & Chen, Z. (2007). Age-related differences in immediate serial recall: Dissociating chunk formation and capacity. *Memory & Cognition, 35*, 724–737.

Nofsinger, J. R. (2001). *Investment madness: How psychology affects your investing...and what to do about it.* New York: Prentice Hall.

Post, T., & Hanewald, K. (2013). Longevity risk, subjective survival expectations, and individual saving behavior. *Journal of Economic Behavior & Organization, 86*, 200–220.

Probst, G., & Bassi, A. (2014). *Tackling complexity: A systemic approach for decision makers.* Sheffield, UK: Greenleaf Publishing Company.

Pronin, E. (2007). Perception and misperception of bias in human judgment. *Trends in Cognitive Sciences, 11*, 37–43.

Rabiner, D., Brown, D., & O'Keeffe, J. (2004). Financial exploitation of older persons. *Journal of Elder Abuse & Neglect, 16*, 65–84.

Rau, P. R., Patel, A., Osobov, I., Khorana, A., & Cooper, M. J. (2003). The game of the name: Valuation effects of name changes in a market turndown. Unpublished working paper.

Salthouse, T. A., & Davis, H. P. (2006). Organization of cognitive abilities and neuropsychological variables across the lifespan. *Developmental Review, 26*, 31–54.

Samanez-Larkin, G. R., Wagner, A. D., & Knutson, B. (2011). Expected value information improves financial risk taking across the adult life span. *Social, Cognitive, and Affective Neuroscience, 2010*(9), 207–217.

Scatinga, L. (2009). *The financial physician: How to cure your money problems and boost your financial health.* Pompton Plains, NJ: Career Press.

Scherpereel, C. M. (2006). Decision orders: a decision taxonomy. *Management Decision, 44*, 123–136.

Shleifer, A. (2000). *Inefficient markets: An introduction to behavioral finance.* New York: Oxford University Press.

Shobe, M. A., & Sturm, S. L. (2007). Youth individual development accounts: Retirement planning initiatives. *Children & Schools, 29*, 172–181.

Simon, H. A. (1973). The structure of ill-structured problems. *Artificial Intelligence, 4*, 181–201.

Sotiropoulos, V., & d'Astous, A. (2013). Attitudinal, self-efficacy, and social norm determinants of young consumers' propensity to overspend on credit cards. *Journal of Consumer Policy, 36*, 179–196. Retrieved from http://link.springer.com/article/10.1007%2Fs10603-013-9223-3#page-1.

Strough, J., Karns, T. E., & Schlosnagle, L. (2011). Decision-making heuristics and biases across the life span. *Annals of the New York Academy of Sciences, 1235*, 57–74.

Su, Y. (2013). Three essays on financial literacy, financial self-awareness, and retirement well-being. *Dissertation Abstracts International Section A, 74.*

Thaler, R. H., & Benartzi, S. (2012). Save more tomorrow™: Using behavioral economics to increase employee saving. In I. M. McDonald (Ed.), *Behavioural macroeconomics* (pp. 283–306). Northampton, MA: Edward Elgar Publishing.

Thaler, R. H., & Sunstein, C. R. (2008). *Nudge: Improving decisions about health, wealth, and happiness*. New Haven, CT: Yale University Press.

Thorndike, E. L. (1920). A constant error in psychological ratings. *Journal of Applied Psychology, 4*, 26–29.

Tymulaa, A., Belmaker, L. A. R., Ruderman, L., Glimcher, P. W., & Levy, I. (2013). Like cognitive function, decision making across the life span shows profound age-related changes. *PNAS, 110*, 17143–17148.

UNESCO. (2004). The plurality of literacy and its implications for policies and programs. *UNESCO Education Sector Position Paper, 13.*

Walsh, D. A., & Hershey, D. A. (1993). Mental models and the maintenance of complex problem-solving skills in old age. In J. Cerella, J. M. Rybash, W. Hoyer, & M. L. Commons (Eds.), *Adult information processing: Limits on loss* (pp. 553–584). San Diego, CA: Academic Press.

Weierich, J. D., Kensinger, E. A., Munnell, A. H., Sass, S. A., Dickerson, B. C., Wright, C. I., et al. (2011). Older and wiser? An affective science perspective on age-related challenges in financial decision making. *Social and Cognitive Affective Neuroscience, 6*, 195–206.

Werbel, J. D., & Danes, S. M. (2010). Work family conflict in new business ventures: The moderating effects of spousal commitment to the new business venture. *Journal of Small Business Management, 48*, 421–440.

Xiao, J., Chen, C., & Chen, F. (2013). *Consumer financial capability and financial satisfaction.* Social Indicators Research.

Yang, T., & DeVaney, S. A. (2012). Determinants of retirement assets and the amount in stock in retirement assets. *Family and Consumer Sciences Research Journal, 41*, 36–55.

Yoon, C., Cole, C. A., & Lee, M. P. (2009). Consumer decision making and aging: Current knowledge and future directions. *Journal of Consumer Psychology, 19*, 2–16.

CHAPTER

17

Aging and Consumer Decision Making

Stephanie M. Carpenter[1], *Carolyn Yoon*[2]

[1]Department of Psychology, University of Michigan, Ann Arbor, MI, USA; [2]Marketing Department, Stephen M. Ross School of Business, University of Michigan, Ann Arbor, MI, USA

Studying consumer behavior across the life span is becoming increasingly important, as the number of consumers over the age of 65 continues to grow dramatically. Recent reports by the U.S. Census Bureau have projected that the older adult population will increase to over 20% of the U.S. population (i.e., 72 million) by the year 2030. This demographic shift highlights the need for more research on aging consumers as the topic is of vital importance to individual consumers and policymakers alike.

In this chapter, we draw on extant literature from consumer behavior, psychology, and related disciplines to provide a review of research findings on decision making by older consumers. First, we review literature that examines how normal aging impacts consumer decision making via changes in cognitive functioning and decision processing. We then describe various factors that moderate the effects of aging on decision making: task environment, context, meaningfulness, personal relevance, and expertise. Finally, we conclude by identifying knowledge gaps and suggesting directions for future research, specifically within the domain of consumer behavior.

AGE DIFFERENCES IN BASIC DECISION SKILLS AND STRATEGIES

Much extant research suggests that normal aging generally leads to systematic declines in cognitive functioning starting from the mid-20s and continuing throughout the adult life span (Park, Lautenschlager, Hedden,

http://dx.doi.org/10.1016/B978-0-12-417148-0.00017-0

Davidson, & Smith, 2002). Tasks that require a great deal of deliberative processing or complex decision making may be more difficult for older adults than for younger adults. Performance on tasks that rely more on affective processing, however, appears to remain largely preserved with age. In the sections that follow, we will briefly outline a few ways in which aging affects basic cognitive and affective processes important to decision making, and the impact of these changes on decision-making skills and strategies.

Aging Influences on Cognitive and Affective Processes

Fluid Mental Abilities and Executive Functioning

Fluid abilities refer to the capacity to process complex, novel, or ambiguous information (Cattell, 1963). They reflect reasoning and problem-solving skills closely linked to executive functioning that involve cognitive control and regulation. Decisions that draw on these abilities show reliable age-related decrements (Bruine de Bruin, Parker, & Fischhoff, 2012).

Basic executive functioning and fluid mental abilities are typically assessed via tasks related to speed of processing, working memory, and inhibitory processes. Speed of processing, or the speed with which one can perform mental operations and process information, is particularly sensitive to age-related declines (Salthouse, 1996), and is correlated with working memory capacity. Working memory is more affected than long-term memory by age-related cognitive declines, and the effects are evident in tasks that require simultaneously holding and processing multiple pieces of information (Hess, 2005; Moscovitch & Winocur, 1995; see Yoon, Cole, & Lee, 2009, for a review). These declines in working memory can have important consequences for complex consumer choices that necessitate the comparison of features or alternatives (Cole & Houston, 1987; Roedder John & Cole, 1986; see also Chapter 7, in this volume).

Inhibition comprises another important aspect of executive functioning, and refers to the ability to shift between task goals, update the contents of working memory, and suppress irrelevant information (e.g., Hedden & Yoon, 2006; West, 1996). Older adults appear to have a diminished ability to inhibit irrelevant information compared to younger adults (Hasher & Zacks, 1988). This suggests that older consumers may be vulnerable to interference effects in shopping environments that are crowded or noisy. Age-related declines in any of these cognitive functions can thus make decision-making tasks more challenging and difficult for older consumers.

Crystallized Mental Abilities and Expertise

Crystallized intelligence relies more on long-term memory and reflects the ability to use experience and knowledge (e.g., vocabulary). In contrast to fluid intelligence, it has been shown to improve with age (Finucane, Mertz, Slovic, & Schmidt, 2005). Expertise is a related factor that should be considered when examining the influence of age-related changes on consumer decision making. Older consumers are likely to have more experience than younger consumers with making decisions in a wide range of consumer domains, and in such cases, age-related decline would not be expected. The effects of consumer expertise will be further addressed later in this chapter.

Affective Decision Processes and Motivation

Older, relative to younger, adults tend to show a shift in attention from more deliberative-focused to more emotion-focused goals (Socioemotional Selectivity Theory of aging; Carstensen, 1992; Carstensen, Isaacowitz, & Charles, 1999). Specifically, older adults' memory for information tends to skew more positive than that of younger adults, a phenomenon referred to as the "positivity effect" or "bias" (Mather & Carstensen, 2005). Younger adults, on the other hand, typically show a greater skew toward a negativity bias. These changes have been explained by shifts across the life span in one's perception of temporal horizon from long to short (Carstensen, 1992), along with a concomitant increased focus on social and emotional goals that can be achieved in the present moment (Charles & Carstensen, 2009). Socioemotional changes in goals among older adults may influence decision-making strategies in important ways by shifting the focus of these strategies from deliberative to emotional.

Systematic versus Heuristic Decision-Making Strategies

A more complete understanding of age differences in consumer decision making also requires consideration of common decision strategies, which can vary from thoughtful and systematic to more heuristic (Tversky & Kahneman, 1974). Framing of decision-relevant information using a positive (e.g., number of lives saved) or negative (e.g., number of lives lost) information frame can lead older adults to use heuristic or biased strategies in their decision making to a greater extent than younger adults (Kim, Goldstein, Hasher, & Zacks, 2005). This occurs presumably as a way for the decision maker to easily manage the decision process without expending too many cognitive resources. That said, inconsistencies do exist in the literature regarding age-related influences on framing (Mikels & Reed, 2009), and more research is needed in this area.

Satisficing is a heuristic, noncompensatory processing strategy that aims at adequate, rather than optimal, decision making (Schwartz et al., 2002). Research has shown that older adults are often more likely than younger adults to examine option information only until they determine that the amount of acquired information is sufficient and acceptable (Chen & Sun, 2003; Peters, 2010; Yoon, Feinberg, & Schwarz, 2010). Younger adults, on the other hand, tend to use more systematic, maximizing strategies when making decisions. Satisficing is thus a decision strategy that older adults may adopt in order to decrease the amount of effort required during more cognitively taxing forms of decision making, or when a decision has few personal implications (Hess, Queen, & Ennis, 2013).

Heuristic processing can have both positive and negative consequences for consumer decision making in older adulthood. For example, a greater reliance on heuristics in older age allows for quick and effective decisions (Yates & Patalano, 1999) when making choices in simple or mundane domains (e.g., grocery or household items). However, older consumers are often faced with much more consequential and novel choices having to do with health care, retirement, and financial planning, all of which typically involve large amounts of complicated information that must be waded through in order for older consumers to arrive at a decision. It is in these more complicated domains that the increased use of heuristic processing by older consumers can become problematic.

While evidence suggests that older adults spontaneously use schema-based and heuristic processing more often than younger adults, asking them to consider the reasons for their decisions also promotes greater use of systematic processing on choice tasks that are sensitive to framing (Kim et al., 2005). This indicates that at least some decision biases to which older adults are susceptible can be overcome with strategies that promote greater systematic information processing.

Taken together, the findings suggest that older consumers are in many cases capable of applying systematic processing strategies when appropriate and necessary, but use them less frequently than younger consumers unless the decision environment encourages or facilitates their use. It will be critical for future work to uncover the ways in which different types of processing strategies can be employed by older consumers to make suitable and effective decisions.

AGE DIFFERENCES IN CONSUMER CHOICE AND DECISION MAKING

Age-related changes in basic processing skills and specific strategies substantially influence how consumers make decisions across the life span. These changes affect a myriad of factors that are crucial to decision making, including brand preferences, choice set sizes, and the use of specific types of decision strategies. They also systematically alter how older consumers evaluate and experience products relative to younger consumers.

A particularly important component of understanding consumer decision making is determining how older adults select options when making choices. Older adults have a preference for, and are more likely to purchase, long-established brands (Lambert-Pandraud, Laurent, & Lapersonne, 2005). This is likely due to a number of factors, including experience with products, product attachment, nostalgia, habit, an aversion to change (Lambert-Pandraud & Laurent, 2010a), and may also be related to the tendency for older adults to satisfice. It may even be the case that forming brand preferences serves as a heuristic strategy.

Another major consideration for older consumers' decision making is the number of options available in one's choice context (Lambert-Pandraud & Lambert, 2010b). Within the domain of health decisions, a number of studies have examined the consequences of the Medicare prescription drug program (Part D) (Abaluck & Gruber, 2009; Tanius, Wood, Hanoch, & Rice, 2009; Wood et al., 2011; see also Chapter 15, in this volume). The Medicare Part D program was created with the intention of maximizing the number of prescription drug choices that would be available to older adults. Research has shown, however, that participants of all ages, including older adults, tend to make better decisions when they have fewer choice options (Tanius et al., 2009; Wood et al., 2011). Further, Abaluck and Gruber (2009) found that older adults tend to focus specifically on a narrow range of dimensions, and the best way to present medical information is to restrict the choice set size to a few options with the lowest average costs. These prior studies suggest that older consumers should be presented with fewer choice options (assuming that these choice options are acceptable along dimensions of importance to older adults) and that choice information be presented in simpler formats to bolster decision performance.

Information search is a cognitively taxing process, and older consumers tend to engage in less search behavior during decision making. Due to the limited amount of time that older consumers spend searching for brand information (Johnson, 1990), they tend to construct smaller consideration sets. Reduced consideration set size is a consequence of a "shrinkage" effect, whereby the decrease in what information is searched for and obtained also leads to the consideration of fewer options (Lambert-Pandraud & Laurent, 2010a). One consequence of these smaller consideration sets is that older adults are more likely to engage in repeat purchasing because they are choosing among only a very small number of options (Lambert-Pandraud et al., 2005). As such, the likelihood of them choosing the same option repeatedly across multiple decision occasions increases, and this leads to brand preferences that are seemingly more stable among older consumers. Another consequence is that older consumers are more likely to eliminate alternatives as soon as any negative information is presented (Riggle & Johnson, 1996).

This preference for smaller consideration sets across the adult life span has been shown to occur linearly and gradually, and across domains (Reed, Mikels, & Löckenhoff, 2013). Although these smaller consideration sets may simplify the decision process, there are sometimes also negative consequences. For instance, searching for too few options (i.e., not searching for all information available) has been shown to lead older adults to perform more poorly than younger adults on sequential decision tasks (Von Helverson & Mata, 2012). This finding was, at least partly, explained by age-related increases in positive affect that arbitrarily lowers the consumer's threshold for what product options are considered attractive.

Mather, Knight, and McCaffrey (2005) provided evidence that when comparing relatively complex options involving a large quantity of information, such as common decisions about apartments, health care plans, or cars, older adults become more feature oriented (i.e., comparing features from the same dimension across options), whereas younger adults become more option oriented (i.e., examining all of the features of one option before moving to the next option). Choice situations that lead older adults to reduce options and minimize the cognitive effort involved in the decision process may arguably translate into a greater focus on the essentials of the decision, such as the experiential benefits offered by the features.

Decisions comprising fewer attributes may indeed improve older adults' decision making (Finucane et al., 2005). Across several real-world decision domains that can require processing large quantities of information (e.g., health, retirement, finances), older adults have been found to be more inconsistent in their decisions and to commit more comprehension errors than younger adults. It must be noted, however, that in domains where consumers are knowledgeable or where self-relevance is particularly high, decision-strategy differences between younger and older adults disappear (Hess et al., 2013; Queen, Hess, Ennis, Dowd, & Gruhn, 2012). This indicates that the decision domain should be taken into consideration when assessing whether older consumers are likely to simplify their choice strategies and in what situations doing so may either help or hinder the decision process.

Related to the motivational tendency toward a positivity bias, older consumers have been found to be more satisfied than younger consumers across a number of product domains. Yoon et al. (2010) examined cross-sectional data from the American Consumer Satisfaction Index (ACSI; Fornell, Johnson, Anderson, Cha, & Bryant, 1996). The ACSI is a database containing information on consumer satisfaction with products and services representing more than 200 companies in 45 industries, as well as some government agencies. Older adults (aged 65 and above) were found to self-report higher satisfaction across a variety of product and service categories (see Yoon et al., 2010, for a review). The phenomenon that emerged was named the "older-and-more-satisfied" effect. The reasons for this robust phenomenon are currently not well understood but are likely to be multicausal. The authors speculated on a number of potential explanations, including (1) older consumers' extensive experience with products and services leading to a better sense of their own preferences, (2) use of a lower comparison standard than younger consumers who may know more about the "latest and greatest" products, and (3) a greater likelihood to satisfice than younger consumers on products or services that meet their basic requirements (Yoon et al., 2010). A better understanding of why this "older-and-more-satisfied" effect occurs would help to expand knowledge on how older consumers make product decisions.

Overall, the reviewed literature highlights the importance of understanding the choice domain when making predictions about the use of different strategies by older consumers. Generally speaking, older consumers tend to prefer smaller, simpler consideration sets and have a tendency toward appraising products more positively, relative to younger consumers. Many age-related effects on consumer decision making, however, become less pronounced when the decision in question is of higher self-relevance, which suggests that not all decision problems will be approached differently by older than younger consumers. The reviewed literature also reveals that not all decision contexts are necessarily more challenging for older than for younger consumers, and points to a number of factors that moderate the observed age-related effects on decision making. In the following section of this chapter, we describe a number of these moderating factors.

MODERATING INFLUENCES ON AGING AND DECISION MAKING

We next consider three broad sets of factors that are known to exert moderating influences on consumer decision making across the life span. These factors include the task environment or context, the meaningfulness or personal relevance of the task, and consumer expertise. Although these factors can influence consumer decision makers of all ages, older adults have been found to be particularly sensitive to the moderating factors described here. First, the task environment or context can greatly affect older consumers, relative to younger consumers. Although a difficult task environment can be particularly challenging, support in the form of environmental cues or decision aids can serve to bolster task performance that leads to more effective decisions. Second, the meaningfulness or personal relevance of the task can aid older consumers insofar as they are inherently more interested in the task domain and motivated to make appropriate decisions. Third, consumer expertise can buffer the effects of age and facilitate effective decision making, although there are some pitfalls associated with an over reliance on experience and familiarity. In addition to describing how these moderating factors influence many of the basic age-related differences in decision making already reviewed, we will also present a number of potential interventions. We now turn to a discussion of each of these factors.

Task Environment or Context

The environment in which a decision is made often has important implications for older decision makers' outcomes (Yoon et al., 2009). In particular, time pressure, distraction, irrelevant information, and environmental support can influence older adults' decision making to an even greater extent than younger consumers. While some of these factors have detrimental effects, others may serve to enhance decision performance.

Time pressure in a decision environment can have a detrimental influence on the decision-making abilities of consumers, especially as they age (Earles, Kersten, Mas, & Miccio, 2004; Park, Iyer, & Smith, 1989). Older consumers under time pressure, especially if they are in unfamiliar settings, are less able to locate their preferred brand and end up purchasing brands they did not intend to purchase (Park et al., 1989). Further, time pressure has been shown to magnify decrements in recall by older adults, as compared to younger adults (Earles et al., 2004). One potential explanation for this age difference is that time pressure activates negative stereotypes about aging, which induces feelings of anxiety among older adults (Earles et al., 2004) and leads to hastier purchase decisions.

Another important factor to consider is the influence of distraction and irrelevant information. Prior findings have documented robust age-related increases in vulnerability to distraction across a variety of tasks (e.g., McDowd & Filion, 1992). For example, older adults report difficulty in locating an object in a cluttered visual field (Kosnik, Winslow, Rasinski, & Sekuler, 1988), respond more slowly, and commit more errors in search tasks when the selection environment contains distracters (e.g., Madden, 1983; Plude & Hoyer, 1986).

Many consumption environments, including supermarkets and shopping malls, are busy and contain distracting information that could presumably influence an older consumers' ability to make a decision. Studies on divided attention have also uncovered age differences in dual-task performance, with magnified age differences as a function of task difficulty (McDowd & Craik, 1988). Decrements in the suppression of task irrelevant information are associated with declines in working memory that are especially prominent when cognitive resources are taxed, but enhancement of task-relevant information may be preserved (Gazzaley, Cooney, Rissman, & Esposito, 2005; Gazzaley, Sheridan, Cooney, & Esposito, 2007). Together, these findings indicate that the relevance of the distracting information to the choice task at hand may have an important influence on whether the information helps or hinders consumer decision making across the adult life span.

Environmental primes, or information automatically activated by environmental context, are especially pertinent for the kinds of decisions that consumers are faced with in daily life. Older adults are more vulnerable than younger adults to the disruptive effects of distraction from task-irrelevant environmental primes and other sources, including irrelevant events from the recent past (Hasher, Lustig, & Zacks, 2007). The explanation given for this sensitivity has been a general inability of older adults to inhibit these irrelevant environmental primes, which suggests there may be negative consequences for older consumers in complex or busy consumption environments such as supermarkets or shopping malls. The diminished inhibitory control experienced by older adults means that irrelevant information remains active in their memory when engaging in subsequent unrelated tasks. It has been shown that this inhibitory deficit can interfere with both older adults' immediate task performance and their downstream performance for up to 15–20 min after initial exposure to the distraction (Hasher et al., 2007). This indicates that irrelevant, distracting information may influence the consumption decisions of older adults to a greater extent than younger adults.

It is noteworthy, however, that emerging evidence suggests there can be some positive downstream consequences to older adults' sustained activation of irrelevant past information. For example, Kim, Hasher, and Zacks (2007) reported superior performance by older adults compared to younger adults on a Remote Associates Task (RAT) after exposure to distracting information on a preceding task (Mednick, 1968). This is particularly interesting because the RAT is considered a measure of cognitive flexibility. In this task, participants are given a set of words (e.g., falling, actor, dust) and are asked to find a new word that can be paired with each word in the triad (e.g., star). Improvement on this task suggests that exposure to this distracting information may boost cognitive flexibility, at least on tasks that involve the processing of associations.

Samanez-Larkin, Wagner, and Knutson (2011) also found that distracting tasks may have less of an influence when the critical information is presented in a simplified format. For example, providing simple expected value information for financial decisions has been shown to improve older adults' decision quality even in the presence of distracting information. One important future direction for research is to further examine how distraction and inhibitory failures lead to performance costs as well as benefits for older adults across a variety of consumption domains.

Recently, Anguera et al. (2013) have provided intriguing evidence that age-related susceptibility to distraction and interference may be reduced for up to 6 months by video game training, which allows participants to exercise cognitive control in multitasking environments. This may prove to be a fruitful avenue for improving the decision-making capabilities of older consumers, but more research is needed to understand the efficacy of such intervention programs. Substantial evidence already exists indicating that cognitive training programs (e.g., ACTIVE trial; Ball et al.,

2002) can be effective at improving and maintaining mental functioning among older adults. More research examining the generalization of such intervention effects to everyday decision making would be informative to our understanding of how older consumers make decisions.

Decision aids represent another category of interventions that may prove especially useful when consumers are faced with distracting contextual and environmental factors (Yoon et al., 2009). The extent to which decision aids can help older consumers, however, has received little research attention. The existing evidence indicates that effective decision aids for older adults can take several forms, including crossing out irrelevant information from preexisting information lists (Cole & Gaeth, 1990) or using visual symbols as a supplement to verbal information (Morrow et al., 2003). The limited empirical evidence regarding this topic has also shown that older adults with higher (vs lower) crystallized and fluid intelligence make greater overall use of decision aids (Johnson, 1997), and that older adults are more likely than younger adults to use memory aids at the end of the decision process, just prior to making the actual decision. Additional research is needed to determine if changes in the point at which different age groups use decision aids is beneficial or detrimental to the decision process. Understanding when and how best to use decision aids across the life span would generate greater insights about the effectiveness of various decision aids.

One especially useful decision-aiding technique for older adults is the task of writing down information, rather than holding it in memory. Cole and Balasubramanian (1993) found that older consumers did not search nutritional information as intensively as younger consumers when shopping for cereal in a grocery store setting. This lack of information search led older consumers to subsequently choose less appropriate cereals. However, when experimenters encouraged participants to write down the information that they acquired during the search process, these age-related differences were eliminated.

The time of day that an older adult is making a decision is also important for complicated and consequential decision making. Older adults, relative to younger adults, are known to show greater improvements in systematic information processing during their peak times of day (Yoon, 1997). This is due to individual differences in circadian arousal patterns that have been found to vary predictably for older and younger adults and, in turn, affect memory and decision-making performance across the life span (May, Hasher, & Stoltzfus, 1993; Yoon, 1997). Older adults tend to reach their peak level of circadian arousal and performance in the morning, whereas younger adults tend to reach it in the afternoon or evening (May et al., 1993; Yoon, 1997). Yoon, Lee, and Dazinger (2007) found that this had downstream consequences for older consumers insofar as they were more likely to be persuaded by heuristic cues at their non-optimal than optimal times of day. This suggests that when making decisions, consumers of all ages, but especially older adults, would be well-advised to take into account time of day; older adults should make complex or deliberative decisions in the morning, whereas younger adults should make these same decisions later in the day.

As indicated here, contextual and environmental factors have a number of consequences for consumer decision making across the life span, and may be especially important to consider for older consumers who are often more sensitive to these effects than younger consumers. Additional research should be conducted to fully understand when these factors lead to both detriments and benefits for consumer decisions, and when training or aiding interventions are likely to be particularly useful for improving the quality of consumer decisions.

Meaningfulness or Personal Relevance

The personal relevance and meaningfulness of a decision is another important factor that can moderate the effects of aging on consumer decision making. As emotion goals change across the life span (Charles & Carstensen, 2009), emotion information may become more meaningful and personally relevant to older than to younger adults. Older adults have been found to be more sensitive to affective and value-based information than younger adults (e.g., Labouvie-Vief & Blanchard-Fields, 1982; Rahhal, May, & Hasher, 2002). Consistent with this finding, as people age, they also become more reliant on affective, experiential, and heuristic forms of processing (e.g., Slovic, Finucane, Peters, & MacGregor, 2002). This may, in turn, shift their decisions to be in favor of more affective and experiential products.

Further, the traditional decision-making literature has largely relied on a strong assumption that deliberative processing abilities are essential for good decision making (Peters, 2010). Predictable declines in deliberative processing that occur with normal aging (Mather, 2006) are thus thought to be detrimental to overall decision quality. However, some research has shown that older adults focus on personally meaningful choice information and rely more on affect than deliberation when making choices (for review, see Peters, Hess, Västfjäll, & Auman, 2007). As is the case with other important factors, the reliance on affect can have both detrimental and supportive effects on older consumers' decision making.

Despite challenges associated with consumer decision making, older adults have been found to rely on a number of strategies for maintaining high levels of decision quality (cf. Peters et al., 2007). Presenting information in more emotion-focused contexts was also found to benefit performance on certain types of information-processing tasks. Mikels et al. (2010) revealed that younger adults had higher decision quality when given deliberative, information-focused instructions, whereas older adults had higher decision quality when given emotion-focused instructions. These findings suggest that older consumers might benefit from decision information presented in a format that promotes the formation of general affective impressions about the options, rather than requiring older adults to rely on memory for specific option details.

Imagery also affords a potentially effective use of systematic processing strategies across the adult life span, and can influence behavior above and beyond the benefits that arise from consumer decision justification (Kim et al., 2005) and from being instructed to think deeply about information during a decision process (Cole & Houston, 1987). Specifically, when instructed to form a mental image representing brand claims, older consumers processed details about the claims more effectively (Law, Hawkins, & Craik, 1998). These findings suggest that cues promoting the use of imagery may boost the meaningfulness and personal relevance of products and enable older consumers to use more systematic processing in decision situations that require careful deliberation and analytical thinking.

Together, these studies suggest that conveying consumer information in ways that encourage imagery and affective processing may improve decision making. It should be noted, however, that although affect can enhance decision-making quality and ability, circumstances exist in which the greater reliance of older adults on affect could lead to negative consequences for decision making (see also Chapter 9, in this volume). For example, older adults may be especially susceptible to affective appeals in advertising and marketing campaigns that provide uninformative or deceptive information, and this will serve to increase the likelihood of falling victim to scams.

Mikels, Cheung, Cone, and Gilovich (2012) have shown that performance on one such decision task, the ratio bias paradigm, actually declines due to overuse of positive affective information among older adults. In their task, participants drew from one of two dishes of jelly beans. One dish had a higher probability of winning, but a higher absolute number of people had won when drawing a jelly bean from the other dish. An overreliance on positive affect led individuals to choose the dish that more people had drawn from, which is the non-optimal choice from a probability standpoint. These results are consistent with Von Helverson and Mata's (2012) finding that age-related increases in positive affect arbitrarily lower a decision maker's threshold for what options are attractive, and thereby lead to poorer performance in sequential decision tasks. This also accords with findings by Bauer, Timpe, Edmonds, Tranel, and Denburg (2012) that older adults make more errors on the Iowa Gambling Task due to disproportionate sensitivity to reward, and with Queen and Hess's (2010) findings that an overreliance on automatic, affective evaluative information leads to non-optimal decisions when the choice requires deliberation (i.e., when the choice options have both positive and negative attributes). Thus, the evidence suggests that a reliance on affect during decision making can have both positive and negative consequences, depending on the type of decision being made.

Further, the influence that socioemotional attention shifts have on emotion goals and temporal horizon has been investigated in studies on information-processing responses to advertising. Older consumers focused more on emotionally meaningful information and goals (Fung & Carstensen, 2003) and subsequently responded more positively to affective advertising appeals than younger consumers (Williams & Drolet, 2005). Older consumers also showed greater liking for and increased recall of information presented in emotional advertisements, and the time horizon perspective moderated these age-related differences. Further, advertisements that were focused on avoiding negative emotions were liked and recalled more among both older and younger consumers when they were experimentally manipulated to have a limited time horizon perspective. These findings highlight the fact that changing temporal horizons, either associated with age or experimentally induced, can affect the extent to which both older and younger adults exhibit positivity and negativity biases.

Based on the evidence presented here, we suggest that older consumers tend to put more effort into decisions that are meaningful or self-relevant, and may be more likely than younger consumers to evaluate advertisements and products more positively. Thus, expanding our knowledge of how meaningfulness and self-relevance influence consumer decision making is of vital importance to understanding how consumers respond to consumer information and products.

Consumer Expertise

Another important factor to consider is the expertise that the consumer brings to the decision context. Consumer expertise is a function of both familiarity (or repeated experience) with a product domain and increasing objective knowledge or skill with making a decision within that domain (Alba & Hutchinson, 1987). After many years of experience and the acquisition of more knowledge, an older adult may be viewed as having gained greater expertise in decisions across many consumer domains. At the same time, there are likely to be domains that pose difficulties for the typical older adult (e.g., high technology).

Familiarity should also be taken into account because older consumers are unlikely to experience difficulties when making decisions involving mundane tasks that are highly familiar (e.g., shopping in a favorite grocery store). Product familiarity often serves to facilitate ease of processing among older consumers because information that is experienced repeatedly is easier to perceive and remember than unfamiliar information. Accordingly, variables that facilitate easy processing of consumer information, including print fonts, layouts, and color contrast, may profoundly influence persuasion among older consumers. This association between ease of processing and perceived familiarity has many important consequences. For example, information that is more familiar is also more likely to be accepted as true. Numerous studies have found that repeating the same statement reliably increases its perceived truth (e.g., Begg, Anas, & Farinacci, 1992; Hasher, Goldstein, & Toppino, 1977). This "illusion of truth" effect is particularly pronounced among older adults (Law et al., 1998), and the reliance on familiarity to infer truth can lead to negative consequences. For instance, being repeatedly exposed to a false health claim leads consumers to misremember that false claim as true later on (Skurnik, Yoon, Park, & Schwarz, 2005).

Although expertise can lead to these negative consequences (Camerer & Johnson, 1991; Shanteau, 1992; Wood & Lynch, 2002), it also has many benefits for consumer decision making. Experts are often confident about their ability to make choices and find information, and this confidence may foster individuals' feelings of self-efficacy and prompt actions or decisions (Bandura, 1976). Greater expertise also facilitates effective decision making by enabling consumers to be more efficient in information search and learning (Brucks, 1985; Johnson & Russo, 1984).

Experience can further promote consumer adaptation, such that older consumers are better able to select strategies to improve their decision making. In fact, the experience and knowledge that older adults acquire over the years may serve to counteract declines in deliberative and cognitive functioning. Research has shown, for example, that older consumers are able to remember the prices of products sold within a grocery store as well as younger consumers, due simply to their extensive experience and familiarity with grocery shopping contexts (Castel, 2005). Such experience effects likely play a large role in helping older adults make successful and satisfying consumption decisions, and future research should explore when experience leads to positive and negative consumption decisions.

Consumer experience within a number of domains leads to the use of strategies that reduce cognitive effort during decision making, including the information search process. As noted earlier, older consumers have been found to seek out less information than younger consumers. They also take longer to process the information they do search for (Johnson, 1990; Mata, Schooler, & Rieskamp, 2007). Older consumers, however, can use adaptive decision strategies within the information-processing contexts. A study instructing participants to make several price inferences indicated that, although older adults indeed sought out less information and took longer to process that information, they also used simpler and less cognitively demanding information-processing strategies (Mata et al., 2007).

This shift in processing strategy actually led older adults to receive higher monetary payoffs than younger adults.

An adaptive shift in strategy selection further influences older consumers' reactions to persuasion. Using in-depth surveys conducted across the adult life span (i.e., ages 18–74), Kirmani and Campbell (2004) showed that older consumers self-reported a wider range of strategies for dealing with persuasion attempts than younger consumers. The authors asserted that this was a consequence of older adults having more exposure to, and thus experience with, advertising and persuasive messages across their lifetime than younger adults. Such findings suggest that older consumers' experience with persuasion attempts may in fact make them relatively resistant to deceptive appeals.

The evidence reviewed here indicates that older adults are able to use adaptive strategies for decision making in consumer domains. This suggests that in many cases, prior knowledge and experience can improve decision making and potentially help older adults counter limitations that result from normal age-related cognitive declines.

CONCLUSIONS

This chapter has reviewed the literature on older consumers' decision making and identified various gaps in knowledge where future research is needed to fully capture the complexity of their decision processes. Future investigations should consider the nature of task or decision environments that have an influence on consumers of all ages and account for older consumers' greater susceptibility to the effects of time pressure and distraction. Detailed and deliberate processing among older consumers could be improved through the provision of environmental supports and decision aids.

Further, more research should focus on decision contexts that are meaningful and relevant to older consumers. Future research should also account for the tendency of older adults to engage in more affective modes of processing strategies, with differential attention paid to positive information. Researchers should take into consideration the importance of familiarity and expertise in older adults' financial, medical, and consumer decisions as aspects of adaptive strategies to complement deliberation. In general, greater research efforts should be directed at uncovering what domains or contexts promote positive and negative decision outcomes. Such research would generate a better understanding of how and when older consumers' decision making could be improved, as well as which decision contexts may be more or less challenging.

Although we are beginning to understand how older consumers adapt their decision and choice strategies to maintain high decision quality and satisfaction, further research on this topic would greatly enhance our understanding of consumer decision making across the life span. It would also be useful to understand what mechanisms underlie the observed "older-and-more-satisfied" effect.

Of additional interest are questions surrounding how older consumers go about making the choices they do. For example, do older consumers rely more on independent and marketer-supplied information, more on informal information sources, or both? Does the decision context or importance influence what information older consumers ultimately rely on? How does this relate to the decreased information search often observed among older consumers?

In terms of the growing field of financial decision making, future research should elucidate what factors render older consumers in a financial domain unable to compensate for age-related cognitive declines even with greater experience. Can these deficits be mitigated in some way?

The discussion within this chapter is by no means exhaustive, and there exist many other areas that are of potential interest to aging and consumer decision making. These include investigations of changes in risky decision making across the life span, changes in goals and motivations that consumers face as they age, and how cultural factors modulate age-related changes in consumer decision making. Further research on these topics will add to the literature on decision quality and provide insights into how decision making can be maintained, or even improved, across the adult life span.

References

Abaluck, J. T., & Gruber, J. (2009). *Choice inconsistencies among the elderly: Evidence from plan choice in the medicare part D program*. The National Bureau of Economic Research Working Paper No. 14759.

Alba, J. W., & Hutchinson, J. W. (1987). Dimensions of consumer expertise. *Journal of Consumer Research, 13*, 411–454.

Anguera, J. A., Boccanfuso, J., Rintoul, J. L., Al-Hashimi, O., Faraji, F., Janowich, J., et al. (2013). Video game training enhances cognitive control in older adults. *Nature, 501*, 97–101.

Ball, K., Berch, D. B., Helmers, K. F., Jobe, J. B., Leveck, M. D., Marsiske, M., & ACTIVE Study Group. (2002). Effects of cognitive training interventions with older adults: a randomized controlled trial. *JAMA, 288*, 2271–2281.

Bandura, A. (1976). Self-reinforcement: theoretical and methodological considerations. *Behaviorism, 4*, 135–155.

Bauer, A. S., Timpe, J. C., Edmonds, E. C., Tranel, D., & Denburg, N. D. (2012). Myopia for the future or hypersensitivity to reward? Age-related changes in decision making on the Iowa gambling task. *Emotion, 13*, 19–24.

Begg, I. M., Anas, A., & Farinacci, S. (1992). Dissocation of processes in belief: Source recollection, statement familiarity, and the illusion of truth. *Journal of Experimental Psychology: General, 12*, 446–458.

Brucks, M. (1985). The effects of product class knowledge on information search behavior. *Journal of Consumer Research, 12*, 1–16.

Bruine de Bruin, W., Parker, A. M., & Fischhoff, B. (2012). Explaining adult age differences in decision-making competence. *Journal of Behavioral Decision Making, 25*, 352–360.

Camerer, C. F., & Johnson, E. J. (1991). The process-performance paradox in expert judgment: How can experts know so much and predict so badly? In K. Anders Ericsson, & Jacqui Smith (Eds.), *Toward a general theory of expertise: Prospects and limits* (pp. 195–217). New York: Cambridge University Press.

Carstensen, L. L. (1992). Social and emotional patterns in adulthood: Support for socioemotional selectivity theory. *Psychology and Aging, 7*, 331–338.

Carstensen, L. L., Isaacowitz, D. M., & Charles, S. T. (1999). Taking time seriously: A theory of socioemotional selectivity. *American Psychologist, 54*, 165–181.

Castel, A. D. (2005). Memory for grocery prices in younger and older adults: The role of schematic support. *Psychology and Aging, Special Issue: Emotion-Cognition Interactions and the Aging Mind, 20*, 718–721.

Cattell, R. B. (1963). Theory of fluid and crystallized intelligence: A critical experiment. *Journal of Educational Psychology, 54*, 1–22.

Charles, S. T., & Carstensen, L. L. (2009). Social and emotional aging. *The Annual Review of Psychology, 61*, 383–409.

Chen, Y., & Sun, Y. (2003). Age differences in financial decision-making: Using simple heuristics. *Educational Gerontology, 29*, 627–635.

Cole, C. A., & Balasubramanian, S. K. (1993). Age differences in consumers' search for information: Public policy implications. *Journal of Consumer Research, 20*, 157–169.

Cole, C. A., & Gaeth, G. J. (1990). Cognitive and age-related differences in the ability to use nutritional information in a complex environment. *Journal of Marketing Research, 27*, 175–184.

Cole, C. A., & Houston, M. J. (1987). Encoding and media effects on consumer learning deficiencies in the elderly. *Journal of Marketing Research, 11*, 551–563.

Earles, J. L., Kersten, A. W., Mas, B. B., & Miccio, D. M. (2004). Aging and memory for self-performed tasks: Effects of task difficulty and time pressure. *Journal of Gerontology: Psychological Sciences, 59B*, 285–293.

Finucane, M. L., Mertz, C. K., Slovic, P., & Schmidt, E. S. (2005). Task complexity and older adults' decision-making competence. *Psychology and Aging, 20*, 71–84.

Fornell, C., Johnson, M. D., Anderson, E. W., Cha, J., & Bryant, B. E. (1996). The American consumer satisfaction index: Nature, purpose, and findings. *Journal of Marketing, 60*, 7–18.

Fung, H. H., & Carstensen, L. L. (2003). Sending memorable messages to the old: Age differences in preferences and memory for advertisements. *Journal of Personality and Social Psychology, 85*, 163–178.

Gazzaley, A., Cooney, J. W., Rissman, J., & Esposito, M. (2005). Top down suppression deficit underlies working memory impairment in normal aging. *Nature Neuroscience, 8*, 1298–1300.

Gazzaley, A., Sheridan, M. A., Cooney, J. W., & Esposito, M. (2007). Age-related deficits in component processes of working memory. *Neuropsychology, 21*, 532–539.

Hasher, L., Goldstein, D., & Toppino, T. (1977). Frequency and the conference of referential validity. *Journal of Verbal Learning and Verbal Behavior, 16*, 107–112.

Hasher, L., Lustig, C., & Zacks, R. (2007). Inhibitory mechanisms and the control of attention. In A. Miyake, A. R. A. Conway, C. Jarrold, M. J. Kane, & J. N. Towse (Eds.), *Variation in working memory* (pp. 227–249). New York, NY: Oxford University Press.

Hasher, L., & Zacks, R. T. (1988). Working memory, comprehension, and aging: A review and a new view. In G. H. Bower (Ed.), *The Psychology of Learning and Motivation*, Vol. 22 (pp. 193–225). New York, NY: Academic Press.

Hedden, T., & Yoon, C. (2006). Individual differences in executive processing predicts susceptibility to interference in verbal working memory. *Neuropsychology, 20*, 511–528.

Hess, T. M. (2005). Memory and aging in context. *Psychological Bulletin, 13*, 383–406.

Hess, T. M., Queen, T. L., & Ennis, G. E. (2013). Age and self-relevance effects on information search during decision making. *Journal of Gerontology: Series B: Psychological Sciences and Social Sciences, 68*, 703–711.

Johnson, M. M. S. (1990). Age differences in decision making: A process methodology for examining strategic information processing. *The Journal of Gerontology: Series B: Psychological Science and Social Sciences, 45*, 75–78.

Johnson, M. M. S. (1997). Individual differences in the voluntary use of a memory aid during decision making. *Experimental Aging Research, 23*, 33–43.

Johnson, E. J., & Russo, J. E. (1984). Product familiarity and learning new information. *Journal of Consumer Research, 11*, 542–550.

Kim, S., Goldstein, D., Hasher, L., & Zacks, R. T. (2005). Framing effects in younger and older adults. *The Journal of Gerontology: Series B: Psychological Science and Social Sciences, 60B*, 215–218.

Kim, S., Hasher, L., & Zacks, R. T. (2007). Aging and benefit of distractibility. *Psychonomic Bulletin & Review, 14*, 301–305.

Kirmani, A., & Campbell, M. C. (2004). Goal seeker and persuasion sentry: How consumer targets respond to interpersonal marketing persuasion. *Journal of Consumer Research, 31*, 573–582.

Kosnik, W., Winslow, L., Rasinski, K., & Sekuler, R. (1988). Visual changes in daily life throughout adulthood. *Journal of Gerontology: Psychological Sciences, 43*, P63–P70.

Labouvie-Vief, G., & Blanchard-Fields, F. (1982). Cognitive ageing and psychological growth. *Ageing and Society, 2*, 183–209.

Lambert-Pandraud, R., & Laurent, G. (2010a). Impact of age on brand choice. In A. Drolet, N. Schwarz, & C. Yoon (Eds.), *The aging consumer: Perspectives from psychology and economics* (pp. 191–208). London: Taylor and Francis.

Lambert-Pandraud, R., & Laurent, G. (2010b). Why do older consumers buy brands? The role of attachment and declining innovativeness. *Journal of Marketing, 74*, 104–121.

Lambert-Pandraud, R., Laurent, G., & Lapersonne, E. (2005). Repeat purchasing of new automobiles by older consumers: Empirical evidence and interpretations. *Journal of Marketing, 69*, 97–103.

Law, S., Hawkins, S. A., & Craik, F. I. M. (1998). Repetition-induced belief in the elderly: Rehabilitating age-related memory deficits. *Journal of Consumer Research, 25*, 91–107.

Madden, D. J. (1983). Aging and distraction by highly familiar stimuli during visual search. *Developmental Psychology, 19*, 499–507.

Mata, R., Schooler, L. J., & Rieskamp, J. (2007). The aging decision maker: Cognitive aging and the adaptive selection of decision strategies. *Psychology and Aging, 22*, 796–810.

Mather, M. (2006). A review of decision making processes: Weighing the risks and benefits of aging. In L. L. Carstensen, & C. R. Hartel (Eds.), *When I'm 64* (pp. 145–173). Washington, DC: The National Academies Press.

Mather, M., & Carstensen, L. L. (2005). Aging and motivated cognition: The positivity effect in attention and memory. *Trends in Cognitive Sciences, 9*, 496–502.

Mather, M., Knight, M., & McCaffrey, M. (2005). The allure of the alignable: Younger and older adults' false memories of choice features. *Journal of Experimental Psychology: General, 134*, 38–51.

May, C. P., Hasher, L., & Stoltzfus, E. R. (1993). Optimal time of day and the magnitude of age differences in memory. *Psychological Science, 4*, 326–330.

McDowd, J. M., & Craik, F. I. (1988). Effects of aging and task difficulty on divided attention performance. *Journal of Experimental Psychology: Human Perception and Performance, 14*, 267–280.

McDowd, J. M., & Filion, D. L. (1992). Aging, selective attention, and inhibitory processes: A psychophysiological approach. *Psychology and Aging, 7*, 65–71.

Mednick, S. A. (1968). The remote associates task. *Journal of Creative Behavior, 2*, 213–214.

Mikels, J. A., Cheung, E., Cone, J., & Gilovich, T. (2012). The dark side of intuition: Aging and increases in nonoptimal intuitive decisions. *Emotion, 13*, 189–195.

Mikels, J. A., Lockenhoff, C. E., Maglio, S. J., Carstensen, L. L., Goldstein, M. K., & Garber, A. (2010). Following your heart or your head: focusing on emotions versus information differentially influences the decision of younger and older adults. *Journal of Experimental Psychology: Applied, 16*, 87–95.

Mikels, J. A., & Reed, A. E. (2009). Monetary losses do not loom larger in later life: Age differences in the framing effect. *Journal of Gerontology: Psychological Sciences, 64B*, 457–460.

Morrow, D. G., Ridolfo, H., Menard, W., Sanborn, A., Stine-Morrow, E., Magnor, C., et al. (2003). Environmental support promotes expertise-based mitigation of age differences on pilot communication tasks. *Psychology and Aging, 18*, 268–284.

Moscovitch, M., & Winocur, G. (1995). Frontal lobes, memory, and aging. *Annals of the New York Academy of Sciences, 789*, 119–150.

Park, C. W., Iyer, E. S., & Smith, D. C. (1989). The effects of situational factors on in-store grocery shopping behavior: The role of store environment and time available for shopping. *Journal of Consumer Research, 15*, 422–433.

Park, D. C., Lautenschlager, G., Hedden, T., Davidson, N. S., & Smith, A. D. (2002). Models of visuospatial and verbal memory across the adult life span. *Psychology and Aging, 17*, 299–320.

Peters. (2010). Aging-related changes in decision making. In A. Drolet, N. Schwarz, & C. Yoon (Eds.), *The aging consumer: Perspectives from psychology and economics* (pp. 75–101). London: Taylor and Francis.

Peters, E., Hess, T. M., Västfjäll, D., & Auman, C. (2007). Adult age differences in dual information processes. *Perspectives on Psychological Science, 2*, 1–23.

Plude, D. J., & Hoyer, W. J. (1986). Age and the selectivity of visual information processing. *Psychology and Aging, 1*, 4–10.

Queen, T. L., & Hess, T. M. (2010). Age differences in the effects of conscious and unconscious thought in decision making. *Psychology and Aging, 25*, 251–261.

Queen, T. L., Hess, T. M., Ennis, G. E., Dowd, K., & Gruhn, D. (2012). Information search and decision making: Effects of age and complexity on strategy use. *Psychology and Aging, 27*, 817–824.

Rahhal, T. A., May, C. P., & Hasher, L. (2002). Truth and character: Sources that older adults can remember. *Psychological Science, 13*, 101–105.

Reed, A. E., Mikels, J. A., & Lockenoff, C. E. (2013). Preference for choice across adulthood: Age trajectories and potential mechanisms. *Psychology and Aging, 28*, 625–632.

Riggle, E. D. B., & Johnson, M. M. S. (1996). Age differences in political decision making: Strategies for evaluating political candidates. *Political Behavior, 18*, 99–118.

Roedder John, D., & Cole, C. A. (1986). Age differences in information processing: Understanding deficits in young and elderly consumers. *Journal of Consumer Research, 13*, 297–315.

Salthouse, T. A. (1996). The processing-speed theory of adult age differences in cognition. *Psychological Review, 103*, 403–428.

Samanez-Larkin, G. R., Wagner, A. D., & Knutson, B. (2011). Expected value information improves financial risk taking across the adult life span. *Social Cognitive and Affective Neuroscience, 6*, 207–217.

Schwartz, B., Ward, A., Monterosso, J., Lyubomirsky, S., White, K., & Lehman, D. R. (2002). Maximizing versus satisficing: Happiness is a matter of choice. *Journal of Personality and Social Psychology, 83*, 1178–1197.

Shanteau, J. (1992). Competence in experts: The role of task characteristics. *Organizational Behavioral and Human Decision Processes, 53*, 252–266.

Skurnik, I., Yoon, C., Park, D. C., & Schwarz, N. (2005). How warnings about false claims become recommendations. *Journal of Consumer Research, 31*, 713–723.

Slovic, P., Finucane, M. L., Peters, E., & MacGregor, D. G. (2002). The affect heuristic. In T. Gilovich, D. Griffin, & D. Kahneman (Eds.), *Heuristics and biases: The psychology of intuitive judgment* (pp. 397–420). New York: Cambridge University Press.

Tanius, B. W., Wood, S., Hanoch, Y., & Rice, T. (2009). Aging and choice: Applications to medicare part D. *Judgment and Decision Making, 4*, 92–101.

Tversky, A., & Kahneman, D. (1974). Judgment under uncertainty: Heurisitics and biases. *Science, 185*, 1124–1131.

Von Helverson, B., & Mata, R. (2012). Losing a dime with a satisfied mind: Positive affect predicts less search in sequential decision making. *Psychology and Aging, 27*, 825–839.

West, R. L. (1996). An application of prefrontal cortex function theory to cognitive aging. *Psychological Bulletin, 120*, 272–292.

Williams, P., & Drolet, A. (2005). Age-related differences in responses to emotional advertisements. *Journal of Consumer Research, 32*, 343–354.

Wood, S., Hanoch, Y., Barnes, A., Liu, P., Cummings, J., Bhattacharya, C., et al. (2011). Numeracy and medicare part D: The importance of choice and literacy for numbers in optimizing decision making for medicare's prescription drug program. *Psychology and Aging, 26*, 295–307.

Wood, S. L., & Lynch, J. G. (2002). Prior knowledge and complacency in new product learning. *Journal of Consumer Research, 29*, 416–426.

Yates, J. F., & Patalano, A. L. (1999). Decision making and aging. In D. C. Park, R. W. Morrell, & K. Shifren (Eds.), *Processing of medical information in aging patients: Cognitive and human factors perspectives* (pp. 31–54). Mahwah, NJ: Lawrence Erlbaum Associates Publishers.

Yoon, C. (1997). Age differences in consumers' processing strategies: An investigation of moderating influences. *Journal of Consumer Research, 24*, 329–342.

Yoon, C., Cole, C. A., & Lee, M. P. (2009). Consumer decision making and aging: Current knowledge and future directions. *Journal of Consumer Psychology, 19*, 2–16.

Yoon, C., Feinberg, F., & Schwarz, N. (2010). Older consumers and satisfaction. In A. Drolet, N. Schwarz, & C. Yoon (Eds.), *The aging consumer: Perspectives from psychology and economics*. London: Taylor and Francis.

Yoon, C., Lee, M. P., & Dazinger, S. (2007). The effects of optimal time of day on persuasion processes in older adults. *Psychology & Marketing, 24*, 475–495.

CHAPTER

18

A Framework for Decision Making in Couples across Adulthood

Tara L. Queen[1], *Cynthia A. Berg*[1], *William Lowrance*[2]

[1]Department of Psychology, University of Utah, Salt Lake City, UT, USA; [2]Huntsman Cancer Institute, University of Utah, Salt Lake City, UT, USA

Couples face a variety of decisions ranging from the mundane, such as which yogurt to buy at the grocery store, to the more substantial, such as whether to purchase a car or what treatment to undergo for a serious illness like cancer. These decisions vary across the life span, with younger couples facing decisions regarding childbearing, midlife couples making decisions about financial planning and managing family, and older adults facing retirement and health decisions. Many of these decisions are seldom made alone and have consequences for the developmental course of couples. Further, the ways in which couples make decisions together earlier in life may set a trajectory for how decisions are made throughout the life span.

Although many life decisions, including financial planning, home buying, and medical decisions, have consequences for the couple (Simpson, Griskevicius, & Rothman, 2012), most of the research on decision making in older adulthood (and much of the decision-making research in general) has focused on the individual. Understanding decision making in couples is likely complex, as the social interactive processes used by couples can vary from highly collaborative, whereby individuals are engaged in affiliative and reciprocal interactions, to one-way directions of influence, to those that are critical and controlling. Research in the fields of economics and marketing has contributed much work on the dynamics of group decision making (e.g., Charness & Sutter, 2012), but interactions between couples in the decision-making process are likely much different than groups comprised of coworkers or unfamiliar individuals.

Aging and Decision Making
http://dx.doi.org/10.1016/B978-0-12-417148-0.00018-2

The existing work on decision making in couples is in its infancy and only scratches the surface of the potential for our understanding of the phenomenon. Much of this work is based on retrospective accounts of decision making and focuses on one part of the decision-making process, such as the final decision, rather than the steps leading toward making the decision or satisfaction with the outcome once the decision is made. Unlike many lab-based decision-making tasks, the everyday decisions couples make are ongoing, as couples move in and out of the decision-making process over time rather than coming to an immediate conclusion (Kirchler, Rodler, Hölzl, & Meier, 2001). The existing literature on decision making in couples focuses heavily on married, heterosexual couples, and thus our review of the literature refers mostly to wife–husband pairs. This focus on heterosexual couples may limit the generalizability of findings from this research and we make suggestions for future directions in our discussion. With this focus on wife–husband pairs, the role of gender in decision making is pervasive in this literature, and a discussion of gender roles as related to various components of decision making within couples is included throughout the chapter.

We present a framework in this chapter for moving the literature forward to extend research on decision making to aging couples. We begin with an overview of our framework, outlining facets of the decision-making process and the individual and contextual factors that affect whether that process is more dyadic or individualistic. We then review relevant literature on dyadic decision making from medicine and marketing and economics, linking these different literatures to the framework. We end the chapter with ideas for future research directions that bridge the gap between the framework and the current literature.

A FRAMEWORK FOR UNDERSTANDING DYADIC DECISION-MAKING PROCESSES

Our framework illustrates how couples move through the decision-making process, bringing their own individual resources to different decision contexts that create the potential for dyadic interactions that vary in their quality and their collaborative versus controlling nature (see Figure 1). As couples make everyday decisions, they may move in and out of dyadic versus individual processes as they identify that a decision needs to be made, search information, make a decision, and reflect on that decision through post-decision processes. Each partner brings to this process her or his individual characteristics and social resources when approaching different decision contexts (see Figure 1). The following framework draws from multiple literature (economic and medical decision making, collaborative problem solving) to address key features of dyadic decision-making processes.

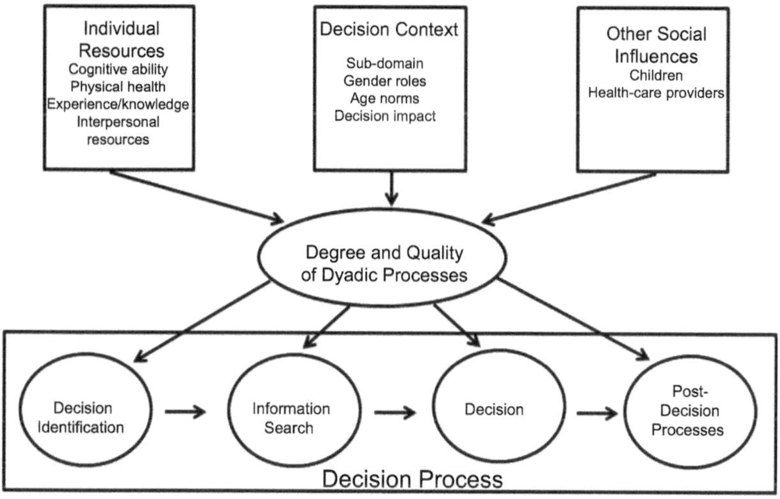

FIGURE 1 Proposed framework for understanding decision-making processes in couples.

The Decision-Making Process

Everyday decision-making processes encompass a number of different phases that couples navigate as they make decisions. We focus here on four main processes: decision identification, information search, the decision, and post-decision phases. The *decision identification phase* (called by Davis and Rigaux (1974) the problem identification phase) occurs as individuals and dyadic units identify that a decision needs to be made. For everyday decisions, this may be as mundane as noting that the household is out of jam and having a brief discussion about what sort of jam the couple wishes to purchase. For more consequential purchasing and medical decisions, this phase may be more elaborate, whereby one member of the couple raises the possibility of a decision or identifies symptoms as abnormal, which initiates a discussion over time regarding the decision and whether to seek expert advice.

The next phase is *information search*, whereby decision makers seek relevant information to guide their decisions. A substantial literature on age differences in individual decision making focuses on this phase of the decision-making process, with age differences noted on the exhaustive/deliberative versus curtailed nature of the search process (Peters, Hess, Västfjäll, & Auman, 2007). Older adults are routinely characterized as seeking out fewer sources of information prior to making a decision (see Peters et al., 2007, for a review), with some debate as to whether such curtailed search is adaptive or maladaptive. Although little research has examined how couples search information, qualitative retrospective research in medical decision making notes that couples frequently search information together to inform final decisions (Maliski, Heilemann, & McCorkel, 2002; Steginga, Occhipinti, Gardiner, Yaxley, & Heathcote, 2002).

After searching information, couples make a *decision*. Much of the decision-making literature has been dominated by dual-process models of decision making (e.g., Epstein, 1994; Reyna, 2004), which contrasts deliberative (analytical, rational weighing of information and alternatives) versus experiential (intuitive judgments tied to emotional feelings and preferences) decision making. Some researchers have hypothesized that older adults are at a disadvantage in decision situations that require careful deliberation (Peters et al., 2007), in part due to age differences in the cognitive abilities (Park, 2000) that may support deliberation such as working memory, executive function, speed of processes, and inhibition (Del Missier, Mäntylä, & Bruine de Bruin, 2010). However, older adults may be advantaged in their recognition of and processing of emotional content, which may contribute to their greater use of experiential decision making (Peters et al., 2007). It has been increasingly recognized that good choices occur when deliberative and experiential processes work in concert (Damasio, 1994).We know of no research that has examined how couples make decisions in terms of deliberative versus heuristic processes. Research on decision-making styles finds that some decision makers are more dependent on other people whereas others prefer to make decisions more intuitively (Scott & Bruce, 1995). Each partner may have a different approach to decision making (e.g., one more deliberative, the other more intuitive) with such discrepancies having implications for dyadic processes, decision quality, and satisfaction with the outcome.

Research on *post-decision processes* has examined satisfaction or regrets regarding the decision, although the focus here has been on an individual's regret rather than regret of both members within the couple. Regret has been studied in the medical decision-making literature, measuring individuals' satisfaction with their chosen medical treatment. In the couple context, regrets versus satisfaction about the decision may be negotiated and discussed, with the possibility that such post-decision processes guide future dyadic processes. For instance, when couples are satisfied with a decision outcome, they are less likely to use coercive strategies in subsequent decision-making scenarios (Su, Fern, & Ye, 2003). The repeated nature of both everyday consumer decisions and more consequential financial and medical decisions highlights the importance of understanding the ways in which individuals within couples navigate the decision-making process and the temporal relations among specific decisions.

Individual, Contextual, and Other Social Influences on the Decision-Making Process

The dyadic decision-making process is affected by a number of individual resources within different decision-making contexts, as well as the participation of others in the social network.

Individual Resources

Each member of the couple brings his or her individual resources in terms of cognitive abilities, general physical health, experience, and emotional/interpersonal abilities to the decision-making context. These individual resources may contribute to the degree to which the couple engages in dyadic decision making and the social interactive process and the effectiveness of dyadic decision making. Cognitive resources have been examined in the individual decision-making literature, with those with higher cognitive ability more likely to engage in greater information search and more deliberative decision-making processes (Meyer, Talbot, & Ranalli, 2007; Zwahr, Park, & Shifren, 1999). Working dyadically with a cognitively capable partner may compensate for the cognitive limitations of the other partner (Berg et al., 2007), leading to more information search. In late life, more general physical health conditions may also affect dyadic decision making. Leventhal, Leventhal, Schaefer, and Easterling (1993) note that the curtailed information search of older adults may come about as a way to conserve more limited physical reserves, suggesting that the dyadic involvement of a more healthy spouse may minimize taxing those resources.

Experience with the decision context may facilitate decision making for older adults, especially when cognitive demands related to the decision are high (Hess & Queen, 2014). Older adults may have expertise in certain life domains. For example, compared to young adults, older adults were better able to tailor their information search (Johnson, Suzanne, & Drungle, 2000) and weigh important information in selecting over-the-counter medications (Stephens & Johnson, 2000). Similarly, individual knowledge of cancer treatments has been associated with older adults making more efficient decisions (Meyer et al., 2007). Although the roles of knowledge and experience have not been explicitly examined in couples' decision making, it is possible that in specific contexts, decisions are deferred to the member of the couple with the most knowledge.

Research on aging and decision making posits that while cognitive ability declines in older age, interpersonal resources, especially the ability to use affective information and regulate emotions in decision making, are maintained (Peters et al., 2007). The ability to deal with interpersonal challenges (including the emotions that may arise) is particularly important to consider in the context of dyadic decision making, where couples are regulating their own emotions together with their partner (Berg, Wiebe, & Butner, 2010). Despite cognitive losses, older adults solve emotionally complex interpersonal problems quite effectively (Blanchard-Fields, 2007), in part by balancing problem-focused strategies (i.e., taking direct action to resolve problems) with emotion-regulation strategies (Watson & Blanchard-Fields, 1998). Older adults' tendency to focus more on emotionally salient information may also affect how they approach information search, attending to more positive rather than negative information, but also tailoring their search patterns depending on for whom they are making a decision (Löckenhoff & Carstensen, 2008).

An important interpersonal resource in the context of couples' decision making is the quality of the relationship. Older adults generally report greater marital satisfaction than couples at other points during the life span (Henry, Berg, Smith, & Florsheim, 2007), and this may contribute to their ability to perceive interpersonal interactions with their spouse in a more positive light (Story et al., 2007). Higher marital satisfaction is associated with perceptions of more frequent collaborative problem solving that is more enjoyable and is perceived to be better at compensating for cognitive limitations (Berg, Schindler, Smith, Skinner, & Beveridge, 2011). A high-quality relationship may also facilitate numerous aspects of the decision-making process as well.

Decision Context

The decision context changes in important ways across adulthood as the types of decisions that individuals make are timed according to the life course. For example, young and middle adulthood are associated with decisions regarding family planning, including whether and when to have children (Walker, 2010) and how to approach infertility. Later in life, couples face retirement decisions and increasing health-related decisions regarding medications (Johnson et al., 2000), diagnostic tests regarding conditions such as cancer (Manne et al., 2012), treatments for chronic illnesses such as diabetes or osteoarthritis, the need for long-term care options (Barnett & Stum, 2012), and end-of-life treatment preferences (Moorman & Inoue, 2013). Couples make consumer decisions across the life span, and an important theme from this literature is that the decision sub-domain may drive the dyadic or individualistic nature of the decision (Davis & Rigaux, 1974). Much of this literature has focused on stereotypical gender roles, finding that men tend to make decisions regarding life insurance and women decisions regarding household products and children's clothing, but collaborate on decisions regarding children's schooling and planning leisure time (Davis & Rigaux, 1974).

Research on decision context has focused on each partner's influence on the decision-making process. Early consumer research characterized influence as existing along gender roles, with men typically wielding more power than women (Davis & Rigaux, 1974). Men's versus women's influence in different contexts may be understood through the distribution of social roles between the genders (Eagly & Wood, 2012). The social roles of breadwinner or caregiver are associated with specialization in specific tasks, which in turn guide how couples work together to divide household labor. These roles seem apparent in research on dyadic decision making, with men likely having more influence in consumer decisions given their financial resources. Contemporary literature, however, finds that women are exerting more influence in consumer decision making and that gender roles are lessening, with husbands exerting more influence in domains in which wives traditionally had influence and vice versa (Belch & Willis, 2001). These changes in influence across time may reflect women's greater participation in the workforce and thereby increases in income, as well as changes in the composition of households (e.g., cohabitation, more blended/step families; Belch & Willis, 2001). However, men's and women's influence is still divided by decision context, often falling along typical gender roles (e.g., men making decisions about automobiles, women making decisions about household appliances and furnishings). In long-term married couples, such gender-based division of decision-making expertise is still apparent (Strough, Cheng, & Swenson, 2002).

Other Social Influences

As couples make both everyday and more consequential decisions, this process frequently involves other important social influences. For instance, when couples make consumer decisions, children are likely an important player in such decision making. Although older research suggests that children have relatively little influence, at least in some contexts (Filiatrault & Ritchie, 1980) more recent research indicates that children have gained influence over family-purchasing decisions over the last several decades, particularly in food choices and less for financially consequential decisions (Shoham & Dalakas, 2005).

Adult children are likely involved in a variety of older adults' decisions; however, this is an area that has received relatively little attention. Circirelli (2006) examined how mother–son and mother–daughter pairs made hypothetical decisions regarding the financial issues of the elderly mother. In these pairs, sons dominated the decision-making process. When there was greater closeness of the parent–child relationship, the elderly mother was more involved in the decision-making process and mothers and adult children expected better outcomes from the decision and less regret. Adult children may also be involved in information search related to medical treatments (e.g., treatments for cancer, whether to have a hip replacement), housing relocation, and end-of-life decisions (Schmid, Allen, Haley, & DeCoster, 2009).

Degree and Quality of Dyadic Decision Making

These contextual and individual factors affect the degree to which couples move through the decision-making process dyadically versus individualistically. For instance, when older adults perceive limitations in their own problem-solving abilities in gender-stereotyped contexts, they prefer solving problems dyadically rather than alone (Strough et al., 2002).

Older women prefer to solve problems involving household repair collaboratively; men prefer to solve problems with meal preparation collaboratively. Dyadic decision making may become more frequent in later adulthood as older adults may utilize a partner for both cognitive and interpersonal support (Berg, Schindler, Smith, & Beveridge, 2011).

Although little research has examined the quality of couples' interactions as they make decisions together, research from the collaborative problem-solving and coping literature is useful in understanding features of interactions that can affect decision outcomes. In general, highly satisfied couples' interactions are characterized by higher levels of warmth and support and lower levels of criticism, hostility, and withdrawal (Fincham, 2003). Further, compared to middle-aged couples, older couples' interactions are characterized by fewer negative and more positive characteristics (Henry et al., 2007; Levenson, Carstensen, & Gottman, 1993). This in part may be due to their greater motivation to seek emotionally meaningful experiences in the context of close relationships (Carstensen, Isaacowitz, & Charles, 1999), which in turn may facilitate their use of dyadic decision making. Older adults are frequently thought to be able to use interpersonal expertise to engage in collaborative problem solving at a more expert level than their younger counterparts (Dixon & Gould, 1996; Johansson, Andersson, & Ronnberg, 2000). Collaborative task performance of married couples is better when dyads utilize positive interactions (warm and affiliative; Berg, Johnson, Meegan, & Strough, 2003) that may involve episodes with a teaching element (Kimbler & Margrett, 2009). Further, collaborative performance in everyday tasks is best when couples adjust the way that they control the interaction such that the more cognitively capable member controls task direction (Berg et al., 2007). Overall, evidence from the collaborative problem-solving literature suggests that older married couples benefit from collaboration especially under demanding cognitive conditions, as they have experience working together (Peter-Wight & Martin, 2011).

Couples' interactions during decision making are associated with the effectiveness and satisfaction with decision outcomes. In a vacation decision-making task, couples who engaged in more highly affiliative interactions across a decision-making and everyday planning task were more likely to search more information prior to making a decision and to make decisions on the basis of comparing features rather than choices (Berg et al., 2003). Similarly, in three family-purchasing decisions (family vacation, dining out, music event), one partner's use of influence was associated with lower satisfaction with the decision by the other partner (Su et al., 2003). These results are consistent with a large literature on the use of control and persuasion tactics that indicates that such tactics may be detrimental to mood and self-esteem (Tucker & Mueller, 2000) as well as to decisions to engage in health-promoting behaviors (Khan, Stephens,

Franks, Rook, & Salem, 2013). Social interactions characterized by hostility, criticism, and control may prevent individuals from engaging in dyadic decision making and may hamper its effectiveness when it does occur. A better understanding of the interpersonal dynamics of couples' decision making may help identify when couples will be successful in making decisions together.

In summary, couples bring individual resources to specific decision-making contexts that affect the degree and quality of collaboration as they identify that a decision needs to be made, search relevant information for making the decision, make the decision, and evaluate their satisfaction with the decision. We next illustrate the value of this framework by reviewing the existing literature on dyadic decision making.

EXISTING LITERATURE ON DYADIC DECISION MAKING

Research on decision making in couples can be found primarily in three areas in the literature: consumer marketing, medical decision making, and retirement research. We will now review this literature, linking the existing research to the framework for dyadic decision making. Although much of this literature has not included older couples, we discuss how these research findings might change as couples age.

Consumer and Financial Decisions

The ways in which couples make consumer and financial decisions have been of particular interest in the field of economics, as such dynamics have implications for marketing and understanding how households choose to spend money. Some of these daily consumer-related decisions may seem mundane, but the ways in which they play out may be informative for understanding how couples approach more life-altering decisions. It is important to recognize the historical context in which the earlier work on consumer decision making in couples was conducted. This topic seemed to be of particular interest in the 1970s and 1980s, and focused heavily on gender roles in family consumer purchases. Although this work may reflect stereotypical views of gender and the marital relationship, it still provides an important perspective on dyadic decision making. The few more contemporary studies we cite suggest that changes in gender roles are being reflected in how couples (generally younger and middle-aged adults) make decisions, but future work should focus on addressing these shifts.

Consumer and financial research has focused on identifying contextual factors that drive which member of the couple has the most influence in making the final decision. In much of the early research on consumer behavior, the wife was thought to be the driving force in everyday household consumer decisions, with researchers going as far as to suggest that "women control 80 percent of every family dollar" (Davis, 1976, p. 246). Such older research suggests that gender-specific roles differ by the type of consumer decision being made. For instance, in a study on family vacation planning decisions, men had more influence in certain aspects of the decision, including the budget, timing of the vacation, and lodging, although the specific destination chosen was shared equally between husbands and wives (Filiatrault & Ritchie, 1980).

An aspect of decision-making influence that has received less attention is how partner influence comes into play when couples are making decisions jointly versus when one member of the couple is making an individual decision. Contemporary research has proposed that a partner's influence in a consumer decision may not always be explicit, but also present through the partner's preferences (Simpson, Griskevicius, & Rothman, 2012). For example, an individual making a decision between brands might remember a partner's preference for one over the other and purchase that specific brand, even though the partner is not present. Partner influence may differ across decision scenarios, acting as a contributing factor in decisions that are made jointly or individually, even when the decision outcome is consumed by oneself or with a partner (Gorlin & Dhar, 2012). This work emphasizes that individual members of a couple rarely make decisions that do not involve some aspect of their partner's influence (or preference). This interdependence relationship presents a unique methodological challenge which may be approached by utilizing dyadic analytic techniques (Simpson et al, 2012) or other statistical models that involve multiple family members (Bagozzi, 2012).

Although one member of the couple may have more influence in a consumer or financial decision, couples are still motivated to seek compromise in order to avoid conflict (Menasco & Curry, 1989). For instance, in a study investigating women and men's likelihood of purchasing long-term care insurance, researchers found that married employees were more likely to purchase insurance if spouses agreed on the fairness of its cost (Barnett & Stum, 2013). Broken down by gender, married women's decisions to purchase insurance were driven by spousal compromise, whereas men's decisions were additionally driven by wives' influence. Wives were hypothesized to be more influential in the decision as they had more experience with insurance (from caring for their own parents) and live longer, making it more beneficial for them to hold such policies. Working women may have more influence in family consumer decisions given their financial contribution (Lee & Beatty, 2002). More current research suggests that partners take turns in exerting influence strategies in family-purchasing decisions (Su et al., 2003).

Although identifying partner roles in consumer decision making may be important from a marketing perspective, from a dyadic decision-making perspective it is valuable to understand how partners work together throughout the course of the decision-making process. The process of couples' consumer decision making, while oftentimes initiated by the member with the most expertise in the decision context, has been shown to be complex, involving many sub-decisions and collaboration at different time points in the decision-making process (Davis, 1970). For example, in one study, husbands and wives were asked to rate their influence (i.e., husband-dominated, wife-dominated, or joint) in several domains of consumer decision making during three phases of the decision-making process: problem recognition, information seeking, and making a final decision (Davis & Rigaux, 1974). In over 60% of the consumer domains, the husband or wife dominance remained the same throughout the decision process. Influence in decision making tends to be driven by specialization, and this seems to have the most influence in the first two stages of decision making. Interestingly, decision making tends to shift to become more shared in the last stage, when individuals are ready to make a final decision. A more recent study aimed to examine how changes in modern family dynamics are reflected in decision-making influence (Belch & Willis, 2001). Women now have more influence in the stages of problem identification and have gained influence in information search and final decision making in specific consumer contexts.

The benefit of specialization (Filiatrault & Ritchie, 1980) in decision making is that it increases the efficiency of daily decision making. Instead of collaborating on all daily consumer or financial decisions, individual members of the couple can be expected to make certain decisions or sub-decisions relatively independently. There is a cost to this approach, however, and one that is particularly relevant to aging. If a partner becomes ill or begins showing signs of dementia, they may no longer be able to make optimal decisions. This may be especially impactful in the realm of finances. In the division of household labor, finances are commonly managed by one person, and if this person develops dementia, the spouse with less financial experience tends to take over responsibility for these decisions (Boyle, 2013). There has been little work in this area, but changes in influence may be an important contributor for understanding the quality of decision making.

In sum, the research on consumer and financial decision making in couples has focused heavily on decision influence. Researchers have begun to examine how couples interact over the course of the decision process, though less is known about the quality of the dyadic process. Additionally, this work typically focuses on younger couples. Future work is needed concerning how individual resources associated with age (e.g., cognitive ability, physical health, interpersonal resources) influence how couples collaborate together to make everyday consumer as well as major financial decisions.

Retirement

The decision to retire marks an important time in later adulthood, involving financial planning and transitioning out of the workforce, both of which have implications for the couple's future. Research on couples' retirement decisions has largely focused on the degree to which couples make decisions together and post-decision processes regarding how satisfied they are with the decision to retire.

Spousal influence is an individual characteristic that has been associated with couples' decisions to retire. While husbands' decisions to retire are less influenced by their wives' upcoming retirement and more aligned with employment policies (Loretto & Vickerstaff, 2013), wives' decisions to retire are quite influenced by their husbands' impending retirement (Smith & Moen, 1998). When one member of the couple retires, the other's retirement shortly follows (Szinovacz & Deviney, 2000), demonstrating the interdependence of the decision to retire. Age cohort differences may also exist in couples' retirement planning, with late baby boomers being more likely than early boomers to make decisions independently and earlier baby boomers making retirement plans more collaboratively (Moen, Huang, Plassmann, & Dentinger, 2006). As may be expected, the couples' joint financial situation is important in the decision to retire, as is the promise of pensions (Szinovacz & Deviney, 2000), with men's retirement more linked to their wives reaching the age of Social Security eligibility and women's retirement more linked to the couples' income. Wives' health was shown to be associated with husbands' decision to retire, with husbands of ailing wives being more likely to make the decision to retire (Szinovacz & Deviney, 2000).

In terms of post-decision processes, gender differences are observed in marital and retirement satisfaction after the retirement decision. Marital quality post-retirement is affected by perceptions of gender roles, in that couples with traditional gender roles (e.g., husband as provider) report lower marital satisfaction when husbands decide to retire before the wife (Szinovacz, 1996). Both marital quality and retirement satisfaction are lower when one spouse retires while the other is working (Szinovacz & Davey, 2005). Additionally, both husbands and wives report lower retirement satisfaction if they rated their spouse as having more household decision-making power than themselves (Szinovacz & Davey, 2005). The effect of spouse influence on retirement satisfaction also varies by gender. In a sample of middle-aged and older retirees and their spouses, women were most satisfied with their retirement when their husband was not influential in their decision (Smith & Moen, 2004). Interestingly, and contrary to previous findings, the opposite was true for the husbands, where retirement satisfaction was higher when wives were influential in their decision. Similar effects were reported for spouse and couple-level retirement satisfaction: it seems most beneficial for women's retirement satisfaction if they feel they had more influence in their decision making.

In sum, retirement decision making is a particularly relevant domain for older couples. Thus far, this literature has examined partner influence and post-decisional outcomes, particularly decision satisfaction. Retirement planning likely occurs earlier in life and understanding the process of setting a retirement plan, deciding on timing, and making the decision to leave the workforce may unfold over the course of many years. Understanding how and when couples begin this decision process may inform how retirement decisions are made later in life.

Medical Decisions

Late adulthood is accompanied by many decisions regarding one's health, and older couples are especially prone to making health decisions jointly (Padula, 1996). Medical decisions are oftentimes overwhelming, both in the amount of information needing to be considered as well as in the emotional impact of receiving a new diagnosis.

Individual cognitive resources play an important role in making health decisions. For example, in a study on women's decisions regarding estrogen replacement therapy, higher cognitive ability was associated with examining and comparing more treatment options and a better-quality decision overall (Zwahr et al., 1999). The role of individual resources has also been observed in dyadic decisions. Couples tend to make end-of-life plans (e.g., creating a living will, appointing a durable health-care power of attorney) collaboratively (Carr & Khodyakov, 2007). Individual factors including age and physical health play important roles in these decisions. Older couples and those in poorer health are more likely to discuss end-of-life preferences, and older age is associated with higher rates of having a living will and an identified power of attorney (Moorman & Inoue, 2013). It is apparent that several different individual resources can impact couples' decision making.

Very few studies have examined the process that couples go through in the context of health decision making, but the involvement of a spouse during different points in the decision-making process may be particularly helpful. For example, a study on men recently diagnosed with prostate cancer demonstrated that following the initial shock of the diagnosis, men involved their wives in an intensive information search in order to better understand treatment options and the course of the disease (Hilton, Crawford, & Tarko, 2000; Maliski et al., 2002). Having the spouse participate in the information-gathering process helped patients reappraise prostate cancer as a less dangerous cancer. Involving others in the decision process is not only helpful for information-gathering purposes, but is also associated with greater well-being and better coping strategies over time (Christie, Meyerowitz,

Giedzinska-Simons, Gross, & Agus, 2009). However, partners may differ in the weight they give information in making a final treatment decision with some evidence that partners may value features such as prognosis, whereas patients focus on their quality of life (Jacobs et al., 2002). Such results emphasize that health-related decisions are not usually made in a single moment, but instead over a longer course of time. For instance, the decisions that couples make concerning cancer treatments can extend over the course of weeks or months (O'Rourke & Germino, 2000).

Couples may vary in how dyadically versus individualistically they approach decision making regarding treatment options. Whereas some partners may be classified as active collaborators, others prefer a more supportive or completely passive role (Schumm, Skea, McKee, & N'Dow, 2010). Although these patterns of partner involvement may reflect how other life decisions were made in the past (Schumm et al., 2010), they may also vary across the decision process. Partners may move in and out of involvement roles depending on where they perceive they are needed most in the decision process as they seek to be involved in ways that are beneficial for the patient (Öhlén, Balneaves, Bottorff, & Brazier, 2006). Partners may play a more active role in the information-seeking phase but fall back to a more supportive role to allow the patient to make an independent final decision. Partners may also be engaged when problems that arise from the illness condition are more severe (Strough, McFall, & Schuller, 2010).

Partners' involvement in cancer treatment information seeking may reflect their individual resources. In a focus group study on prostate cancer patients, some wives reported being involved in information seeking both to support their husbands and to diminish their own anxiety (Feltwell & Rees, 2004). Other women reported avoiding involvement also to reduce anxiety and to maintain a normal lifestyle. The ways in which partners chose to be involved seemed to also reflect how they were coping with the cancer diagnosis. Further, spousal influence may reflect their expertise with the content of the decision. In making prostate cancer decisions, wives who were more direct in their opinions tended to have a medical background, bringing expertise into the decision process (O'Rourke & Germino, 2000).

An important social influence in health decision making is the healthcare provider (Adelman, Greene, & Ory, 2000; Rini et al., 2011), although the patient–partner–provider triad has not been examined. The majority of adults prefer to have a collaborative relationship with their doctors when making difficult medical decisions (Singh et al., 2010). The nature of patient–provider interactions may vary across the life span and across medical conditions. Older adults may experience a less collaborative relationship with their provider than younger adults, with the provider being more directive about what the patient should do (Step, Siminoff, & Rose, 2009). Viewing the health-care provider as the expert may contribute to patients taking a less active role in the decision-making process and viewing treatment decisions as made largely by the physician (Cohen & Britten, 2003). Perceptions that one is a collaborator with one's health-care provider in making difficult medical treatment decisions is associated with greater satisfaction with the treatment decision, especially for younger patients (Fischer et al., 2006). However, decision confidence may be highest among patients who report making the final decision themselves (Zikmund-Fisher et al., 2010). Programs such as the Shared Decision-Making Program, authorized by the Affordable Care Act, are designed to inform medical treatment decision making by enhancing communication between patients and physicians and may be useful in promoting shared decision making (Informed Medical Decisions Foundation, 2014).

Health professionals may need to be more aware of the involvement of partners, balancing the need for patient autonomy together with family involvement (Ho, 2008). The delivery of information around treatment may need to be tailored to both patients and partners' information-seeking preferences (Schumm et al., 2010). Focus group interviews have revealed that patients often feel overwhelmed, distressed, and rushed during their appointments at oncology clinics, making it difficult to ask questions and retain answers (Harden et al., 2002). These findings have led nursing researchers to suggest providing patients and their partners with a private, less busy setting where they can ask questions after their appointment. Recognizing both patient and partner information-seeking preferences and understanding how the environment can influence decision making are first steps in creating ways for patients and their spouses to make more informed health decisions.

In sum, compared to the consumer and financial decision-making domains, research on health decision making in couples has examined several components of the proposed framework. Researchers have found that partners are actively involved in the decision process, and that patients value their participation during certain points. Although researchers have begun to examine individual resources such as cognitive ability and physical health in couples' decision making, less is known about the roles of these resources in dyadic decision making. Future research should attend to understanding the dynamics of these resources when couples make decisions together.

FUTURE DIRECTIONS

Adults across the life span face many decisions that affect not only the individual, but most especially the intimate partner. Older adults face many difficult and consequential decisions. Understanding how couples approach these decisions together would help move the aging and decision-making literature forward. Little research has been conducted examining decision making at the couple level, with several avenues of research needed to understand more fully the ways in which couples navigate life's important decisions.

First, more research is needed that examines the dyadic decision-making process as it unfolds over time and how it may vary by context. As noted above, most everyday and more consequential decisions occur over weeks and months, and understanding how couples move in and out of dyadic processes would help to address when intimate partners can be most helpful. The advice-seeking literature suggests that partners may be most helpful in the information-gathering phase (Bonaccio & Dalal, 2006). Individuals may seek others' advice for reasons such as sharing the accountability of an outcome, ensuring the quality of the decision, and gaining new information or a new perspective on the decision-making situation. Some of the research on treatment decision making has implicitly begun examining this, by pinpointing where in the decision process partners become involved (e.g., Feltwell & Rees, 2004). Advice seeking from a partner may change over the life span, as couples build on their experience in making decisions together. The tendency to seek advice may differ across decision contexts, where more advice may be sought when a partner has more expertise or influence. Context may also influence the stage in the process where advice is preferred or perceived as helpful. For example, in treatment decisions, advice may be most needed in the information-seeking phase compared to the final decision-making phase, where the patient may prefer to be responsible for making the decision that affects his or her own body. In the case of retirement, women are more satisfied with their decision when their husbands are less involved, suggesting that advice in that context is less helpful or needed (Smith & Moen, 2004). Understanding at what point advice is most desired and how that varies by context would lend a more complete picture to how couples make more substantial life decisions.

Second, our framework proposes that individual resources, including cognitive ability, personal experience, and physical health, contribute to the degree and quality of older couples' collaborative decision making. Research on collaborative problem solving suggests that spouses help compensate for partners' cognitive losses (Berg et al., 2007), but less is known about how collaboration may be beneficial in decision-making situations. In our review of work on financial decision making, we highlight the costs of decision-making specialization within couples and discuss how a partner may have to take over decision making in a less familiar context when a spouse falls ill (Boyle, 2013). The results of this work suggest that once an individual loses the ability to make decisions, a partner will step in and take over. Less is known, however, about the transition to this point. How do couples navigate that transition together, and what makes collaborative decision making successful in those situations? Future work may build on the collaborative problem-solving work to examine how couples make important decisions together when individual resources are declining.

Last, research on dyadic decision making must also take into account the changing nature of gender roles and family norms as well as the changing demographics occurring within families. Gender roles, women's financial roles within the family, children's influence, and the composition of couples (heterosexual as compared to same-sex couples) have changed greatly since the early work on couples' consumer decision making (Davis & Rigaux, 1974) and contribute to different patterns of the dyadic decision-making process. For instance, same-sex couples tend to display less role specialization compared to different-sex couples, at least until having children (Giddings, Nunley, Schneebaum, & Zietz, 2014), potentially having implications for how household decisions are made. In different-sex married couples, the older partner often has more bargaining power (i.e., influence). These role differences have implications for how couples make important life decisions together. Further, many more couples are choosing to cohabitate rather than marry (Copen, Daniels, & Mosher, 2013), with some research suggesting that couples in such relationships approach mutual decisions differently (Razzouk, Seitz, & Capo, 2007). Oreffice (2011) finds that in same-sex and different-sex cohabitating households, the younger or wealthier partner displays more influence in decision making. Cohabitating couples may keep financial resources more independent than married couples, with greater collaboration in decision making when resources have to be pooled. Research on decision making between same-sex and cohabitating couples is currently sparse; future research is needed to understand if and how same-sex and cohabitating couples approach decision making differently from opposite-sex, married couples.

CONCLUSION

Although researchers have begun to consider decision making within the social context of intimate partners, there is great opportunity for expanding upon this knowledge base. The proposed framework illustrates how couples may move in and out of individualistic and dyadic processes as they identify that a decision needs to be made, gather information relevant to the decision, make the decision, and deal with post-decision processes. The framework further identifies how characteristics of the individual, decision context, and other social partners influence this process. As couples across the life span, and especially in late life, make decisions that chart their life-course trajectory, it is important to understand how dyads can optimize such decisions in a way that provides the greatest satisfaction.

References

Adelman, R. D., Greene, M. G., & Ory, M. G. (2000). Communication between older patients and their physicians. *Clinics in Geriatric Medicine, 16*, 1–24.

Bagozzi, R. P. (2012). Alternative approaches for thinking about and modeling consumer decisions in relationships. *Journal of Consumer Psychology, 22*, 315–319.

Barnett, A. E., & Stum, M. S. (2012). Couples managing the risk of financing long-term care. *Journal of Family and Economic Issues, 33*, 363–375.

Barnett, A. E., & Stum, M. S. (2013). Spousal decision making and long-term care insurance. *Journal of Financial Counseling and Planning, 24*, 5–19.

Belch, M. A., & Willis, L. A. (2001). Family decision at the turn of the century: Has the changing structure of households impacted the family decision-making process? *Journal of Consumer Behaviour, 2*, 111–124.

Berg, C. A., Johnson, M. M. S., Meegan, S. P., & Strough, J. (2003). Collaborative problem-solving interactions in young and old married couples. *Discourse Processes, 15*, 33–58.

Berg, C. A., Schindler, I., Smith, T. W., Skinner, M., & Beveridge, R. M. (2011). Perceptions of the cognitive compensation and interpersonal enjoyment functions of collaboration among middle-aged and older married couples. *Psychology and Aging, 26*, 167–173.

Berg, C. A., Smith, T. W., Ko, K., Story, N., Beveridge, R., Allen, N., et al. (2007). Task control and cognitive abilities of self and spouse in collaboration in middle-aged and older couples. *Psychology and Aging, 22*, 420–427.

Berg, C. A., Wiebe, D. J., & Butner, J. (2010). Affect covariation in marital couples dealing with stressors surrounding prostate cancer. *Gerontology, 57*, 167–172.

Blanchard-Fields, F. (2007). Everyday problem solving and emotion an adult developmental perspective. *Current Directions in Psychological Science, 16*, 26–31.

Bonaccio, S., & Dalal, R. S. (2006). Advice taking and decision-making: An integrative literature review, and implications for the organizational sciences. *Organizational Behavior and Human Decision Processes, 101*, 127–151.

Boyle, G. (2013). 'She's usually quicker than the calculator': Financial management and decision-making in couples living with dementia. *Health and Social Care in the Community, 21*, 554–562.

Carr, D., & Khodyakov, D. (2007). End-of-life health care planning among young-old adults: An assessment of psychosocial influences. *The Journals of Gerontology Series B: Psychological Sciences and Social Sciences, 62*, S135–S141.

Carstensen, L., Isaacowitz, D. M., & Charles, C. T. (1999). Taking time seriously: A theory of socioemotional selectivity. *American Psychologist, 54*, 165–181.

Charness, G., & Sutter, M. (2012). Groups make better self-interested decisions. *The Journal of Economic Perspectives, 26*, 157–176.

Christie, K. M., Meyerowitz, B. E., Giedzinska-Simons, A., Gross, M., & Agus, D. B. (2009). Predictors of affect following treatment decision-making for prostate cancer: Conversations, cognitive processing, and coping. *Psycho-Oncology, 18*, 508–514.

Circirelli, V. G. (2006). Caregiving decision making by older mothers and adult children: Process and expected outcome. *Psychology and Aging, 21*, 209–221.

Cohen, H., & Britten, N. (2003). Who decides about prostate cancer treatment? A qualitative study. *Family Practice, 20*, 724–729.

Copen, C. E., Daniels, K., & Mosher, W. D. (2013). First premarital cohabitation in the United States: 2006–2010 National Survey of Family Growth. *National Health Statistics Report, 64*, 1–15.

Damasio, A. R. (1994). *Descartes' error: Emotion, reason, and the human brain*. New York: Putnam.

Davis, H. L. (1970). Dimensions of marital roles in consumer decision making. *Journal of Marketing Research, 7*, 168–177.

Davis, H. L. (1976). Decision making within the household. *Journal of Consumer Research, 2*, 241–260.

Davis, H. L., & Rigaux, B. P. (1974). Perception of marital roles in decision processes. *Journal of Consumer Research, 1*, 51–62.

Del Missier, F., Mäntylä, T., & Bruine de Bruin, W. (2010). Executive functions in decision making: An individual differences approach. *Thinking and Reasoning, 16*, 69–97.

Dixon, R. A., & Gould, O. N. (1996). Adults telling and retelling stories collaboratively. In P. B. Baltes, & U. M. Staudinger (Eds.), *Interactive minds: Life-span perspectives on the social foundation of cognition* (pp. 221–241). New York: Cambridge University Press.

Eagly, A. H., & Wood, W. (2012). Social role theory. *Handbook of Theories in Social Psychology, 2*, 458–476.

Epstein, S. (1994). Integration of the cognitive and the psychodynamic unconscious. *American Psychologist, 49*, 709–724.

Feltwell, A. K., & Rees, C. E. (2004). The information-seeking behaviours of partners of men with prostate cancer: A qualitative pilot study. *Patient Education and Counseling, 54*, 179–185.

Filiatrault, P., & Ritchie, J. B. (1980). Joint purchasing decisions: a comparison of influence structure in family and couple decision-making units. *Journal of Consumer Research, 7*, 131–140.

Fincham, F. D. (2003). Marital conflict: correlates, structure, and context. *Current Directions in Psychological Science, 12*, 23–27.

Fischer, M., Visser, A., Voerman, B., Garssen, B., van Andel, G., & Bensing, J. (2006). Treatment decision making in prostate cancer: Patients' participation in complex decisions. *Patient Education and Counseling, 63*, 308–313.

Giddings, L., Nunley, J. M., Schneebaum, A., & Zietz, J. (2014). Birth cohort and the specialization gap between same-sex and different-sex couples. *Demography, 51*, 509–534.

Gorlin, M., & Dhar, R. (2012). Bridging the gap between joint and individual decisions: Deconstructing preferences in relationships. *Journal of Consumer Psychology, 22*, 320–323.

Harden, J., Schafenacker, A., Northouse, L., Mood, D., Smith, D., Pienta, K., & Baranowski, K. (2002). Couples experiences with prostate cancer: focus group research. *Oncology Nursing Forum, 29*, 701–709.

Henry, N. J. M., Berg, C. A., Smith, T. W., & Florsheim, P. (2007). Positive and negative characteristics of marital interaction and their association with marital satisfaction in middle-aged and older couples. *Psychology and Aging, 22*, 428–441.

Hess, T. M., & Queen, T. L. (2014). Aging influences on judgment and decision processes: Interactions between ability and experience. In P. Verhaeghen, & C. Hertzog (Eds.), *The Oxford handbook of emotion, social cognition, and problem solving in adulthood* (pp. 238–255). New York, NY: Oxford University Press.

Hilton, B. A., Crawford, J. A., & Tarko, M. A. (2000). Men's perspectives on individual and family coping with their wives' breast cancer and chemotherapy. *Western Journal of Nursing Research, 22*, 438–459.

Ho, A. (2008). Relational autonomy or undue pressure? Family's role in medical decision-making. *Scandinavian Journal of Caring Sciences, 22*, 128–135.

Informed Medical Decisions Foundation. (2014). Retrieved April 2, 2014.

Jacobs, J. R., Banthia, R., Sadler, G. R., Varni, J. W., Malcarne, V. L., Greenbergs, H. L., & Johnstone, P. A. (2002). Problems associated with prostate cancer: Differences of opinion among health care providers, patients, and spouses. *Journal of Cancer Education, 17*, 33–36.

Johansson, O., Andersson, J., & Ronnberg, J. (2000). Do elderly couples have a better prospective memory than other elderly people when they collaborate? *Applied Cognitive Psychology, 14*, 121–133.

Johnson, M. S., Suzanne, C., & Drungle, M. (2000). Purchasing over-the-counter medications: the influence of age and familiarity. *Experimental Aging Research, 26*, 245–261.

Khan, C. M., Stephens, M. A. P., Franks, M. M., Rook, K. S., & Salem, J. K. (2013). Influences of spousal support and control on diabetes management through physical activity. *Health Psychology, 32*, 739–747.

Kimbler, K. J., & Margrett, J. A. (2009). Older adults' interactive behaviors during collaboration on everyday problems: Linking process and outcome. *International Journal of Behavioral Development, 33*, 531–542.

Kirchler, E., Rodler, C., Hölzl, E., & Meier, K. (2001). *Conflict and decision-making in close relationships. Love, money and daily routines*. Philadelphia, PA: Psychology Press.

Lee, C. K., & Beatty, S. E. (2002). Family structure and influence in family decision making. *Journal of Consumer Marketing, 19*, 24–41.

Levenson, R. W., Carstensen, L. L., & Gottman, J. M. (1993). Long-term marriage: age, gender, and satisfaction. *Psychology and Aging, 8*, 301–313.

Leventhal, E. A., Leventhal, H., Schaefer, P., & Easterling, D. (1993). Conservation of energy, uncertainty reduction, and swift utilization of medical care among the elderly. *Journals of Gerontology, Series B: Psychological Sciences and Social Sciences, 48*, 78–86.

Löckenhoff, C. E., & Carstensen, L. L. (2008). Decision strategies in health care choices for self and others: Older but not younger adults make adjustments for the age of the decision target. *The Journals of Gerontology Series B: Psychological Sciences and Social Sciences, 63*, P106–P109.

Loretto, W., & Vickerstaff, S. (2013). The domestic and gendered context for retirement. *Human Relations, 66*, 65–86.

Maliski, S. L., Heilemann, M. V., & McCorkel, R. (2002). From "death sentence" to "good cancer". *Nursing Research, 51*, 391–397.

Manne, S., Etz, R. S., Hudson, S. V., Medina-Forrester, A., Boscarino, J. A., Bowen, D. J., et al. (2012). A qualitative analysis of couples' communication regarding colorectal cancer screening using the Interdependence Model. *Patient Education and Counseling, 87*, 18–22.

Menasco, M. B., & Curry, D. J. (1989). Utility and choice: An empirical study of wife/husband decision making. *Journal of Consumer Research, 16*, 87–97.

Meyer, B. J., Talbot, A. P., & Ranalli, C. (2007). Why older adults make more immediate treatment decisions about cancer than younger adults. *Psychology and Aging, 22*, 505–524.

Moen, P., Huang, Q., Plassmann, V., & Dentinger, E. (2006). Deciding the future: Do daul-earner couples plan together for retirement? *American Behavioral Scientist, 49*, 1422–1443.

Moorman, S. M., & Inoue, M. (2013). Persistent problems in end-of-life planning among young- and middle-aged american couples. *Journals of Gerontology Series B: Psychological Sciences and Social Sciences, 68*, 97–106.

Öhlén, J., Balneaves, L. G., Bottorff, J. L., & Brazier, A. S. (2006). The influence of significant others in complementary and alternative medicine decisions by cancer patients. *Social Science & Medicine, 63*, 1625–1636.

Oreffice, S. (2011). Sexual orientation and household decision making: same-sex couples' balance of power and labor supply choices. *Labour Economics, 18*, 145–158.

O'Rourke, M. E., & Germino, B. B. (2000). From two perspectives to one choice: Blending couple and individual views of prostate cancer treatment selection. *Journal of Family Nursing, 6*, 231–251.

Padula, C. (1996). Older couples' decision making on health issues. *Western Journal of Nursing Research, 18*, 675–687.

Park, D. C. (2000). The basic mechanisms accounting for age-related decline in cognitive function. In D. C. Park, & N. Schwarz (Eds.), *Cognitive aging: A primer* (pp. 3–21). Philadelphia, PA: Psychology Press.

Peter-Wight, M., & Martin, M. (2011). When 2 is better than 1 + 1: Older spouses' individual and dyadic problem solving. *European Psychologist, 16*, 288–294.

Peters, E., Hess, T. M., Västfjäll, D., & Auman, C. (2007). Adult age differences in dual information processes: Implications for the role of affective and deliberative processes in older adults' decision making. *Perspectives on Psychological Science, 2*, 1–23.

Razzouk, N., Seitz, V., & Capo, K. P. (2007). A comparison of consumer decision-making behavior of married and cohabiting couples. *Journal of Consumer Marketing, 24*, 264–274.

Reyna, V. F. (2004). How people make decisions that involve risk a dual-processes approach. *Current Directions in Psychological Science, 13*, 60–66.

Rini, C., Jandorf, L., Goldsmith, R. E., Manne, S. L., Harpaz, N., & Itzkowitz, S. H. (2011). Interpersonal influences on patients' surgical decision making: The role of close others. *Journal of Behavioral Medicine, 34*, 396–407.

Schmid, B., Allen, R. S., Haley, P. P., & DeCoster, J. (2009). Family matters: Dyadic agreement in end-of-life medical decision making. *The Gerontologist, 50*, 226–237.

Schumm, K., Skea, Z., McKee, L., & N'Dow, J. (2010). 'They're doing surgery on two people': A meta-ethnography of the influences on couples' treatment decision making for prostate cancer. *Health Expectations, 13*, 335–349.

Scott, S. G., & Bruce, R. A. (1995). Decision-making style: The development and assessment of a new measure. *Educational and Psychological Measurement, 55*, 818–831.

Shoham, A., & Dalakas, V. (2005). He said, she said... they said: parents and children's assessment of children's influence on family consumption decisions. *Journal of Consumer Marketing, 22*, 152–160.

Simpson, J. A., Griskevicius, V., & Rothman, A. J. (2012). Consumer decisions in relationships. *Journal of Consumer Psychology, 22*, 304–314.

Singh, J. A., Sloan, J. A., Atherton, P. J., Smith, T., Hack, T. F., Huschka, M. M., & Degner, L. F. (2010). Preferred roles in treatment decision making among patients with cancer: A pooled analysis of studies using the control preferences scale. *American Journal of Managed Care, 16*, 688–696.

Smith, D. B., & Moen, P. (1998). Spousal influence on retirement: His, her, and their perceptions. *Journal of Marriage and Family, 60*, 734–744.

Smith, D. B., & Moen, P. (2004). Retirement satisfaction for retirees and their spouses: Do gender and the retirement decision-making process matter? *Journal of Family Issues, 25*, 262–285.

Steginga, S. K., Occhipinti, S., Gardiner, R. A., Yaxley, J., & Heathcote, P. (2002). Making decisions about treatment for localized prostate cancer. *BJU International, 89*, 255–260.

Stephens, E. C., & Johnson, M. M. (2000). Dr. Mom and other influences on younger and older adults' OTC medication purchases. *Journal of Applied Gerontology, 19*, 441–459.

Step, M. M., Siminoff, L. A., & Rose, J. H. (2009). Differences in oncologist communication across age groups and contributions to adjuvant decision outcomes. *Journal of the American Geriatrics Society, 57*, s279–s282.

Story, T. N., Berg, C. A., Smith, T., Beveridge, R., Henry, N. A., et al. (2007). Positive sentiment bias in middle and older married couples. *Psychology and Aging, 22*, 719–727.

Strough, J., Cheng, S., & Swenson, L. M. (2002). Preferences for collaborative and individual everyday problem solving in later adulthood. *International Journal of Behavioral Development, 26*, 26–35.

Strough, J., McFall, J. P., & Schuller, K. L. (2010). Endorsement of interpersonal strategies for dealing with hypothetical everyday arthritis problems as a function of marital status, gender, and problem severity. *The International Journal of Aging and Human Development, 70*, 39–59.

Su, C., Fern, E. F., & Ye, K. (2003). A temporal dynamic model of spousal family purchase-decision behavior. *Journal of Marketing Research, 40*, 268–281.

Szinovacz, M. E. (1996). Couples' employment/retirement patterns and perceptions of marital quality. *Research on Aging, 18*, 243–268.

Szinovacz, M. E., & Davey, A. (2005). Retirement and marital decision making: Effects on retirement satisfaction. *Journal of Marriage and Family, 67*, 387–398.

Szinovacz, M. E., & Deviney, S. (2000). Marital characteristics and retirement decisions. *Research on Aging*, *22*, 470–498.

Tucker, J. S., & Mueller, J. S. (2000). Spouses' social control of health behaviors: Use and effectiveness of specific strategies. *Personality and Social Psychology Bulletin*, *26*, 1120–1130.

Walker, E. L. (2010). *Complete without kids: An insider's guide to childfree living by choice or by chance*. Greenleaf Book Group.

Watson, T. L., & Blanchard-Fields, F. (1998). Thinking with your head and your heart: Age differences in everyday problem-solving strategy preferences. *Aging, Neuropsychology, and Cognition*, *5*, 225–240.

Zikmund-Fisher, B. J., Couper, M. P., Singer, E., Levin, C. A., Fowler, F. J., Ziniel, S., et al. (2010). The decisions study: A nationwide survey of United States adults regarding 9 common medical decisions. *Medical Decision Making*, *30*, 20S–34S.

Zwahr, M. D., Park, D. C., & Shifren, K. (1999). Judgments about estrogen replacement therapy: the role of age, cognitive abilities, and beliefs. *Psychology and Aging*, *14*, 179–191.

Index

Note: Page numbers followed by "b", "f" and "t" indicate boxes, figures and tables respectively.

A

AAED. *See* Age-associated executive dysfunction (AAED)
Acute coronary syndrome (ACS), 301
Adaptive decision making
  age differences implications, strategy selection and execution, 120–121
  aging and strategy use. *See* Strategy use
  cognitive control and reward processing, 108–109
  core cognitive abilities, 105
  lifespan changes
    decomposition of, 105–106, 107f
    ecological rationality, 105–106
    mediating mechanism, 106–108
    strategies, definition, 106
    strategy selection and execution, 108
Adaptive toolbox, 272–273
Adult Decision-Making Competence (A-DMC), 130, 236–238, 238f
Affect, 3–5, 10, 67, 69–71, 118, 133–134, 141, 150, 172–178, 191–192, 194–196, 201–202, 238–239, 266–267, 275–276, 287, 298, 305, 321, 341, 354, 362–363, 372, 375–379
Affect heuristic, 175–176, 239, 248
Affective enhancement perspectives, 202–203
Affordable Care Act, 270
Age-associated executive dysfunction (AAED), 80, 96–97
Age-associated memory impairment (AAMI), 96–97
Alternative shift, 272
Ambiguous symptoms, 297
American Consumer Satisfaction Index (ACSI), 356–357
Anchoring strategy, 112
Applied decision-making research, 11–12
  cohort-based effects, 7
  context-specific investigations, 5–6
  financial fraud, 7–8
  health literacy, 6–7
  social context features, 7–8
Arithmetic, 106, 109–113
Arithmetic strategy use
  anchoring strategy, 112
  behavioral patterns and prevailing explanations, 109–110
  choice/no-choice method, 112
  computational estimation task, 113
  cost–benefit calculus, 114
  environment favoring complex strategies, 118–119
  environment/task adaptivity, 116
  exhaustive verification strategy, 111–112
  general executive control process, 113
  in memory, 110–111
  meta-analysis, 119–120
  model-free learning, 118
  numerosity estimation tasks, 112
  perceptual strategy, 112
  plausibility strategy, 111–112
  prototypical decision strategies, 114, 115t
  reward processing, 118
  rounding-up and rounding-down strategies, 113
  take-the-best strategy, 116–118, 117f
  too-much-choice hypothesis, 119–120
Asthma, 299–300
Attribute shift strategy, 272

B

Balloon Analog Risk Task, 136
Behavioral decision-making, 4, 235–237, 240, 243, 247
"Benign senescent forgetfulness", 96–97

C

CAM. *See* Complementary and alternative medical treatments (CAM)
Causal perceptions, 287

Certainty effect, 193–194
CHF. *See* Congestive heart failure (CHF)
Choice set size
decision making, numeracy in, 317–319
preference for choice, 319–321
Cognition, 3–5, 33, 106, 169–172, 218–219, 240, 263
cognitive abilities, 149–150
cognitive capabilities and decision making, adult lifespan
documented cognitive aging pattern, 152–153
fluid intelligence, 151, 152f–153f
meta-analysis, 150
complementary cognitive capabilities
crystallized intelligence, 154–155
debt literacy, 154
decision quality, 153–154
domain-general crystallized intelligence, 156
financial domain-specific crystallized intelligence, 156
financial literacy, 154
framing effects and under/over-confidence, 155
job performance, 157
multiple pathway model, 154, 155f
temporal discounting, 154
U-shaped age–price curve, 155–156
practical decision making, domain-specific experience
additional knowledge, 160
context-specific decision making, 160–161
domain-specificity, 157–158
marketplace expertise, 159
"person-context", 159–160
query theory, 160
public policy and effective decision environments
domain-specific knowledge, 161–162
maximize impact, crystallized intelligence, 162–163
minimize impact, fluid decline, 163–164
Cognitive abilities, 80, 312
Cognitive aging, 1, 3–4, 18–20, 42–43, 54, 108–109, 131, 152–153, 190
Cognitive biases, insidious aspect of, 339–340
Cognitive capabilities
crystallized intelligence, 154–155
debt literacy, 154
decision quality, 153–154
domain-general crystallized intelligence, 156
financial domain-specific crystallized intelligence, 156
financial literacy, 154
framing effects and under/over-confidence, 155
job performance, 157
multiple pathway model, 154, 155f
temporal discounting, 154
U-shaped age–price curve, 155–156
Cognitive control, 9, 42–43, 54, 108–109, 113, 137, 352, 359–360
Cognitive-experiential self-theory (CEST), 173–174
Cognitive and noncognitive factors, 141
Cohort effects, 132, 250–251
Collaborative decision making, in couples
dyadic decision-making processes, 373f
consumer and financial decisions, 379–381
decision context, 376–377
decision identification phase, 373
degree and quality, 377–379
individual resources, 375–376
information search, 373
medical decisions, 383–385
post-decision processes, 374
retirement, 382–383
social influences, 377
heterosexual couples, 372
life decisions, 371
Common-Sense Model (CSM), 285, 286f
description of, 303–305
representations in, 287–288
selective evidence, executive function in, 295–303
action plans and planning, 295–296
chronic illness management, 299–302
everyday health threats, decisions to prevent and manage, 296–299
life-threatening illnesses and end-of-life decisions, 302–303
Complementary and alternative medical treatments (CAM), 298–299
Computational modeling, 65, 68–69, 74
Congestive heart failure (CHF), 301–302
Conservation motivation, 294–295
Consumer choice
ACSI, 356–357
cognitive and affective processes
affective decision processes, 353
crystallized mental abilities, 352–353

executive functioning, 352
expertise, 352–353
fluid mental abilities, 352
motivation, 353
systematic *vs.* heuristic decision-making strategies, 353–354
consumer expertise
consumer experience, 364–365
familiarity, 363–364
illusion of truth effect, 363–364
factors, 357
information search, 355
meaningfulness/personal relevance
deliberative processing, 361
imagery, 362
temporal horizon, 363
Medicare Part D program, 355
moderating influences
consumer expertise, 363–365
factors, 357
meaningfulness/personal relevance, 361–363
task environment/context, 358–361
older-and-more-satisfied effect, 356–357, 365–366
studies, 90–92, 91f
task environment/context
decision aids, 360
primes, 358–359
RAT, 359
time pressure, 358
Contextual perspective, 5, 7, 11–12, 189–191, 204–205
Cost–benefit decision making
age-related memory impairment, 31–33
age-related neurodegenerative conditions, 33–34
animal models, advantages, 17–18
cognitive aging, 18
homologous brain systems, 33
intertemporal choice section
"adjusting" procedures, 22
attenuated delay discounting, 22, 23f
corticostriatal circuits, 28
D2 dopamine receptor mRNA expression, 27
delay discounting, 21–22
delayed rewards, 25
"fixed-delay" procedures, 22
food rewards, 22–24
intertemporal choice task, 22, 23f
neurotransmitter dopamine, 26–27
phasic dopamine signals, 26–27
prefrontal cortico-striatal activity, 26
reward-related neural activation, 26
single-unit neural activity, 25
time valuation and perception, age influences, 24
neural circuitry, 19–20, 20f
primary *vs.* secondary reinforcers, 20–21
probabilistic (risky) decision making, 28–31, 30f
reinforcers, 20–21
risky-choice behavior, 33
Counterfactual thinking. *See* if only error
Crystallized intelligence/mental abilities, 151–152, 152f–153f, 157–158, 241, 330–332, 352–353
CSM. *See* Common-Sense Model (CSM)

D

Decision aids, 158, 163, 247–248, 360
Decision identification phase, 373
Decision-making competence, 130, 236–238
A-DMC component tasks, 236–238, 238f
affect, 239
and age, 240–241
age-related declines, 239
behavioral decision research, 237–238
components, 236–237, 237t
deliberation, 238–239
and age, 240
descriptive accounts, 236
dual-process models, 239
effective interventions development, 247–248
elements of, 248–249
experience and age, 241–242
intra-individual changes, 250–251
lab to life link, 246–247
middle-aged adults, 250
motivational model
and affect, 243–245
contextually embedded process, 242–243
and deliberation, 245
developmental changes recognization, 242–243
dual-process theories, 243
and experience, 245–246
individual characteristics, 242–243
lifespan theories, 243
personal characteristics and features, 242–243
process model, 242–243, 242f
normative theories, 236
prescriptive approaches, 236

Decision rules, 118, 130–132, 170–171, 339
Development/life-span developmental, 7, 105–108, 156, 178, 189–190, 214, 235, 242–243, 312, 315
Delay discounting/intertemporal discounting, 21–28, 23f, 32–33
Diabetes, 299–300
Dopamine, 26–28, 41–43, 54, 62–65
Domain-specific knowledge, 330–332
Dual-process perspectives, 4, 173, 178, 190–205, 239, 243, 312–314
  decision making, 190–192
  prospect theory, 192–205
    probability weighting, 193–200
    value, 200–205, 201f
Dyadic decision-making processes, 373f
  consumer and financial decisions, 379–381
  decision context, 376–377
  decision identification phase, 373
  degree and quality, 377–379
  individual resources, 375–376
  information search, 373
  medical decisions, 383–385
  post-decision processes, 374
  retirement, 382–383
  social influences, 377

E

Electronic Health Record (EHR) systems, 268–269
Emotion, 3–4, 6, 10, 72–73, 80–82, 92–94, 134, 136–138, 170–172, 219–220, 243–245, 266, 285, 305, 361, 374
  adult lifespan, decision making across, 178–182
    affective aspects, age differences in, 179
    deliberative aspects, age differences in, 178
    gains and losses, risky decisions involving, 181
  cognition and motivation, age-related changes in, 170–172
  judgment and decision making, theoretical perspectives on, 172–178
    appraisal-tendency framework, 177
    cognitive-experiential self-theory, 173–174
    dual process models, 173
    heuristic affect, 175–176
    risk-as-feelings hypothesis, 176
  signaling, 96
End of life decisions, 302–303
Episodic memory
  executive control process, 134
  familiarity-based strategies, 135
  global/gist-based judgments/impressions, 134
  IGT, 136
  process simulation, 136–137
  Recognizing Social Norms task, 134–135
  self-initiated processing and recoding operations, 132–133
Exhaustive verification strategy, 111–112
Experience/Expertise, 157–161, 241–242, 330, 352–353, 363–365
Experience-rich and affect-based strategies, 226

F

Financial decision making, 92–93, 93f
  choice preference, cognitive ability effect on, 314–316
    methods, 315
    results, 315–316
  choice preference and size, 310–312
  choice set size and preference, additional factors in, 319–321
  dual-process models and implications for, 312–314
  fluid abilities/crystallized abilities and financial knowledge, 330–332
  individuals make suboptimal decisions, reasons for, 336
    compromise performance, decision biases for, 338–340
    insufficient basic cognitive abilities and resources, 338
    interventions designed, 342–344
    situational and contextual influences, 340–341
    task familiarity and financial literacy, 336–338
  nature of, 332–336
  numeracy and choice set size, 317–319
Fluid intelligence/mental abilities, 151–152, 154–156, 161–162, 240, 330–332, 352
Framing effects, 4–5, 93–94, 130, 175, 179–181, 203–205, 208, 236–237, 339, 353
Fraud victimization, 80
Frontal aging hypothesis, 83–84
Future time perspective, 171–172, 204–205, 222–223, 225, 243–245, 363

G

Gist/Gist-based strategies, 173, 239, 275–276
Good enough decisions, 3–4

H

Health decisions
  modeling health preferences themes, 284–285
  processes underlying modeling and actions, 285–295
Health literacy (HL), process-knowledge model of, 263–264, 263f
Heuristic processing, 354
Hindsight bias, 134

I

If only error, 248–249
Illness
  acute, 300
  chronic, 294–295, 297–302
Illusion of truth, 363–364
Implicit and nondeclarative memory, 138–139
Impossibility effect, 193–194
In situ hybridization procedures, 27
Integral affect, 172–173
Intellectual abilities (IQ), 317
Intertemporal choice section, 220–222, 236–237, 248–249
  "adjusting" procedures, 22
  ad libitum access, 47
  attenuated delay discounting, 22, 23f
  behavioral and neural effects, 46–47
  cognitive control, 45
  corticostriatal circuits, 28
  D2 dopamine receptor mRNA expression, 27
  delay discounting, 21–22
  delayed rewards, 25
  "fixed-delay" procedures, 22
  food rewards, 22–24
  intertemporal choice task, 22, 23f
  neurotransmitter dopamine, 26–27
  phasic dopamine signals, 26–27
  prefrontal cortico-striatal activity, 26
  reward-related neural activation, 26
  single-unit neural activity, 25
  in situ hybridization procedures, 27
  time valuation and perception, age influences, 24
  ventral striatal signal, 45, 46f
Intuition, 180–181
Iowa Gambling Task (IGT), 84–85
  behavior, 85–86, 86f
  framing effects, 93–94
  hypersensitivity to reward, 87–88
  psychophysiological, 86–87
Iowa Scales of Personality Change (ISPC), 95

L

Language comprehension, 264–267
  affect, 266
  illness representation, 266–267
  knowledge, 265–266
  processing capacity, 264–265
  processing capacity/knowledge and affect, interplay of, 267
Literacy deficits, 337–338

M

Medical/health decisions, 262–267, 285–295, 383–385
Medicare Modernization Act, 270
Medicare Part D program, 246, 355
Medical literacy, 304–305
Memory-based theories, 127
Midlevel tasks, 335
Motivation, 170–172, 203–204, 219–220, 242–246
Motivational model
  and affect, 243–245
  contextually embedded process, 242–243
  and deliberation, 245
  developmental changes recognization, 242–243
  dual-process theories, 243
  and experience, 245–246
  individual characteristics, 242–243
  lifespan theories, 243
  personal characteristics and features, 242–243
  process model, 242–243, 242f
Motivational influences, dual-process perspectives on. *See* Socioemotional selectivity theory
decision making, 190–192
prospect theory, 192–205
Mouselab, 319–320
Myocardial infarction (MI), 288

N

National Research Council, 3–4
Neurobiological mechanisms, 2–3, 8–9, 18, 20–22, 28, 45–47, 63–64

Neuroimaging, 19–20, 28, 45, 50–51, 65, 72
Neuroscience
feedback-driven learning, 41
frontostriatal and fronto-medial-temporal networks, 54
frontostriatal neural circuitry, 41–43, 42f
frontostriatal systems, 53
gains and losses, 44
intertemporal decision making
ad libitum access, 47
behavioral and neural effects, 46–47
cognitive control, 45
ventral striatal signal, 45, 46f
intertemporal delays, 53–54
learning
functional connectivity, 52
learning-based risky-decision task, 52
meta-analysis, 50
prediction errors, 50–51
structural integrity, 51–52, 51f
valence effects, 50
perspectives, 1–2
risky decision making, 47–50, 49f
ventromedial frontostriatal neural systems, 41
Noncompensatory strategies, 271–272
Nondeclarative memory process, 141–142
Nonmemory-related cognitive abilities, 79
Numeracy, 245, 317–319
Neuroimaging studies
behavioral disparities, 89–90
fluorodeoxyglucose-positron emission tomography, 88
impaired decision-making abilities, 89
older impaired vs. older unimpaired decision makers, 89

O

Older-and-more-satisfied effect, 356–357, 365–366
Overconfidence, 130–132, 236–237, 237t

P

Patient-centered models, 266–267
Perceptual strategy, 112
Personality traits, 94–95
Phineas Gage, prefrontal sector, 81
Plausibility strategy, 111–112
Positivity effect, 3, 137, 171, 176–177, 180, 219–220, 224, 275, 353
Prefrontal cortex, 41–43, 42f, 51–52, 51f, 62–63, 68
Probabilistic decision making, 28–31
Prospect theory, 192–205
probability weighting, 193–200
value, 200–205, 201f
Prostate specific antigen (PSA) test, 303
Public policy and effective decision environments, 96–97, 161–164, 184
domain-specific knowledge, 161–162
maximize impact, crystallized intelligence, 162–163
minimize impact, fluid decline, 163–164

R

Randomized assignment, 342–343
Rapid Estimate of Adult Literacy in Medicine (REALM), 262–263
Rat/rodent, 17–22, 33
Ratio bias, 174
Rational/normative decision making, 4–5
Recognizing Social Norms task, 134–135
Reinforcement learning types
hybrid reinforcement learning algorithm, 69–71, 70f
model-free choice behavior, 69–71, 70f
model-free learning, 68–69
second-stage options, 69–71
2-stage Markov decision task, 69–71, 70f
Remote Associates Task (RAT), 359
Retirement, 246–247, 330, 332–334, 343
Rewards, 41–48
Risk, 5, 7–8, 28–31, 47–50, 61, 95, 97, 109, 136, 150–151, 155, 172–174, 176–178, 181, 191–192, 197–198, 204, 236–237, 277, 285, 318, 334–335, 340–341, 366
Risk-as-feelings hypothesis, 176
Risk perception, 140–141, 236–237
Rounding-up and rounding-down strategies, 113

S

Selection, Optimization, and Compensation model, 191–192
Selective engagement theory, 192, 203–204
Self-assessments of health (SAH), 292
Self-diagnosis, 289
Semantic memory, 140–141
Skin conductance rate, 86–87
Social norms, 236–237, 237t
Socioemotional selectivity theory (SST), 171–172, 191–192, 199–200, 219–220, 222–224, 243, 353
Somatic marker hypothesis (SMH), 81–82
SST. *See* Socioemotional selectivity theory (SST)

Striatum, 41–42, 42f, 45, 52–53, 62–64
Sunk cost, 140–141, 236–237, 244–245
Systematic errors, 338–339

T

Temporal difference (TD) learning
avoidance learning, 67–68
blood oxygenation level-dependent signal, 67–68
learning rate, 67
prediction error, 67
reinforcement learning theory, 66–67, 66f
Test of Functional Health Literacy in Adults (TOFHLA), 262–263
Temporal horizons, 10, 223, 225, 243–245, 249, 353, 363
Textbase, 264–265
The Paradox of Choice (Schwartz), 310
Time-lines set, 287
Time
age-related decline, dopamine system, 65
cognitive function, 63
D1 receptor density, 62–63
presynaptic markers, 62–63
reinforcement learning, 63–64
reward-related evoked potential components, 63–64
ameliorate learning deficits, 72–74
dopaminergic teaching signals, 66
fluid cognitive functions, 61
meta-analytic data, 62
model-based decision mechanisms, 71–72
model-free decision mechanisms, 71–72
in neurophysiological mechanisms, 65
reduced error-related negativity, 65–66
reinforcement learning types
hybrid reinforcement learning algorithm, 69–71, 70f
model-free choice behavior, 69–71, 70f
model-free learning, 68–69
second-stage options, 69–71
2-stage Markov decision task, 69–71, 70f
TD learning. *See* Temporal difference (TD) learning
Time horizons, 137, 171–172, 214–217, 223, 225–226, 243
Time perception, age differences, 225
actuarial life expectancy and prior experience, 217–218
cognition, 218–219
decision outcomes, 222–223
decision processing and strategies, 223–225
end-of-life decisions, 213
experience-rich and affect-based strategies, 226
global time horizons and mental representations
future anhedonia, 217
qualitative characteristics, 215–216
temporal extension, 214–215
intertemporal choice, 220–222
joint decision-making scenarios, 226
lifespan developmental research, 214
motivation and emotion, 219–220
TOFHLA. *See* Test of Functional Health Literacy in Adults (TOFHLA)

U

Uncertainty, 12, 47–48, 61–62, 71–72, 81–82, 177, 301, 332–334
age-related decline, dopamine system, 65
cognitive function, 63
D1 receptor density, 62–63
presynaptic markers, 62–63
reinforcement learning, 63–64
reward-related evoked potential components, 63–64
ameliorate learning deficits, 72–74
dopaminergic teaching signals, 66
fluid cognitive functions, 61
meta-analytic data, 62
model-based decision mechanisms, 71–72
model-free decision mechanisms, 71–72
in neurophysiological mechanisms, 65
reduced error-related negativity, 65–66
reinforcement learning types
hybrid reinforcement learning algorithm, 69–71, 70f
model-free choice behavior, 69–71, 70f
model-free learning, 68–69
second-stage options, 69–71
2-stage Markov decision task, 69–71, 70f
TD learning. *See* Temporal difference (TD) learning

V

Visuo-spatial memory process, 141–142

W

Working memory, 128–129, 129t, 352
A-DMC, 130
competitive structural equation modeling, 131
data collection, 132
dual-task experiments, 129–130
mediation models, 131
mediation testing, 132

Kolibri 360 GmbH
Ferdinand-Jühlke-Straße 7
99095 Erfurt, Deutschland
produktsicherheit@kolibri360.de